KNAT: Full Study Guide for the Kaplan Nursing Admissions Test

To obtain permission(s) to use the material from this work for any purpose including workshops or seminars, please submit a written request to

Smart Edition Media
36 Gorham Street
Suite 1
Cambridge, MA 02138
800-496-5994

Email: info@smarteditionmedia.com

Library of Congress Cataloging-in-Publication Data
Smart Edition Media.
KNAT: Full Study Guide for the Kaplan Nursing Admissions Test
ISBN: Print: 978-1-949147-00-1, 1st edition

1. KNAT Exam
2. Study Guides
3. Kaplan Nursing Admissions Test
4. College Preparation
5. Careers

Disclaimer:

Printed in the United States of America

KNAT: Full Study Guide for the Kaplan Nursing Admissions Test/Smart Edition Media.

ISBN: Print: 978-1-949147-00-1
        Ebook: 978-1-949147-29-2

Print and digital composition by Book Genesis, Inc.

KNAT Practice Online

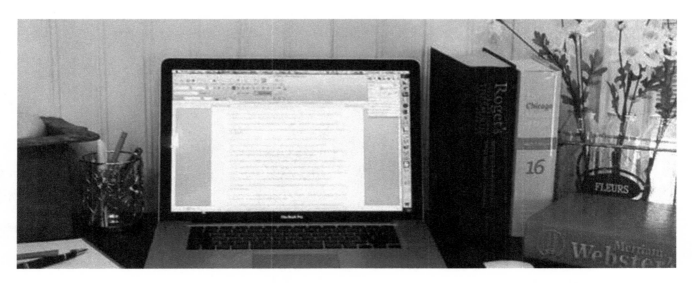

Smart Edition Media's Online Learning Resources allow you the flexibility to study for your exam on your own schedule and are the perfect companion to help you reach your goals! You can access online content with an Internet connection from any computer, laptop, or mobile device.

Online Learning Resources

Designed to enable you to master the content in quick bursts of focused learning, these tools cover a complete range of subjects, including:

- English Language Arts
- Reading
- Math
- Science
- Writing

Our online resources are filled with test-taking tips and strategies, important facts, and practice problems that mirror questions on the exam.

Online Sample Tests & Flashcards

Access additional full-length practice tests online!

Use these tests as a diagnostic tool to determine areas of strength and weakness before embarking on your study program or to assess mastery of skills once you have completed your studies.

FLASHCARDS **GAMES** **QUIZZES** **TESTS**

Go to the URL: **https://smarteditionmedia.com/pages/knat-online-resources** and follow the password/login instructions.

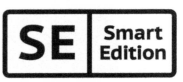

TABLE OF CONTENTS

Introduction

An Overview of the KNAT Exam

The KNAT is a college admissions examination that is often selected by nursing schools and programs during the application process as a requirement for admission. The KNAT consists of 91 multiple choice questions in the core subject areas of English, math, and science to help determine a student's mastery of basic skills, as well as predict a student's ability to handle a nursing program course of study.

About This Book

This book provides you with an accurate and complete representation of the KNAT test and includes instructional content on the three core sections on the exam. The reviews in this book are designed to provide the information and strategies you need to do well on the exam. The full-length practice test in the book is based on the KNAT and contains questions similar to those you can expect to encounter on the official test. A detailed answer key follows each practice quiz and test. These answer keys provide explanations designed to help you completely understand the test material. Each explanation references the book chapter to allow you to go back to that section for additional review, if necessary.

Online Sample Tests

The purchase of this book grants you access to two additional full-length practice tests online. You can locate these exams on the Smart Edition Media website.

Go to the URL: https://smarteditionmedia.com/pages/knat-online-resources and follow the password/login instructions.

How to Use This Book

Studies show that most people begin preparing for college-entry exams approximately 8 weeks before their test date. If you are scheduled to take your test in sooner than 8 weeks, do not despair! Smart Edition Media has designed this study guide to be flexible to allow you to concentrate on areas where you need the most support.

Whether you have 8 weeks to study – or much less than that – we urge you to take one of the online practice tests to determine areas of strength and weakness, if you have not done so already. These tests can be found in your online resources.

Once you have completed a practice test, use this information to help you create a study plan that suits your individual study habits and time frame. If you are short on time, look at your diagnostic test results to determine which subject matter could use the most attention and focus the majority of your efforts on those areas. While this study guide is organized to follow the order of the actual test, you are not required to complete the book from beginning to end, in that exact order.

How This Book Is Organized

Take a look at the Table of Contents. Notice that each **Section** in the study guide corresponds to a subtest of the exam. These sections are broken into **Chapters** that identify the major content categories of the exam.

Each chapter is further divided into individual **Lessons** that address the specific content and objectives required to pass the exam. Some lessons contain embedded example questions to assess your comprehension of the content "in the moment." All lessons contain a bulleted list called "**Let's Review.**" Use this list to refresh your memory before taking a practice quiz, test, or the actual exam. A **Practice Quiz**, designed to check your progress as you move through the content, follows each chapter.

Whether you plan on working through the study guide from cover to cover, or selecting specific sections to review, each chapter of this book can be completed in one sitting. If you must end your study session before finishing a chapter, try to complete your current lesson in order to maximize comprehension and retention of the material.

Study Strategies and Tips

MAKE STUDY SESSIONS A PRIORITY.

- Use a calendar to schedule your study sessions. Set aside a dedicated amount of time each day/week for studying. While it may seem difficult to manage, given your other responsibilities, remember that in order to reach your goals, it is crucial to dedicate the time now to prepare for this test. A satisfactory score on your exam is the key to unlocking a multitude of opportunities for your future success.

- Do you work? Have children? Other obligations? Be sure to take these into account when creating your schedule. Work around them to ensure that your scheduled study sessions can be free of distractions.

> **TIPS FOR FINDING TIME TO STUDY.**
> - Wake up 1-2 hours before your family for some quiet time
> - Study 1-2 hours before bedtime and after everything has quieted down
> - Utilize weekends for longer study periods
> - Hire a babysitter to watch children

TAKE PRACTICE TESTS

- Smart Edition Media offers practice tests, both online and in print. Take as many as you can to help be prepared. This will eliminate any surprises you may encounter during the exam.

KNOW YOUR LEARNING STYLE

- Identify your strengths and weaknesses as a student. All students are different and everyone has a different learning style. Do not compare yourself to others.
- Howard Gardner, a developmental psychologist at Harvard University, has studied the ways in which people learn new information. He has identified seven distinct intelligences. According to his theory:

"we are all able to know the world through language, logical-mathematical analysis, spatial representation, musical thinking, the use of the body to solve problems or to make things, an understanding of other individuals, and an understanding of ourselves. Where individuals differ is in the strength of these intelligences - the so-called profile of intelligences -and in the ways in which such intelligences are invoked and combined to carry out different tasks, solve diverse problems, and progress in various domains."

- Knowing your learning style can help you to tailor your studying efforts to suit your natural strengths.
- What ways help you learn best? Videos? Reading textbooks? Find the best way for you to study and learn/review the material

WHAT IS YOUR LEARNING STYLE?

- **Visual-Spatial** – Do you like to draw, do jigsaw puzzles, read maps, daydream? Creating drawings, graphic organizers, or watching videos might be useful for you.
- **Bodily-kinesthetic** – Do you like movement, making things, physical activity? Do you communicate well through body language, or like to be taught through physical activity? Hands-on learning, acting out, role playing are tools you might try.
- **Musical** – Do you show sensitivity to rhythm and sound? If you love music, and are also sensitive to sounds in your environments, it might be beneficial to study with music in the background. You can turn lessons into lyricsor speak rhythmically to aid in content retention.
- **Interpersonal** – Do you have many friends, empathy for others, street smarts, and interact well with others? You might learn best in a group setting. Form a study group with other students who are preparing for the same exam. Technology makes it easy to connect, if you are unable to meet in person, teleconferencing or video chats are useful tools to aid interpersonal learners in connecting with others.
- **Intrapersonal** – Do you prefer to work alone rather than in a group? Are you in tune with your inner feelings, follow your intuition and possess a strong will, confidence and opinions? Independent study and introspection will be ideal for you. Reading books, using creative materials, keeping a diary of your progress will be helpful. Intrapersonal learners are the most independent of the learners.
- **Linguistic** – Do you use words effectively, have highly developed auditory skills and often think in words? Do you like reading, playing word games, making up poetry or stories? Learning tools such as computers, games, multimedia will be beneficial to your studies.
- **Logical-Mathematical** – Do you think conceptually, abstractly, and are able to see and explore patterns and relationships? Try exploring subject matter through logic games, experiments and puzzles.

CREATE THE OPTIMAL STUDY ENVIRONMENT

- Some people enjoy listening to soft background music when they study. (Instrumental music is a good choice.) Others need to have a silent space in order to concentrate. Which do you prefer? Either way, it is best to create an environment that is free of distractions for your study sessions.
- Have study guide – Will travel! Leave your house: Daily routines and chores can be distractions. Check out your local library, a coffee shop, or other quiet space to remove yourself from distractions and daunting household tasks will compete for your attention.
- Create a Technology Free Zone. Silence the ringer on your cell phone and place it out of reach to prevent surfing the Web, social media interactions, and email/texting exchanges. Turn off the television, radio, or other devices while you study.
- Are you comfy? Find a comfortable, but not *too* comfortable, place to study. Sit at a desk or table in a straight, upright chair. Avoid sitting on the couch, a bed, or in front of the TV. Wear clothing that is not binding and restricting.
- Keep your area organized. Have all the materials you need available and ready: Smart Edition study guide, computer, notebook, pen, calculator, and pencil/eraser. Use a desk lamp or overhead light that provides ample lighting to prevent eye-strain and fatigue.

HEALTHY BODY, HEALTHY MIND

- Consider these words of wisdom from Buddha, "To keep the body in good health is a duty – otherwise we shall not be able to keep our mind strong and clear."

KEYS TO CREATING A HEALTHY BODY AND MIND:

- Drink water – Stay hydrated! Limit drinks with excessive sugar or caffeine.
- Eat natural foods – Make smart food choices and avoid greasy, fatty, sugary foods.
- Think positively – You can do this! Do not doubt yourself, and trust in the process.
- Exercise daily – If you have a workout routine, stick to it! If you are more sedentary, now is a great time to begin! Try yoga or a low-impact sport. Simply walking at a brisk pace will help to get your heart rate going.
- Sleep well – Getting a good night's sleep is important, but too few of us actually make it a priority. Aim to get eight hours of uninterrupted sleep in order to maximize your mental focus, memory, learning, and physical wellbeing.

FINAL THOUGHTS

- Remember to relax and take breaks during study sessions.
- Review the testing material. Go over topics you already know for a refresher.
- Focus more time on less familiar subjects.

EXAM PREPARATION

In addition to studying for your upcoming exam, it is important to keep in mind that you need to prepare your mind and body as well. When preparing to take an exam as a whole, not just studying, taking practice exams, and reviewing math rules, it is critical to prepare your body in order to be mentally and physically ready. Often, your success rate will be much higher when you are *fully* ready.

Here are some tips to keep in mind when preparing for your exam:

SEVERAL WEEKS/DAYS BEFORE THE EXAM

- Get a full night of sleep, approximately 8 hours
- Turn off electronics before bed
- Exercise regularly
- Eat a healthy balanced diet, include fruits and vegetable
- Drink water

THE NIGHT BEFORE

- Eat a good dinner
- Pack materials/bag, healthy snacks, and water

- Gather materials needed for test: your ID and receipt of test. You do not want to be scrambling the morning of the exam. If you are unsure of what to bring with you, check with your testing center or test administrator.
- Map the location of test center, identify how you will be getting there (driving, public transportation, uber, etc.), when you need to leave, and parking options.
- Lay your clothes out. Wear comfortable clothes and shoes, do not wear items that are too hot/cold
- Allow minimum of ~8 hours of sleep
- Avoid coffee and alcohol
- Do not take any medications or drugs to help you sleep
- Set alarm

THE DAY OF THE EXAM

- Wake up early, allow ample time to do all the things you need to do and for travel
- Eat a healthy, well-rounded breakfast
- Drink water
- Leave early and arrive early, leave time for any traffic or any other unforeseeable circumstances
- Arrive early and check in for exam. This will give you enough time to relax, take off coat, and become comfortable with your surroundings.

Take a deep breath, get ready, go! You got this!

SECTION I. WRITING

CHAPTER 1 CONVENTIONS OF STANDARD ENGLISH

SPELLING

Spelling correctly is important to accurately convey thoughts to an audience. This lesson will cover (1) vowels and consonants, (2) suffixes and plurals, (3) homophones and homographs.

Vowels and Consonants

Vowels and **consonants** are different speech sounds in English.

The letters A, E, I, O, U and sometimes Y are **vowels** and can create a variety of sounds. The most common are short sounds and long sounds. Long **vowel** sounds sound like the name of the letter such as the *a* in late. Short **vowel** sounds have a unique sound such as the *a* in cat. A rule for **vowels** is that when two vowels are walking, the first does the talking as in pain and meat.

Consonants include the other twenty-one letters in the alphabet. **Consonants** are weak letters and only make sounds when paired with **vowels**. That is why words always must have a **vowel**. This also means that **consonants** need to be doubled to make a stronger sound like sitting, grabbed, progress. Understanding general trends and patterns for **vowels** and **consonants** will help with spelling. The table below represents the difference between short and long **vowels** and gives examples for each.

	Symbol	Example Words
Short a	a	Cat, mat, hat, pat
Long a	ā	Late, pain, pay, they, weight, straight
Short e	e	Met, said, bread
Long e	ē	Breeze, cheap, dean, equal
Short i	i	Bit, myth, kiss, rip
Long i	ī	Cry, pie, high
Short o	o	Dog, hot, pop
Long o	ō	Snow, nose, elbow
Short u	u	Run, cut, club, gum
Long u	ū	Duty, rule, new, food
Short oo	oo	Book, foot, cookie
Long oo	ōō	Mood, bloom, shoot

Suffixes and Plurals

A **suffix** is a word part that is added to the ending of a root word. A **suffix** changes the meaning and spelling of words. There are some general patterns to follow with **suffixes**.

- Adding -er, -ist, or -or changes the root to mean *doer* or *performer*

    - Paint → Painter
    - Abolition → Abolitionist
    - Act → Actor

- Adding -ation or -ment changes the root to mean *an action* or *a process*

    - Ador(e) → Adoration
    - Develop → Development

- Adding -ism changes the root to mean *a theory or ideology*

    - Real → Realism

- Adding -ity, -ness, -ship, or -tude changes the root to mean *a condition, quality, or state*

    - Real → Reality
    - Sad → Sadness
    - Relation → Relationship
    - Soli(tary) → Solitude

Plurals are similar to suffixes as letters are added to the end of the word to signify more than one person, place, thing, or idea. There are also general patterns to follow when creating **plurals**.

- If a word ends in -s,-ss,-z,-zz,-ch, or -sh, add -es.

    - Bus → Buses

- If a word ends in a -y, drop the -y and add -ies.

    - Pony → Ponies

- If a word ends in an -f, change the f to a v and add -es.

    - Knife → Knives

- For all other words, add an -s.

    - Dog → Dogs

Homophones and Homographs

A **homophone** is a word that has the same sound as another word, but does not have the same meaning or spelling.

- To, too, and two
- There, their, and they're
- See and sea

A **homograph** is a word that has the same spelling as another word, but does not have the same sound or meaning.

- Lead (to go in front of) and lead (a metal)
- Bass (deep sound) and bass (a fish)

Let's Review!

- Vowels include the letters A, E, I, O, U and sometimes Y and have both short and long sounds.
- Consonants are the other twenty-one letters and have weak sounds. They are often doubled to make stronger sounds.
- Suffixes are word parts added to the root of a word and change the meaning and spelling.
- To make a word plural, add -es, -ies, -ves, or -s to the end of a word.
- Homophones are words that have the same sound, but not the same meaning or spelling.
- Homographs are words that have the same spelling, but not the same meaning or sound.

CAPITALIZATION

Correct capitalization helps readers understand when a new sentence begins and the importance of specific words. This lesson will cover the capitalization rules of (1) geographic locations and event names, (2) organizations and publication titles, (3) individual names and professional titles, and (4) months, days, and holidays.

Geographic Locations and Event Names

North, east, south, and west are not capitalized unless they relate to a **definite region**.

- Go north on I-5 for 200 miles.
- The West Coast has nice weather.

Words like northern, southern, eastern, and western are also not capitalized unless they describe **people or the cultural and political activities of people**.

- There is nothing interesting to see in eastern Colorado.
- Midwesterners are known for being extremely nice.
- The Western states almost always vote Democratic.

These words are not capitalized when placed before a name or region unless it is part of the **official name**.

- She lives in southern California.
- I loved visiting Northern Ireland.

Continents, countries, states, cities, and **towns** need to be capitalized.

- Australia has a lot of scary animals.
- Not many people live in Antarctica.
- Albany is the capital of New York.

Historical events should be capitalized to separate the specific from the general.

- The bubonic plague in the Middle Ages killed a large portion of the population in Europe.
- The Great Depression took place in the early 1930s.
- We are living in the twenty-first century.

Organizations and Publication Titles

The **names of national organizations** need to be capitalized. Short prepositions, articles, and conjunctions within the title are not capitalized unless they are the first word.

- The National American Woman Suffrage Association was essential in passing the Nineteenth Amendment.
- The House of Representatives is one part of Congress.

- The National Football League consists of thirty-two teams.

The **titles of books, chapters, articles, poems, newspapers, and other publications** should be capitalized.

- Her favorite book is *A Wrinkle in Time.*
- I do the crossword in *The New York Times* every Sunday.
- *The Jabberwocky* by Lewis Carroll has many silly sounding words.

Individual Names and Professional Titles

People's names as well as their **familial relationship title** need to be capitalized.

- Barack Obama was our first African American president.
- Uncle Joe brought the steaks for our Memorial Day grill.
- Aunt Sarah lives in California, but my other aunt lives in Florida.

Professional titles need to be capitalized when they precede a name, or as a direct address. If it is after a name or is used generally, titles do not need to be capitalized.

- Governor Cuomo is trying to modernize the subway system in New York.
- Andrew Cuomo is the governor of New York.
- A governor runs the state. A president runs the country.
- Thank you for the recommendation, Mr. President.
- I need to see Doctor Smith.
- I need to see a doctor.

Capitalize the **title of high-ranking government officials** when an individual is referred to.

- The Secretary of State travels all over the world.
- The Vice President joined the meeting.

With **compound titles**, the prefixes or suffixes do not need to be capitalized.

- George W. Bush is the ex-President of the United States.

Months, Days, and Holidays

Capitalize **all months of the year** (January, February, March, April, May, June, July, August, September, October, November, December) and **days of the week** (Sunday, Monday, Tuesday, Wednesday, Thursday, Friday, Saturday).

- Her birthday is in November.
- People graduate from college in May or June.
- Saturdays and Sundays are supposed to be fun and relaxing.

Holidays are also capitalized.

- Most kids' favorite holiday is Christmas.
- The new school year usually starts after Labor Day.
- It is nice to go to the beach over Memorial Day weekend.

The **seasons** are not capitalized.

- It gets too hot in the summer and too cold in the winter.
- The flowers and trees bloom so beautifully in the spring.

Let's Review!

- Only capitalize directional words like north, south, east, and, west when they describe a definite region, people, and their political and cultural activities, or when it is part of the official name.
- Historical periods and events are capitalized to represent their importance and specificity.
- Every word except short prepositions, conjunctions, and articles in the names of national organizations are capitalized.
- The titles of publications follow the same rules as organizations.
- The names of individual people need to be capitalized.
- Professional titles are capitalized if they precede a name or are used as a direct address.
- All months of the year, days of the week, and holidays are capitalized.
- Seasons are not capitalized.

PUNCTUATION

Punctuation is important in writing to accurately represent ideas. Without correct punctuation, the meaning of a sentence is difficult to understand. This lesson will cover (1) periods, question marks, and exclamation points, (2) commas, semicolons, and colons, and (3) apostrophes, hyphens, and quotation marks.

Terminal Punctuation Marks: Periods, Question Marks, and Exclamation Points

Terminal punctuation is used at the end of a sentence. Periods, question marks, and exclamation points are the three types of terminal punctuation.

Periods (.) mark the end of a declarative sentence, one that states a fact, or an imperative sentence, one that states a command or request). Periods can also be used in abbreviations.

- Doctors save lives.
- She has a B.A. in Psychology.

Question Marks (?) signify the end of a sentence that is a question. Where, when, who, whom, what, why, and how are common words that begin question sentences.

- Who is he?
- Why is the sky blue?
- Where is the restaurant?

Exclamation Points (!) indicate strong feelings, shouting, or emphasize a feeling.

- Watch out!
- I hate you!
- That is incredible!

Internal Punctuation: Commas, Semicolons, and Colons

Internal punctuation is used within a sentence to help keep words, phrases, and clauses in order. These punctuation marks can be used to indicate elements such as direct quotations and definitions in a sentence.

A **comma (,)** signifies a small break within a sentence and separates words, clauses, or ideas.

Commas are used before conjunctions that connect two independent clauses.

- I ate some cookies, and I drank some milk.

Commas are also used to set off an introductory phrase.

- After the test, she grabbed dinner with a friend.

Short phrases that emphasis thoughts or emotions are enclosed by **commas**.

- The school year, thankfully, ends in a week.

Commas set off the words yes and no.

- Yes, I am available this weekend.
- No, she has not finished her homework.

Commas set off a question tag.

- It is beautiful outside, isn't it?

Commas are used to indicate direct address.

- Are you ready, Jack?
- Mom, what is for dinner?

Commas separate items in a series.

- We ate eggs, potatoes, and toast for breakfast.
- I need to grab coffee, go to the store, and put gas in my car.

Semicolons (;) are used to connect two independent clauses without a coordinating conjunction like *and* or *but*. A **semicolon** creates a bond between two sentences that are related. Do not capitalize the first word after the **semicolon** unless it is a word that is normally capitalized.

- The ice cream man drove down my street; I bought a popsicle.
- My mom cooked dinner; the chicken was delicious.
- It is cloudy today; it will probably rain.

Colons (:) introduce a list.

- She teaches three subjects: English, history, and geography.

Within a sentence, **colons** can create emphasis of a word or phrase.

- She had one goal: pay the bills.

More Internal Punctuation: Apostrophes, Hyphens, and Quotation Marks

Apostrophes (') are used to indicate possession or to create a contraction.

- Bob has a car - Bob's car is blue.
- Steve's cat is beautiful.

For plurals that are also possessive, put the **apostrophe** after the s.

- Soldiers' uniforms are impressive.

Make contractions by combining two words.

- I do not have a dog - I don't have a dog
- I can't swim.

Its and it's do not follow the normal possessive rules. Its is possessive while it's means "it is."

- It's a beautiful day to be at the park.
- The dog has many toys, but its favorite is the rope.

Hyphens (-) are mainly used to create compound words.

- The documentary was a real eye-opener for me.
- We have to check-in to the hotel before midnight.
- The graduate is a twenty-two-year-old woman.

Quotation Marks (") are used when directly using another person's words in your own writing. Commas and periods, sometimes question marks and exclamation points, are placed within **quotation marks**. Colons and semicolons are placed outside of the **quotation marks**, unless they are part of the quoted material. If quoting an entire sentence, capitalize the first word. If it is a fragment, do not capitalize the first word.

- Ernest Hemingway once claimed, "There is nothing noble in being superior to your fellow man; true nobility is being superior to your former self."
- Steve said, "I will be there at noon."

An indirect quote which paraphrases what someone else said does not need **quotation marks**.

- Steve said he would be there at noon.

Quotation marks are also used for the titles of short works such as poems, articles, and chapters. They are not italicized.

- Robert Frost wrote "The Road Not Taken."

Let's Review!

- **Periods (.)** signify the end of a sentence or are used in abbreviations.
- **Question Marks (?)** are also used at the end of a sentence and distinguish the sentence as a question.
- **Exclamation Points (!)** indicate strong feelings, shouting, or emphasis and are usually at the end of the sentence.
- **Commas (,)** are small breaks within a sentence that separate clauses, ideas, or words. They are used to set off introductory phrases, the words yes and no, question tags, indicate direct address, and separate items in a series.
- **Semicolons (;)** connect two similar sentences without a coordinating conjunctions such as and or but.
- **Colons (:)** are used to introduce a list or emphasize a word or phrase.
- **Apostrophes (')** indicate possession or a contraction of two words.
- **Hyphens (-)** are used to create compound words.
- **Quotation Marks (")** are used when directly quoting someone else's words and to indicate the title of poems, chapters, and articles.

CHAPTER 1 CONVENTIONS OF STANDARD ENGLISH
PRACTICE QUIZ

1. Which word(s) in the following sentence should NOT be capitalized?

   Can You Speak German?

   A. You and Speak

   B. Can and German

   C. Can, You, and Speak

   D. You, Speak, and German

2. Fill in the blank with the correctly capitalized form.

   Every week, they get together to watch _____.

   A. *the bachelor*   C. *The bachelor*

   B. *The Bachelor*   D. *the Bachelor*

3. Choose the correct sentence.

   A. They used to live in the pacific northwest.

   B. They used to live in the Pacific northwest.

   C. They used to live in the pacific Northwest.

   D. They used to live in the Pacific Northwest.

4. What is the sentence with the correct use of punctuation?

   A. Offcampus apartments are nicer.

   B. Off campus apartments are nicer.

   C. Off-campus apartments are nicer.

   D. Off-campus-apartments are nicer.

5. Which of the following sentences is correct?

   A. I asked Scott, How was your day?

   B. Scott said, it was awesome.

   C. He claimed, "My history presentation was great!"

   D. I said, That's wonderful!

6. What is the mistake in the following sentence?

   The highestranking officer can choose his own work, including his own hours.

   A. *Highestranking* needs a hyphen.

   B. There should be a comma after *officer*.

   C. There should be no comma after *work*.

   D. There should be a semicolon after *work*.

7. Which of the following spellings is correct?

   A. Busines   C. Buseness

   B. Business   D. Bussiness

8. What is the correct plural of morning?

   A. Morning   C. Morninges

   B. Mornings   D. Morningies

9. On Earth, _____ are seven continents.

   A. their   C. theer

   B. there   D. they're

Chapter 1 Conventions of Standard English
Practice Quiz — Answer Key

1. A. *You and Speak.* Can is the first word in the sentence and needs to be capitalized. German is a nationality and needs to be capitalized. The other two words do not need to be capitalized. **See Lesson: Capitalization.**

2. B. *The Bachelor.* The names of TV shows are capitalized. *The* is capitalized here because it is the first word in the name. **See Lesson: Capitalization.**

3. D. *They used to live in the Pacific Northwest.* Specific geographic regions are capitalized. **See Lesson: Capitalization.**

4. C. *Off-campus apartments are nicer.* Hyphens are often used for compound words that are placed before the noun to help with understanding. **See Lesson: Punctuation.**

5. C. *He claimed, "My history presentation was great!"* Quotation marks enclose direct statements. **See Lesson: Punctuation.**

6. A. *Highestranking needs a hyphen.* Hyphens are used for compound words that describe a person or object. **See Lesson: Punctuation.**

7. B. *Business* is the only correct spelling. **See Lesson: Spelling.**

8. B. For most words ending in consonants, just add -s. **See Lesson: Spelling.**

9. B. *There* describes a place or position and is correctly spelled. **See Lesson: Spelling.**

CHAPTER 2 PARTS OF SPEECH

NOUNS

In this lesson, you will learn about nouns. A noun is a word that names a person, place, thing, or idea. This lesson will cover (1) the role of nouns in sentences and (2) different types of nouns.

Nouns and Their Role in Sentences

A **noun** names a person, place, thing, or idea.

Some examples of nouns are:

- Gandhi
- New Hampshire
- garden
- happiness

A noun's role in a sentence is as **subject** or **object**. A subject is the part of the sentence that does something, whereas the object is the thing that something is done to. In simple terms, the subject acts, and the object is acted upon.

Look for the nouns in these sentences.

1. The Louvre is stunning. (subject noun: The Louvre)
2. Marco ate dinner with Sara and Petra. (subject noun: Marco; object nouns: dinner, Sara, Petra)

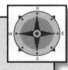

KEEP IN MIND . . .
The subjects *I* and *we* in the two sentences to the left are pronouns, not nouns.

3. Honesty is the best policy. (subject noun: honesty; object noun: policy)
4. After the election, we celebrated our new governor. (object nouns: governor, election)
5. I slept. (0 nouns)

Look for the nouns in these sentences.

1. Mrs. Garcia makes a great pumpkin pie. (subject noun: Mrs. Garcia; object noun: pie)
2. We really need to water the garden. (object noun: garden)
3. Love is sweet. (subject noun: love)
4. Sam loves New York in the springtime. (subject noun: Sam; object nouns: New York, springtime)
5. Lin and her mother and father ate soup, fish, potatoes, and fruit for dinner. (subject nouns: Lin, mother, father; object nouns: soup, fish, potatoes, fruit, dinner)

Why isn't the word *pumpkin* a noun in the first sentence? *Pumpkin* is often a noun, but here it is used as an adjective that describes what kind of *pie*.

Why isn't the word *water* a noun in the second sentence? Here, *water* is an **action verb**. To *water the garden* is something we do.

How is the word *love* a noun in the third sentence and not in the fourth sentence? *Love* is a noun (thing) in sentence 3 and a verb (action) in the sentence 4.

How many nouns can a sentence contain? As long as the sentence remains grammatically correct, it can contain an unlimited number of nouns.

> **BE CAREFUL!**
> Words can change to serve different roles in different sentences. A word that is usually a noun can sometimes be used as an adjective or a verb. Determine a word's function in a sentence to be sure of its part of speech.

Types of Nouns

A. Singular and Plural Nouns

Nouns can be **singular** or **plural**. A noun is singular when there is only one. A noun is plural when there are two or more.

- The book has 650 pages.

Book is a singular noun. *Pages* is a plural noun.

Often, to make a noun plural, we add *-s* at the end of the word: *cat/cats*. This is a **regular** plural noun. Sometimes we make a word plural in another way: *child/children*. This is an **irregular** plural noun. Some plurals follow rules, while others do not. The most common rules are listed here:

> **KEEP IN MIND . . .**
> **Some nouns are countable,** and others are not. For example, we eat *three blueberries*, but we **do not** drink *three milks*. Instead, we drink *three glasses of milk* or *some milk*.

Singular noun	Plural noun	Rule for making plural
star	stars	for most words, add *-s*
box	boxes	for words that end in *-j*, *-s*, *-x*, *-z*, *-ch* or *-sh*, add *-es*
baby	babies	for words that end in *-y*, change *-y* to *-i* and add *-es*
woman	women	irregular
foot	feet	irregular

B. Common and Proper Nouns

Common nouns are general words, and they are written in lowercase. **Proper nouns** are specific names, and they begin with an uppercase letter.

Examples:

Common noun	Proper noun
ocean	Baltic Sea
dentist	Dr. Marx
company	Honda
park	Yosemite National Park

C. Concrete and Abstract Nouns

Concrete nouns are people, places, or things that physically exist. We can use our senses to see or hear them. *Turtle, spreadsheet,* and *Australia* are concrete nouns.

Abstract nouns are ideas, qualities, or feelings that we cannot see and that might be harder to describe. *Beauty, childhood, energy, envy, generosity, happiness, patience, pride, trust, truth,* and *victory* are abstract nouns.

Some words can be either concrete or abstract nouns. For example, the concept of *art* is abstract, but *art* that we see and touch is concrete.

- We talked about *art*. (abstract)
- She showed me the *art* she had created in class. (concrete)

Let's Review!

- A noun is a person, place, thing, or idea.
- A noun's function in a sentence is as subject or object.
- Common nouns are general words, while proper nouns are specific names.
- Nouns can be concrete or abstract.

PRONOUNS

A pronoun is a word that takes the place of or refers to a specific noun. This lesson will cover (1) the role of pronouns in sentences and (2) the purpose of pronouns.

Pronouns and Their Role in Sentences

A **pronoun** takes the place of a noun or refers to a specific noun.

Subject, Object, and Possessive Pronouns

A pronoun's role in a sentence is as **subject**, **object**, or **possessive**.

Subject Pronouns	Object Pronouns	Possessive Pronouns
I	me	my, mine
you	you	your, yours
he	her	his
she	him	her, hers
it	it	its
we	us	ours
they	them	their, theirs

In simple sentences, subject pronouns come before the verb, object pronouns come after the verb, and possessive pronouns show ownership.

Look at the pronouns in these examples:

- <u>She</u> forgot <u>her</u> coat. (subject: she; possessive: her)
- <u>I</u> lent <u>her</u> <u>mine</u>. (subject: I; object: her; possessive: mine)
- <u>She</u> left <u>it</u> at school. (subject: she; object: it)
- <u>I</u> had to go and get <u>it</u> the next day. (subject: I; object: it)
- <u>I</u> will never lend <u>her</u> something of <u>mine</u> again! (subject: I; object: her; possessive: mine)

BE CAREFUL!

It is easy to make a mistake when you have multiple words in the role of subject or object.

Correct	Incorrect	Why?
John and I went out.	*John and me* went out.	*John and I* is a subject. *I* is a subject pronoun; *me* is not.
Johan took *Sam and me* to the show.	Johan took *Sam and I* to the show.	*Sam and me* is an object. *Me* is an object pronoun; *I* is not.

Relative Pronouns

Relative pronouns connect a clause to a noun or pronoun.

These are some relative pronouns:

who, whom, whoever, whose, that, which

- Steve Jobs, *who founded Apple*, changed the way people use technology.

The pronoun *who* introduces a clause that gives more information about Steve Jobs.

- This is the movie *that Emily told us to see*.

The pronoun *that* introduces a clause that gives more information about the movie.

Other Pronouns

Some other pronouns are:

this, that, what, anyone, everything, something

> **DID YOU KNOW?**
> Pronouns can sometimes refer to general or unspecified things.

Look for the pronouns in these sentences.

- What is that?
- There is something over there!
- Does anyone have a pen?

Pronouns and Their Purpose

The purpose of a pronoun is to replace a noun. Note the use of the pronoun *their* in the heading of this section. If we did not have pronouns, we would have to call this section *Pronouns and Pronouns' Purpose*.

What Is an Antecedent?

A pronoun in a sentence refers to a specific noun, and this noun called the **antecedent**.

- John Hancock signed the Declaration of Independence. He signed it in 1776.

The antecedent for *he* is John Hancock. The antecedent for *it* is the Declaration of Independence.

> **BE CAREFUL!**
> Look out for unclear antecedents, such as in this sentence:
>
> - Take the furniture out of the room and paint *it*.
>
> What needs to be painted, the furniture or the room?

Find the pronouns in the following sentence. Then identify the antecedent for each pronoun.

Erin had an idea *that she* suggested to Antonio: "*I'*ll help *you* with *your* math homework if *you* help *me* with *my* writing assignment."

Pronoun	Antecedent
that	idea
she	Erin
I	Erin
you	Antonio
your	Antonio's
you	Antonio
me	Erin
my	Erin's

What Is Antecedent Agreement?

A pronoun must agree in **gender** and **number** with the antecedent it refers to. For example:

- Singular pronouns *I, you, he, she*, and *it* replace singular nouns.
- Plural pronouns *you, we*, and *they* replace plural nouns.
- Pronouns *he, she*, and *it* replace masculine, feminine, or neutral nouns.

Correct	Incorrect	Why?
<u>Students</u> should do <u>their</u> homework every night.	<u>A student</u> should do <u>their</u> homework every night.	The pronoun *their* is plural, so it must refer to a plural noun such as *students*.
When <u>an employee</u> is sick, <u>he or she</u> should call the office.	When <u>an employee</u> is sick, <u>they</u> should call the office.	The pronoun *they* is plural, so it must refer to a plural noun. *Employee* is not a plural noun.

Let's Review!

- A pronoun takes the place of or refers to a noun.
- The role of pronouns in sentences is as subject, object, or possessive.
- A pronoun must agree in number and gender with the noun it refers to.

ADJECTIVES AND ADVERBS

An **adjective** is a word that describes a noun or a pronoun. An **adverb** is a word that describes a verb, an adjective, or another adverb.

Adjectives

An **adjective** describes, modifies, or tells us more about a **noun** or a **pronoun**. Colors, numbers, and descriptive words such as *healthy*, *good*, and *sharp* are adjectives.

> **KEEP IN MIND . . .**
> Adjectives typically come **before the noun** in English. However, with **linking verbs** (non-action verbs such as *be, seem, look*), the adjective may come **after the verb** instead. Think of it like this: a linking verb **links** the adjective to the noun or pronoun.

Look for the adjectives in the following sentences:

	Adjective	Noun or pronoun it describes
I rode the blue bike.	blue	bike
It was a long trip.	long	trip
Bring two pencils for the exam.	two	pencils
The box is brown.	brown	box
She looked beautiful.	beautiful	she
That's great!	great	that

Multiple adjectives can be used in a sentence, as can multiple nouns. Look at these examples:

	Adjectives	Noun or pronoun it describes
The six girls were happy, healthy, and rested after their long beach vacation.	six, happy, healthy, rested; long, beach	girls; vacation
Leo has a good job, but he is applying for a better one.	good; better	job; one

> **KEEP IN MIND . . .**
> Note comparative and superlative forms of adjectives, such as:
>
> fast, faster, fastest
>
> far, farther, farthest
>
> good, better, best
>
> bad, worse, worst

Articles: *A, An, The*

Articles are a unique part of speech, but they work like adjectives. An article tells more about a noun. *A* and *an* are **indefinite** articles. Use *a* before a singular **general** noun. Use *an* before a singular general noun that begins with a vowel.

The is a **definite** article. Use *the* before a singular or plural **specific** noun.

Look at how articles are used in the following sentences:

- I need *a* pencil to take *the* exam. (any pencil; specific exam)
- Is there *a* zoo in town? (any zoo)
- Let's go to *the* zoo today. (specific zoo)
- Can you get me *a* glass of milk? (any glass)
- Would you bring me *the* glass that's over there? (specific glass)

Adverbs

An **adverb** describes, modifies, or tells us more about a **verb**, an **adjective**, or another **adverb**. Many adverbs end in *-ly*. Often, adverbs tell when, where, or how something happened. Words such as *slowly, very*, and *yesterday* are adverbs.

Adverbs that Describe Verbs

Adverbs that describe verbs tell something more about the action.

Look for the adverbs in these sentences:

	Adverb	Verb it describes
They walked quickly.	quickly	walked
She disapproved somewhat of his actions, but she completely understood them.	somewhat; completely	disapproved; understood
The boys will go inside if it rains heavily.	inside; heavily	go; rains

Adverbs that Describe Adjectives

Adverbs that describe adjectives often add intensity to the adjective. Words like *quite, more*, and *always* are adverbs.

Look for the adverbs in these sentences:

	Adverb	Adjective it describes
The giraffe is very tall.	very	tall
Do you think that you are more intelligent than them?	more	intelligent
If it's really loud, we can make the volume slightly lower.	really; slightly	loud; lower

Adverbs that Describe Other Adverbs

Adverbs that describe adverbs often add intensity to the adverb.

Look for the adverbs in these sentences:

	Adverb	Adverb it describes
The mouse moved too quickly for us to catch it.	too	quickly
This store is almost never open.	almost	never
Those women are quite fashionably dressed.	quite	fashionably

Adjectives vs. Adverbs

Not sure whether a word is an adjective or an adverb? Look at these examples.

	Adjective	Adverb	Explanation
fast	You're a *fast* driver.	You drove *fast*.	The adjective *fast* describes *driver* (noun); the adverb *fast* describes *drove* (verb).
early	I don't like *early* mornings!	Try to arrive *early*.	The adjective *early* describes *mornings* (noun); the adverb *early* describes *arrive* (verb).
good/well	They did *good* work together.	They worked *well* together.	The adjective *good* describes *work* (noun); the adverb *well* describes *worked* (verb).
bad/badly	The dog is *bad*.	The dog behaves *badly*.	The adjective *bad* describes *dog* (noun); the adverb *badly* describes *behaves* (verb).

Let's Review!

- An **adjective** describes, modifies, or tells us more about a **noun** or a **pronoun**.
- An **adverb** describes, modifies, or tells us more about a **verb**, an **adjective**, or another **adverb**.

BE CAREFUL!

When an adverb ends in -*ly*, add *more* or *most* to make comparisons.

Correct: The car moved *more slowly*.

Incorrect: The car moved *slower*.

CONJUNCTIONS AND PREPOSITIONS

A **conjunction** is a connector word; it connects words, phrases, or clauses in a sentence. A **preposition** is a relationship word; it shows the relationship between two nearby words.

Conjunctions

A **conjunction** connects words, phrases, or clauses.

And, so, and *or* are conjunctions.

> **KEEP IN MIND . . .**
>
> A clause is a phrase that has a subject and a verb.
>
> Some clauses are **independent**. An independent clause can stand alone.
>
> Some clauses are **dependent**. A dependent clause relies on another clause in order to make sense.

Types of Conjunctions

- **Coordinating** conjunctions connect two words, phrases, or independent clauses. The full list of coordinating conjunctions is: *and, or, but, so, for, nor, yet.*
- **Subordinating** conjunctions connect a main (independent) clause and a dependent clause. The conjunction may show a relationship or time order for the two clauses. Some subordinating conjunctions are: *after, as soon as, once, if, even though, unless.*
- **Correlative** conjunctions are pairs of conjunctions that work together to connect two words or phrases. Some correlative conjunctions are: *either/or, neither/nor, as/as.*

Example	Conjunction	What it is connecting
Verdi, Mozart, **and** *Wagner* are famous opera composers.	and	three nouns
Would you like *angel food cake, chocolate lava cake,* **or** *banana cream pie* for dessert?	or	three noun phrases
I took the bus to work, **but** *I walked home.*	but	two independent clauses
It was noisy at home, **so** *we went to the library.*	so	two independent clauses
They have to clean the house **before** *the realtor shows it.*	before	a main clause and a dependent clause
Use **either** *hers* **or** *mine.*	either/or	two pronouns
After *everyone leaves,* make sure you lock up.	after	a main clause and a dependent clause
I'd **rather** *fly* **than** *take the train.*	rather/than	two verb phrases
As soon as *they announced the winning number,* she looked at her ticket and shouted, "Whoopee!"	as soon as	a main clause and a dependent clause

> **DID YOU KNOW?**
>
> In the last example above, "*Whoopee!*" is an interjection. An **interjection** is a short phrase or clause that communicates emotion.
>
> Some other interjections are:
>
> - *Way to go!*
> - *Yuck.*
> - *Hooray!*
> - *Holy cow!*
> - *Oops!*

Prepositions

A **preposition** shows the relationship between two nearby words. Prepositions help to tell information such as direction, location, and time. *To, for,* and *with* are prepositions.

KEEP IN MIND . . .
Some prepositions are more than one word. *On top of* and *instead of* are prepositions.

Example	Preposition	What it tells us
The desk is in the classroom.	in	location
We'll meet you at 6:00.	at	time
We'll meet you at the museum.	at	place
The book is on top of the desk.	on top of	location

Prepositional Phrases

A preposition must be followed by an **object of the preposition**. This can be a noun or something that serves as a noun, such as a pronoun or a gerund.

DID YOU KNOW?
A gerund is the *-ing* form a verb that serves as a noun. *Hiking* is a gerund in this sentence:

I wear these shoes for *hiking*.

A **prepositional phrase** is a preposition plus the object that follows it.

Look for the prepositional phrases in the following examples. Note that a sentence can have more than one prepositional phrase.

Example	Preposition	Object of the preposition
The tiny country won the war *against all odds*.	against	all odds
Look *at us*!	at	us
Why don't we go swimming *instead of sweating in this heat*?	instead of; in	sweating; this heat
Aunt Tea kept the trophy *on a shelf of the cabinet between the sofas in the living room*.	on; of; between; in	a shelf; the cabinet; the sofas; the living room

> **BE CAREFUL!**
> Sometimes a word looks like a preposition but is actually part of the verb. In this case, the verb is called a phrasal verb, and the preposition-like word is called a particle. Here is an example:
>
> - *Turn on* the light. (*Turn on* has a meaning of its own; it is a phrasal verb. *On* is a particle here, rather than a preposition.)
> - Turn *on that street*. (*On that street* shows location; it is a prepositional phrase. *On* is a preposition here.)

Let's Review!

- A **conjunction** connects words, phrases, or clauses. *And, so,* and *or* are conjunctions.
- A **preposition** shows the relationship between two nearby words. *To, for,* and *with* are prepositions.
- A **prepositional phrase** includes a preposition plus the object of the preposition.

VERBS AND VERB TENSES

A **verb** is a word that describes a **physical or mental action** or a **state of being**. This lesson will cover the role of verbs in sentences, verb forms and tenses, and helping verbs.

The Role of Verbs in Sentences

A verb describes an action or a state of being. A complete sentence must have at least one verb.

Verbs have different tenses, which show time.

Verb Forms

Each verb has three primary forms. The **base form** is used for simple present tense, and the **past form** is used for simple past tense. The **participle form** is used for more complicated time situations. Participle form verbs are accompanied by a helping verb.

Base Form	Past Form	Participle Form
end	ended	ended
jump	jumped	jumped
explain	explained	explained
eat	ate	eaten
take	took	taken
go	went	gone
come	came	come

Some verbs are **regular**. To make the **past** or **participle** form of a regular verb, we just add *-ed*. However, many verbs that we commonly use are **irregular**. We need to memorize the forms for these verbs.

In the chart above, *end, jump,* and *explain* are regular verbs. *Eat, take, go,* and *come* are irregular.

Using Verbs

A simple sentence has a **subject** and a **verb**. The subject tells us who or what, and the verb tells us the action or state.

Example	Subject	Verb	*Explanation/Time*
They ate breakfast together yesterday.	They	ate	*happened yesterday*
I walk to school.	I	walk	*happens regularly*
We went to California last year.	We	went	*happened last year*
She seems really tired.	She	seems	*how she seems right now*
The teacher is sad.	teacher	is	*her state right now*

You can see from the examples in this chart that **past tense verbs** are used for a time in the past, and **present tense verbs** are used for something that happens regularly or for a state or condition right now.

Often a sentence has more than one verb. If it has a connector word or more than one subject, it can have more than one verb.

- The two cousins <u>live</u>, <u>work</u>, and <u>vacation</u> together. (3 verbs)
- The girls <u>planned</u> by phone, and then they <u>met</u> at the movies. (2 verbs)

BE CAREFUL!
When you have more than one verb in a sentence, make sure both verb tenses are correct.

Helping Verbs and Progressive and Perfect Tenses

Helping Verbs

A **helping verb** is a supporting verb that accompanies a main verb.

Questions, negative sentences, and certain time situations require helping verbs.

forms of helping verb "to be"	forms of helping verb "to have"	forms of helping verb "to do"	some modals (used like helping verbs)
am, are, is, was, were, be, being, been	have, has, had, having	do, does, did, doing	will, would, can, could, must, might, should

Here are examples of helping verbs in questions and negatives.

- Where *is* he *going*?
- *Did* they *win*?
- I *don't want* that.
- The boys *can't* go.

Progressive and Perfect Tenses

Helping verbs accompany main verbs in certain time situations, such as when an action is or was ongoing, or when two actions overlap in time. To form these tenses, we use a **helping verb** with the **base form plus -ing** or with the **participle form** of the main verb.

The **progressive tense** is used for an action that is or was ongoing. It takes base form of the main verb plus *-ing*.

Example sentence	Tense	Explanation/Time
I <u>am taking</u> French this semester.	Present progressive	*happening now, over a continuous period of time*
I <u>was working</u> when you stopped by.	Past progressive	*happened over a continuous period of time in the past*

The **perfect tense** is used to cover two time periods. It takes the *participle* form of the main verb.

Example sentence	Tense	*Explanation/Time*
I have lived here for three years.	Present perfect	*started in the past and continues to present*
I had finished half of my homework when my computer stopped working.	Past perfect	*started and finished in the past, overlapping in time with another action*

Sometimes we use both the **progressive** and **perfect** tenses together.

Example sentence	Tense	*Explanation/Time*
I have been walking for hours!	Present perfect progressive	*started in the past, took place for a period of time, and continues to present*
She had been asking for a raise for months before she finally received one.	Past perfect progressive	*started in the past, took place for a period of time, and ended*

Let's Review!

- A verb describes an action or state of being.
- Each verb has three primary forms: base form, past form, and participle form.
- Verbs have different tenses, which are used to show time.
- Helping verbs are used in questions, negative sentences, and to form progressive and perfect tenses.

Chapter 2 Parts of Speech Practice Quiz

1. Select the part of speech of the underlined word in the following sentence.

   She did quite well on the exam.

   A. Noun   C. Adjective

   B. Adverb   D. Preposition

2. Select the noun that the underlined adjectives describe.

   Two weeks after his surgery, Henry felt strong and healthy.

   A. weeks   C. surgery

   B. his   D. Henry

3. Which word is an adverb that describes the underlined verb?

   The man spoke to us wisely.

   A. man   C. us

   B. to   D. wisely

4. Identify the conjunction in the following sentence.

   He is sick, yet he came to work.

   A. is   C. came

   B. yet   D. to

5. Which is not a prepositional phrase?

   Keep me informed about the status of the problem throughout the day.

   A. Keep me informed

   B. about the status

   C. of the problem

   D. throughout the day

6. How many prepositions are in the following sentence?

   The athletes traveled from Boston to Dallas for the competition.

   A. 0   C. 2

   B. 1   D. 3

7. Which words in the following sentence are proper nouns?

   Matthew had a meeting with his supervisor on Tuesday.

   A. Matthew, meeting

   B. Matthew, Tuesday

   C. meeting, supervisor

   D. supervisor, Tuesday

8. How many plural nouns are in the following sentence?

   Marie's father's appendix was taken out.

   A. 0   C. 2

   B. 1   D. 3

9. Which of the following words is an abstract noun?

   A. Car   C. Ruler

   B. Tent   D. Health

10. Which word in the following sentence is a pronoun?

    To whom should the applicant address the letter?

    A. To   C. whom

    B. the   D. should

11. **Which pronoun correctly completes the following sentence?**

    Nigel introduced Van and ____ to the new administrator.

    A. I   C. she

    B. me   D. they

12. **Select the noun to which the underlined pronoun refers.**

    Greta Garbo, <u>who</u> performed in both silent and talking pictures, is my favorite actress.

    A. actress   C. performed

    B. pictures   D. Greta Garbo

13. **How many verbs are in the following sentence?**

    They toured the art museum and saw the conservatory.

    A. 0   C. 2

    B. 1   D. 3

14. **Which word in the following sentence is a helping verb?**

    They did not ask for our help.

    A. did   C. for

    B. ask   D. our

15. **Select the correct verb form to complete the following sentence.**

    William didn't think he would enjoy the musical, but he ____.

    A. do   C. liked

    B. did   D. would

Chapter 2 Parts of Speech Practice Quiz — Answer Key

1. **B.** *Quite* is an adverb that describes the adverb *well*. **See Lesson: Adjectives and Adverbs.**

2. **D.** These adjectives describe *Henry*. **See Lesson: Adjectives and Adverbs.**

3. **D.** *Wisely* is an adverb that describes the verb *spoke*. **See Lesson: Adjectives and Adverbs.**

4. **B.** *Yet* is a conjunction. **See Lesson: Conjunctions and Prepositions.**

5. **A.** *Keep me informed* does not contain a preposition. *About, of,* and *throughout* are prepositions. **See Lesson: Conjunctions and Prepositions.**

6. **D.** *From, to,* and *for* are prepositions. **See Lesson: Conjunctions and Prepositions.**

7. **B.** *Matthew* and *Tuesday* are proper nouns. **See Lesson: Nouns.**

8. **A.** *Marie's* and *father's* are possessive; neither is plural. *Appendix* is a singular noun. **See Lesson: Nouns.**

9. **D.** *Health* is an abstract noun; it does not physically exist. **See Lesson: Nouns.**

10. **C.** *Whom* is a pronoun. **See Lesson: Pronouns.**

11. **B.** An object pronoun must be used here. **See Lesson: Pronouns.**

12. **D.** *Who* is a relative pronoun that refers to the subject *Greta Garbo*. **See Lesson: Pronouns.**

13. **C.** *Toured* and *saw* are verbs. **See Lesson: Verbs and Verb Tenses.**

14. **A.** *Did* is a helping verb; *ask* is the main verb. **See Lesson: Verbs and Verb Tenses.**

15. **B.** *Did* can be used here, for a shortened form of *did enjoy it*. **See Lesson: Verbs and Verb Tenses.**

CHAPTER 3 KNOWLEDGE OF LANGUAGE

TYPES OF SENTENCES

Sentences are a combination of words that communicate a complete thought. Sentences can be written in many ways to signal different relationships among ideas. This lesson will cover (1) simple sentences (2) compound sentences (3) complex sentences (4) parallel structure.

Simple Sentences

A **simple sentence** is a group of words that make up a **complete thought**. To be a complete thought, simple sentences must have one **independent clause**. An independent clause contains a single **subject** (who or what the sentence is about) and a **predicate** (a **verb** and something about the subject.)

Let's take a look at some simple sentences:

Simple Sentence	Subject	Predicate	Complete Thought?
The car was fast.	car	was fast (verb = was)	Yes
Sally waited for the bus.	Sally	waited for the bus (verb = waited)	Yes
The pizza smells delicious.	pizza	smells delicious (verb = smells)	Yes
Anton loves cycling.	Anton	loves cycling (verb = loves)	Yes

It is important to be able to recognize what a simple sentence is in order to avoid **run-ons** and **fragments**, two common grammatical errors.

A **run-on** is when two or more independent clauses are combined without proper punctuation:

FOR EXAMPLE

Gregory is a very talented actor he was the lead in the school play.

If you take a look at this sentence, you can see that it is made up of 2 independent clauses or simple sentences:

1. *Gregory is a very talented actor*
2. *he was the lead in the school play*

You <u>cannot</u> have two independent clauses running into each other without proper punctuation.

You can fix this run-on in the following way:

Gregory is a very talented actor. He was the lead in the school play.

A **fragment** is a group of words that looks like a sentence. It starts with a capital letter and has end punctuation, but when you examine it closely you will see it is not a complete thought.

Let's put this information all together to determine whether a group of words is a simple sentence, a run-on, or a fragment:

Group of Words	Category
Mondays are the worst they are a drag.	Run-On: These are two independent clauses running into one another without proper punctuation. FIX: *Mondays are the worst. They are a drag.*
Because I wanted soda.	Fragment: This is a dependent clause and needs more information to make it a complete thought. FIX: *I went to the store because I wanted soda.*
Ereni is from Greece.	Simple Sentence: YES! This is a simple sentence with a subject (*Ereni*) and a predicate (*is from Greece*), so it is a complete thought.
While I was apple picking.	Fragment: This is a dependent clause and needs more information to make it a complete thought. FIX: *While I was apple picking, I spotted a bunny.*
New York City is magical it is my favorite place.	Run-On: These are two independent clauses running into one another without proper punctuation. FIX: *New York City is magical. It is my favorite place.*

Compound Sentences

A **compound sentence** is a sentence made up of two independent clauses connected with a **coordinating conjunction**.

Let's take a look at the following sentence:

Joe waited for the bus, but it never arrived.

If you take a close look at this compound sentence, you will see that it is made up of two independent clauses:

1. *Joe waited for the bus*
2. *it never arrived*

The word *but* is the coordinating conjunction that connects these two sentences. Notice that the coordinating conjunction has a comma right before it. This is the proper way to punctuate compound sentences.

Here are other examples of compound sentences:

FOR EXAMPLE

I want to try out for the baseball team, and I also want to try out for track.

*Sally can play the clarinet in the band, **or** she can play the violin in the orchestra.*

*Mr. Henry is going to run the half marathon, **so** he has a lot of training to do.*

All these sentences are compound sentences since they each have two independent clauses joined by a comma and a coordinating conjunction.

The following is a list of **coordinating conjunctions** that can be used in compound sentences. You can use the mnemonic device "FANBOYS" to help you remember them:

For

And

Nor

But

Or

Yet

So

Think back to Section 1: Simple Sentences. You learned about run-ons. Another way to fix run-ons is by turning the group of words into a compound sentence:

RUN-ON: *Gregory is a very talented actor he was the lead in the school play.*

FIX: *Gregory is a very talented actor, **so** he was the lead in the school play.*

Complex Sentences

A **complex** sentence is a sentence that is made up of an independent clause and one or more dependent clauses connected to it.

Think back to Section 1 when you learned about fragments. You learned about a **dependent clause**, the part of a sentence that cannot stand by itself. These clauses need other information to make them complete.

You can recognize a dependent clause because they always begin with a **subordinating conjunction**. These words are a key ingredient in complex sentences.

Here is a list of **subordinating conjunctions**:

after	although	as	because	before
despite	even if	even though	if	in order to
that	once	provided that	rather than	since
so that	than	that	though	unless
until	when	whenever	where	whereas
wherever	while	why		

Let's take a look at a few complex sentences:

> **FOR EXAMPLE**
>
> ***Since the alarm clock didn't go off, I was late for class.***
>
> This is an example of a complex sentence because it contains:
>
> A dependent clause: *Since the alarm clock didn't go off*
> An independent clause: *I was late for class*
> A subordinating conjunction: *since*
>
> ***Sarah studied all night for the exam even though she did not receive an A.***
>
> This is an example of a complex sentence because it contains:
>
> A dependent clause: *even though she did not receive an A*
> An independent clause: *Sarah studied all night*
> A subordinating conjunction: *even though*
>
> ***NOTE:*** *To make a complex sentence, you can either start with the dependent clause or the independent clause. When beginning with the dependent clause, you need a comma after it. When beginning with an independent clause, you do not need a comma after it.*

Parallel Structure

Parallel structure is the repetition of a grammatical form within a sentence to make the sentence sound more harmonious. Parallel structure comes into play when you are making a list of items. Stylistically, you want all the items in the list to line up with each other to make them sound better.

Let's take a look at when to use parallel structure:

1. Use parallel structure with verb forms:

    In a sentence listing different verbs, you want all the verbs to use the same form:

    Manuel likes hiking, biking, and mountain climbing.

    In this example, the words *hiking, biking* and *climbing* are all gerunds (having an -ing ending), so the sentence is balanced since the words are all using the gerund form of the verb.

    Manuel likes to hike, bike, and mountain climb.

In this example, the words *hike, bike* and *climb* are all infinitives (using the basic form of the verb), so the sentence is balanced.

You do not want to mix them up:

Manuel likes hiking, biking, and to mountain climb.

This sentence **does not** use parallel structure since *hiking* and *biking* use the gerund form of the verb and *to mountain climb* uses the infinitive form.

2. Use parallel structure with active and passive voice:

    In a sentence written in the **active voice**, the subject performs the action:

    Sally kicked the ball.

    Sally, the subject, is the one doing the action, kicking the ball.

    In a sentence written in the **passive voice**, the subject is acted on by the verb.

    The ball was kicked by Sally.

    When using parallel structure, you want to make sure your items in a list are either all in **active voice**:

    Raymond baked, frosted, and decorated the cake.

    Or all in **passive voice**:

    The cake was baked, frosted, and decorated by Raymond.

    You do not want to mix them up:

    The cake was baked, frosted, and Raymond decorated it.

    This sentence **does not** use parallel structure because it starts off with passive voice and then switches to active voice.

3. Use parallel structure with the length of terms within a list:

    When making a list, you should either have all short individual terms or all long phrases.

    Keep these consistent by either choosing short, individual terms:

    Cassandra is bold, courageous, and strong.

    Or longer phrases:

    Cassandra is brave in the face of danger, willing to take risks, and a force to be reckoned with.

    You do not want to mix them up:

    Cassandra is bold, courageous, and a force to be reckoned with.

This sentence **does not** use parallel structure because the first two terms are short, and the last one is a longer phrase.

Let's Review!

- A simple sentence consists of a clause, which has a single subject and a predicate.
- A compound sentence is made up of two independent clauses connected by a coordinating conjunction.
- A complex sentence is made up of a subordinating conjunction, an independent clause and one or more dependent clauses connected to it.
- Parallel structure is the repetition of a grammatical form within a sentence to make the sentence sound more harmonious.

TYPES OF CLAUSES

There are four types of clauses that are used to create sentences. Sentences with several clauses, and different types of clauses, are considered complex. This lesson will cover (1) independent clauses, (2) dependent clauses and subordinate clauses, and (3) coordinate clauses.

Independent Clause

An **independent clause** is a simple sentence. It has a subject, a verb, and expresses a complete thought.

- Steve went to the store.
- She will cook dinner tonight.
- The class was very boring.
- The author argues that listening to music helps productivity.

Two **independent clauses** can be connected by a semicolon. There are some common words that indicate the beginning of an **independent clause** such as: moreover, also, nevertheless, however, furthermore, consequently.

- I wanted to go to dinner; however, I had to work late tonight.
- She had a job interview; therefore, she dressed nicely.

Dependent and Subordinate Clauses

A **dependent clause** is not a complete sentence. It has a subject and a verb but does not express a complete thought. **Dependent clauses** are also called **subordinate clauses**, because they depend on the **independent or main clause** to complete the thought. A sentence that has both at least one **independent clause** and one **subordinate clause** are considered complex.

Subordinate clauses can be placed before or after the **independent clause**. When the **subordinate clause** begins the sentence, there should be a comma before the **main clause**. If the **subordinate clause** ends the sentence, there is no need for a comma.

Dependent clauses also have common indicator words. These are often called **subordinating conjunctions** because they connect a **dependent clause** to an **independent clause**. Some of these include: although, after, as, because, before, if, once, since, unless, until, when, whether, and while. Relative pronouns also signify the beginning of a **subordinate clause**. These include: that, which, who, whom, whichever, whoever, whomever, and whose.

- When I went to school...
- Since she joined the team...
- After we saw the play...
- *Because she studied hard*, she received an A on her exam.
- *Although the professor was late*, the class was very informative.
- I can't join you *unless I finish my homework*.

Coordinate Clause

A **coordinate clause** is a sentence or phrase that combines clauses of equal grammatical rank (verbs, nouns, adjectives, phrases, or independent clauses) by using a coordinating conjunction (and, but, for, nor, or so, yet). **Coordinating conjunctions** cannot connect a **dependent or subordinate clause** and an **independent clause.**

- She woke up, and he went to bed.
- We did not have cheese, so I went to the store to get some.
- Ice cream and candy taste great, but they are not good for you.
- Do you want to study, or do you want to go to Disneyland?

Let's Review!

- An **independent clause** is a simple sentence that has a noun, a verb, and a complete thought. Two **independent clauses** can be connected by a semicolon.
- A **dependent or subordinate clause** depends on the main clause to complete a thought. A **dependent or subordinate clause** can go before or after the **independent clause** and there are indicator words that signify the beginning of the **dependent or subordinate clause.**
- A **coordinate clause** connects two verbs, nouns, adjectives, phrases, or **independent clauses** using a **coordinating conjunction** (and, but, for, nor, or, so, yet).

SUBJECT AND VERB AGREEMENT

Every sentence must include a **subject** and a **verb**. The subject tells **who or what**, and the verb describes an **action or condition**. Subject and verb agree in number and person.

Roles of Subject and Verb

A complete sentence includes a **subject** and a **verb**. The verb is in the part of the sentence called the **predicate**. A predicate can be thought of as a verb phrase.

Simple Sentences

A sentence can be very simple, with just one or two words as the **subject** and one or two words as the **predicate**.

Sometimes, in a command, a subject is "understood," rather than written or spoken.

BE CAREFUL!

It's is a contraction of *it is*.

Its (without an apostrophe) is the possessive of the pronoun *it*.

Look at these examples of short sentences:

Sentence	Subject	Predicate, with main verb(s) underlined
I ate.	I	<u>ate</u>
They ran away.	They	<u>ran</u> away
It's OK.	It	<u>is</u> OK
Go and find the cat!	(You)	<u>go</u> and <u>find</u> the cat

Complex Sentences

Sometimes a subject or predicate is a long phrase or clause.

Some sentences have more than one subject or predicate, or even a predicate within a predicate.

Sentence	Subject(s)	Predicate(s), with main verb(s) underlined
My friend from work had a bad car accident.	My friend from work	<u>had</u> a bad car accident
John, his sister, and I plan to ride our bikes across the country this summer.	John, his sister, and I	<u>plan</u> to ride our bikes across the country this summer
I did so much for them, and they didn't even thank me.*	I; they	<u>did</u> so much for them; didn't even <u>thank</u> me
She wrote a letter that explained the problem.**	She	<u>wrote</u> a letter that explained the problem

*This sentence consists of two clauses, and each clause has its own subject and its own predicate.

**In this sentence, *that explained the problem* is part of the predicate, and it is also a relative clause with own subject and predicate.

Subject and Verb Agreement

Subjects and verbs must agree in **number** and **person**. This means that different subjects take different forms of a verb.

With **regular** verbs, simply add *-s* to the singular third person verb, as shown below:

	Singular		Plural	
	Subject	Verb	Subject	Verb
(first person)	I	play	we	play
(second person)	you	play	you	play
(third person)	he/she/it	plays	they	play

Some verbs are **irregular**, so simply adding *-s* doesn't work. For example:

verb	form for third person singular subject
have	has
do	does
fix	fixes

Look for subject-verb agreement in the following sentences:

- *I* usually <u>eat</u> a banana for breakfast.
- *Marcy* <u>does</u> well in school.
- The *cat* <u>licks</u> its fur.

Subject-Verb Agreement for the Verb *Be*

Present		Past	
I am	we are	I was	we were
you are	you are	you were	you were
he/she/it is	they are	they were	they were

Things to Look Out For

Subject-verb agreement can be tricky. Be careful of these situations:

- **Sentences with more than one subject:** If two subjects are connected by *and*, the subject is **plural**. When two singular subjects are connected by *neither/nor*, the subject is **singular**.

Sandra and Luiz <u>shop</u>. (plural)
Neither Sandra nor Luiz <u>has</u> money. (singular)

- **Collective nouns:** Sometimes a noun stands for a group of people or things. If the subject is **one group**, it is considered **singular**.

Those students are still on chapter three. (plural)
That class is still on chapter three. (singular)

- ***There is*** and ***there are:*** With pronouns such as *there*, *what*, and *where*, the verb agrees with the noun or pronoun that follows it.

There's a rabbit! (singular)
Where are my shoes? (plural)

- **Indefinite pronouns:** Subjects such as *everybody*, *someone*, and *nobody* are **singular**. Subjects such as *all*, *none*, and *any* can be either **singular or plural**.

Everyone in the band plays well. (singular)
All of the students are there. (plural)
All is well. (singular)

Let's Review!

- Every sentence has a subject and a verb.
- The predicate is the part of the sentence that contains the verb.
- The subject and verb must agree in number and person.
- The third person singular subject takes a different verb form.

MODIFIERS

A modifier is a word, phrase, or clause that adds detail or changes (modifies) another word in the sentence. Descriptive words such as adjectives and adverbs are examples of modifiers.

The Role of Modifiers in a Sentence

Modifiers make a sentence more descriptive and interesting.

Look at these simple sentences. Notice how much more interesting they are with modifiers added.

Simple sentence	With modifiers added
I drove.	I drove my family along snowy roads to my grandmother's house.
They ate.	They ate a fruit salad of blueberries, strawberries, peaches, and apples.
The boy looked.	The boy in pajamas looked out the window at the birds eating from the feeder.
He climbed.	He climbed the ladder to fix the roof.

Look at the modifiers in bold type in the following sentences. Notice how these words add description to the basic idea in the sentence.

	Modifier	Word it Modifies	Type
The hungry man ate **quickly.**	1. the; 2. hungry; 3. quickly	1. man 2. man; 3. ate	1. article 2. adjective; 3. adverb
The small child, **who had scraped his knee,** cried **quietly.**	1. the; 2. small; 3. who had scraped his knee; 4. quietly	1. child; 2. child; 3. child; 4. cried	1. article; 2. adjective; 3. adjective clause; 4. adverb
The horse **standing near the fence** is **beautiful.**	1. the; 2. standing near the fence; 3. beautiful	1. horse; 2. horse; 3. horse	1. article; 2. participle phrase; 3. adjective
Hana and Mario stood **by the lake** and watched **a gorgeous** sunset.	1. by the lake; 2. a; 3. gorgeous	1. stood; 2. sunset; 3. sunset	1. prepositional phrase; 2. article; 3. adjective
They tried **to duck out of the way as the large spider dangled from the ceiling.**	1. to duck out of the way; 2. as the large spider dangled; 3. from the ceiling	1. tried; 2. duck; 3. dangled	1. infinitive phrase; 2. adverb clause; 3. prepositional phrase

DID YOU KNOW?

Adjectives and adverbs are not the only modifiers. With a participle phrase, **an -ing verb** can act as a modifier. For example, *eating from the feeder* modifies *the birds*. With an infinitive, *to* **plus the main form of a verb** can act as a modifier. For example, *to fix the roof* modifies *climbed*.

Misplaced and Dangling Modifiers

A **misplaced modifier** is a modifier that is placed incorrectly in a sentence, so that it modifies the wrong word.

A **dangling modifier** is a modifier that modifies a word that should be included in the sentence but is not.

Look at these examples.

- First, notice the modifier, in bold.
- Next, look for the word it modifies.

Incorrect	Problem	How to fix it	Correct
Sam wore his new shirt to school, **which was too big for him.**	Misplaced modifier. Notice the placement of the modifier **which was too big for him.** It is placed after the word *school*, which makes it seem like *school* is the word it describes. However, this was not the writer's intention. The writer intended for **which was too big for him** to describe the word *shirt*.	The modifier needs to be placed after the word *shirt*, rather than after the word *school*.	Sam wore his new shirt, **which was too big for him**, to school.
Running down the hallway, Maria's bag of groceries fell.	Dangling modifier. The modifier **running down the hallway** is placed before the phrase *Maria's bag of groceries*, which makes it seem this is what it describes. However, this was not the writer's intention; the *bag of groceries* cannot run! The correct reference would be the noun *Maria*, which was omitted from the sentence completely.	The modifier must reference *Maria*, rather than *Maria's bag of groceries*. This can be fixed by adding the noun *Maria* as a subject.	**Running down the hallway,** Maria dropped her bag of groceries.
With a leash on, my sister walked the dog.	Misplaced modifier. The modifier **with a leash on** is placed before *my sister*, which makes it seem like she is wearing a leash.	Move the modifier so that it is next to *the dog*, rather than *my sister*.	My sister walked the dog, **who had a leash on.**

Let's Review!

- A modifier is a word, phrase, or clause that adds detail by describing or modifying another word in the sentence.
- Adverbs, adjectives, articles, and prepositional phrases are some examples of modifiers.
- Misplaced and dangling modifiers have unclear references, leading to confusion about the meaning of a sentence.

DIRECT OBJECTS AND INDIRECT OBJECTS

A direct or indirect object has a relationship with the action verb that precedes it. A direct object directly receives the action of the verb. An indirect object indirectly receives the action.

Direct and Indirect Objects in a Sentence

An **object** in grammar is something that is acted on. The **subject** does the action; the **object** receives it.

An object is usually a noun or a pronoun.

There are three types of objects:

- direct object
- indirect object
- object of the preposition

KEEP IN MIND . . .
When there is an **indirect object**, it will be placed between the verb and the direct object.

Many sentences have a direct object. Some sentences also have an indirect object.

Look at these examples:

- Kim threw *the ball*. *The ball* is the direct object. *Ask yourself:* What did she throw?
- Kim threw *Tommy* the ball. *Tommy* is the indirect object. *Ask yourself:* Who did she throw it to?

Look for the objects in the sentences below.

Sentence	Direct Object	Indirect Object	Be careful!
Her mom poured her a glass of milk.	a glass of milk (*ask:* what did she pour?)	her (*ask:* who did she pour it for?)	The indirect object, when there is one, can be found between the verb and the direct object.
They work hard.			Not all sentences have objects. Here, *hard* is not an object. It is not the recipient of *work*. Instead, it is a modifier; it describes the work.
Kazu bought Katrina a present.	a present (*ask:* what did he buy?)	Katrina (*ask:* whom did he buy it for?)	
Kazu bought a present for Katrina.	a present (*ask:* what did he buy?)		Don't confuse indirect objects with prepositional phrases. *For* is a preposition, so *Katrina* is the object of the preposition; it is not an indirect object.

KNAT: Full Study Guide for the Kaplan Nursing Admissions Test.

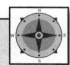

BE CAREFUL!

Some verbs can never take **direct objects**. These are:

- **Linking verbs** such as *is* and *seem*.
- **Intransitive verbs** such as *snore, go, sit*, and *die*.
- *Ask yourself:* Can you *snore* something? No. Therefore, this verb cannot take a direct object.

Let's Review!

- A direct object directly receives the action of the verb.
- An indirect object indirectly receives the action of the verb.
- An indirect object comes between the verb and the direct object.

KEEP IN MIND . . .

If there is a preposition, the object is the **object of the preposition** rather than an **indirect object**.

Compare these two sentences:

- She made *me* dinner. (*Me* is an indirect object.)
- She made dinner *for me*. (*For me* is a prepositional phrase.)

Chapter 3 Knowledge of Language Practice Quiz

1. Identify the direct object in the following sentence.

   Paulo accidentally locked his keys in his car.

   A. Paulo   C. his keys
   B. accidentally   D. his car

2. Select the word that is an object of the underlined verb.

   The graduates <u>held</u> lit candles.

   A. The   C. lit
   B. graduates D. candles

3. Select the verb that acts on the underlined direct object in the following sentence.

   We have no choice but to sit here and wait for these cows to cross <u>the road</u>!

   A. have   C. wait
   B. sit   D. cross

4. Which modifier, if any, modifies the underlined word in the following sentence?

   We always visit the <u>bakery</u> on the corner when we are in town.

   A. always   C. when we are in town
   B. on the corner
                      D. No modifier describes it.

5. Identify the dangling or misplaced modifier, if there is one.

   Having been repaired, we can drive the car again.

   A. Having been repaired
   B. we can drive
   C. the car again
   D. There is no dangling or misplaced modifier.

6. Which ending does <u>not</u> create a sentence with a dangling modifier?

   Trying to earn some extra money, ____.

   A. the new position paid more
   B. he got a second job
   C. the job was difficult
   D. it was an extra shift

7. Select the "understood" subject with which the underlined verb must agree.

   <u>Watch</u> out!

   A. You   C. I
   B. He   D. Out

8. How many verbs must agree with the underlined subject in the following sentence?

   <u>Kareem Abdul-Jabbar</u>, my favorite basketball player, dribbles, shoots, and scores to win the game!

   A. 0   C. 2
   B. 1   D. 3

9. Select the correct verb to complete the following sentence.

    Our family ____ staying home for the holidays this year.

    A. is   C. am

    B. be   D. are

10. Fill in the blank with the correct subordinating conjunction.

    You cannot go to the movies with your friends _____ you finish your homework.

    A. if   C. since

    B. once   D. unless

11. Identify the dependent clause in the following sentence.

    We decided to take our dog to the park although it was hot outside.

    A. We decided to take our dog

    B. to the park

    C. although it was hot outside

    D. to take our dog

12. Identify the independent clause in the following sentence.

    After eating dinner, the couple went on a stroll through the park.

    A. After eating dinner

    B. the couple went on a stroll through the park

    C. through the park

    D. went on a stroll

13. Which of the following is an example of a simple sentence?

    A. Tamara's sporting goods store.

    B. Tamara has a sporting goods store in town.

    C. Tamara has a sporting goods store it is in town.

    D. Tamara's sporting goods store is in town, and she is the owner.

14. Which of the following uses a conjunction to combine the sentences below so the focus is on puppies requiring a lot of work?

    Puppies are fun-loving animals. They do require a lot of work.

    A. Puppies are fun-loving animals; they do require a lot of work.

    B. Puppies are fun-loving animals, so they do require a lot of work.

    C. Since puppies are fun-loving animals they do require a lot of work.

    D. Although puppies are fun-loving animals, they do require a lot of work.

15. Which of these options would complete the following sentence to make it a compound sentence?

    The class of middle school students

    _____.

    A. served food at

    B. served food at a soup kitchen

    C. served food at a soup kitchen, and they enjoyed the experience

    D. served food at a soup kitchen even though they weren't required to

CHAPTER 3 KNOWLEDGE OF LANGUAGE PRACTICE QUIZ — ANSWER KEY

1. C. *His keys* is the direct object of the verb *locked*. **See Lesson: Direct Objects and Indirect Objects.**

2. D. *Candles* is the direct object of the verb *held*. **See Lesson: Direct Objects and Indirect Objects.**

3. D. *The road* is a direct object of the verb *cross*. **See Lesson: Direct Objects and Indirect Objects.**

4. B. *On the corner* modifies *bakery*. **See Lesson: Modifiers.**

5. A. *Having been repaired* is placed where it references *we*, but it should reference *the car*. **See Lesson: Modifiers.**

6. B. Of these choices, *trying to earn some extra money* can only reference *he*. **See Lesson: Modifiers.**

7. A. In a command like this one, the "understood" subject is *you*. **See Lesson: Subject and Verb Agreement.**

8. D. The verbs *dribbles, shoots,* and *scores* must agree with the subject *Kareem Abdul-Jabbar*. **See Lesson: Subject and Verb Agreement.**

9. A. The subject *family* is singular and takes the verb *is*. **See Lesson: Subject and Verb Agreement.**

10. D. The word "unless" signifies the beginning of a dependent clause and is the only conjunction that makes sense in the sentence. **See Lesson: Types of Clauses.**

11. C. *Although it was hot outside* is dependent because it does not express a complete thought and relies on the independent clause. The word "although" also signifies the beginning of a dependent clause. **See Lesson: Types of Clauses.**

12. B. The couple went on a stroll through the park. It is independent because it has a subject, verb, and expresses a complete thought. **See Lesson: Types of Clauses.**

13. B. This is a simple sentence since it contains one independent clause consisting of a simple subject and a predicate. **See Lesson: Types of Sentences.**

14. D. The subordinate conjunction "although" combines the sentences and puts the focus on puppies requiring a lot of work. **See Lesson: Types of Sentences.**

15. C. This option would make the sentence a compound sentence. **See Lesson: Types of Sentences.**

CHAPTER 4 VOCABULARY ACQUISITION

ROOT WORDS, PREFIXES, AND SUFFIXES

A root word is the most basic part of a word. You can create new words by: adding a prefix, a group of letters placed before the root word; or a suffix, a group of letters placed at the end of a root word. In this lesson you will learn about root words, prefixes, suffixes, and how to determine the meaning of a word by analyzing these word parts.

Root Words

Root words are found in everyday language. They are the most basic parts of words. Root words in the English language are mostly derived from Latin or Greek. You can add beginnings (prefixes) and endings (suffixes) to root words to change their meanings. To discover what a root word is, simply remove its prefix and/or suffix. What you are left with is the root word, or the core or basis of the word.

At times, root words can be stand-alone words.

Here are some examples of stand-alone root words:

STAND-ALONE ROOT WORDS	MEANINGS
dress	*clothing*
form	*shape*
normal	*typical*
phobia	*fear of*
port	*carry*

Most root words, however, are **not** stand-alone words. They are not full words on their own, but they still form the basis of other words when you remove their prefixes and suffixes.

Here are some common root words in the English language:

ROOT WORDS	MEANINGS	EXAMPLES
ami, amic	*love*	amicable
anni	*year*	anniversary
aud	*to hear*	auditory
bene	*good*	beneficial
biblio	*book*	bibliography
cap	*take, seize*	capture
cent	*one hundred*	century
chrom	*color*	chromatic

ROOT WORDS	MEANINGS	EXAMPLES
chron	*time*	chronological
circum	*around*	circumvent
cred	*believe*	credible
corp	*body*	corpse
dict	*to say*	dictate
equi	*equal*	equality
fract; rupt	*to break*	fracture
ject	*throw*	eject
mal	*bad*	malignant
min	*small*	miniature
mort	*death*	mortal
multi	*many*	multiply
ped	*foot*	pedestrian
rupt	*break*	rupture
sect	*cut*	dissect
script	*write*	manuscript
sol	*sun*	solar
struct	*build*	construct
terr	*earth*	terrain
therm	*heat*	thermometer
vid, vis	*to see*	visual
voc	*voice; to call*	vocal

Prefixes

Prefixes are the letters added to the **beginning** of a root word to make a new word with a different meaning.

Prefixes on their own have meanings, too. If you add a prefix to a root word, it can change its meaning entirely.

Here are some of the most common prefixes, their meanings, and some examples:

PREFIX	MEANING	EXAMPLE
auto	*self*	autograph
con	*with*	conclude
hydro	*water*	hydrate
im, in, non, un	*not*	unimportant
inter	*between*	international
mis	*incorrect, badly*	mislead

PREFIX	MEANING	EXAMPLE
over	*too much*	over-stimulate
post	*after*	postpone
pre	*before*	preview
re	*again*	rewrite
sub	*under, below*	submarine
trans	*across*	transcribe

Let's look back at some of the root words from Section 1. By adding prefixes to these root words, you can create a completely new word with a new meaning:

ROOT WORD	PREFIX	NEW WORD	MEANING
dress (*clothing*)	un (*remove*)	**un**dress	*remove clothing*
sect (*cut*)	inter (*between*)	**inter**sect	*cut across or through*
phobia (*fear*)	hydro (*water*)	**hydro**phobia	*fear of water*
script (*write*)	post (*after*)	**post**script	*additional remark at the end of a letter*

Suffixes

Suffixes are the letters added to the **end** of a root word to make a new word with a different meaning.

Suffixes on their own have meanings, too. If you add a suffix to a root word, it can change its meaning entirely.

Here are some of the most common suffixes, their meanings, and some examples:

SUFFIX	MEANING	EXAMPLE
able, ible	*can be done*	agreeable
an, ean, ian	*belonging or relating to*	European
ed	*happened in the past*	jogged
en	*made of*	wooden
er	*comparative (more than)*	stricter
est	*comparative (most)*	largest
ful	*full of*	meaningful
ic	*having characteristics of*	psychotic
ion, tion, ation, ition	*act, process*	hospitalization
ist	*person who practices*	linguist
less	*without*	artless
logy	*study of*	biology

Let's look back at some of the root words from Section 1. By adding suffixes to these root words, you can create a completely new word with a new meaning:

ROOT WORD	SUFFIX	NEW WORD	MEANING
aud (*to hear*)	logy (*study of*)	audio**logy**	*the study of hearing*
form (*shape*)	less (*without*)	form**less**	*without a clear shape*
port (*carry*)	able (*can be done*)	port**able**	*able to be carried*
normal (*typical*)	ity (*state of*)	normal**ity**	*condition of being normal*

Determining Meaning

Knowing the meanings of common root words, prefixes, and suffixes can help you determine the meaning of unknown words. By looking at a word's individual parts, you can get a good sense of its definition.

If you look at the word *transportation*, you can study the different parts of the word to figure out what it means.

If you were to break up the word you would see the following:

PREFIX: *trans = across*	ROOT: *port = carry*	SUFFIX: *tion = act or process*

If you put all these word parts together, you can define transportation as: *the act or process of carrying something across*.

Let's define some other words by looking at their roots, prefixes and suffixes:

WORD	PREFIX	ROOT	SUFFIX	WORKING DEFINITION
indestructible	in (*not*)	struct (*build*)	able (*can be done*)	Not able to be "un" built (torn down)
nonconformist	non (*not*) con (*with*)	form (*shape*)	ist (*person who practices*)	A person who can not be shaped (someone who doesn't go along with the norm)
subterranean	sub (*under, below*)	terr (*earth*)	ean (*belonging or relating to*)	Relating or belonging to something under the earth

Let's Review!

- A root word is the most basic part of a word.
- A prefix is the letters added to beginning of a root word to change the word and its meaning.
- A suffix is the letters added to the end of a root word to change the word and its meaning.
- You can figure out a word's meaning by looking closely at its different word parts (root, prefixes, and suffixes).

CONTEXT CLUES AND MULTIPLE MEANING WORDS

Sometimes when you read a text, you come across an unfamiliar word. Instead of skipping the word and reading on, it is important to figure out what that word means so you can better understand the text. There are different strategies you can use to determine the meaning of unfamiliar words. This lesson will cover (1) how to determine unfamiliar words by reading context clues, (2) multiple meaning words, and (3) using multiple meaning words properly in context.

Using Context Clues to Determine Meaning

When reading a text, it is common to come across unfamiliar words. One way to determine the meaning of unfamiliar words is by studying other context clues to help you better understand what the word means.

Context means the other words in the sentences around the unfamiliar word.

You can look at these other words to find **clues** or **hints** to help you figure out what the word means.

FOR EXAMPLE

Look at the following sentence:

Some of the kids in the cafeteria _ostracized_ Janice because she dressed differently; they never allowed her to sit at their lunch table, and they whispered behind her back.

If you did not know what the word _ostracized_ meant, you could look at the **other words** for **clues** to help you.

Here is what we know based on the clues in the sentence:

- Janice dressed differently
- Some kids did not allow her to sit at their table
- They whispered behind her back

We know that the kids **never allowed her to sit at their lunch** table and that they **whispered behind her back**. If you put all these clues together, you can conclude that the other students were **mistreating** Janice by **excluding** her.

Therefore, based on these context clues, _ostracized_ means "excluded from the group."

Here's another example:

> **EXAMPLE 2**
>
> Look at this next sentence:
>
> Louis's teacher was offended because after she called on him he gave a *flippant* response instead of a serious answer.
>
> If you did not know what the word *flippant* meant, you could look at the **other words** for **clues** to help you.
>
> Here is what we know based on the clues in the sentence:
>
> • Louis's teacher was offended
> • He gave a flippant response instead of a serious answer
>
> We know that Louis said something that **offended** his teacher. Another keyword in this sentence is the word **instead**. This means that **instead of a serious answer** Louis gave the **opposite** of a serious answer.
>
> Therefore, based on these context clues, *flippant* means "lacking respect or seriousness."

Multiple Meaning Words

Sometimes when we read words in a text, we encounter words that have **multiple meanings**.

Multiple meaning words are words that have **more than one definition** or meaning.

> **FOR EXAMPLE**
>
> The word **current** is a multiple meaning word. Here are the different definitions of *current*:
>
> CURRENT:
>
> 1. adj: happening or existing in the present time
>   Example: *It is important to keep up with <u>current</u> events so you know what's happening in the world.*
> 2. noun: the continuous movement of a body of water or air in a certain direction
>   Example: *The river's <u>current</u> was strong as we paddled down the rapids.*
> 3. noun: a flow of electricity
>   Example: *The electrical <u>current</u> was very weak in the house.*

Here are some other examples of words with multiple meanings:

Multiple Meaning Word	Definition #1	Definition #2	Definition #3
Buckle	noun: a metal or plastic device that connects one end of a belt to another	verb: to fasten or attach	verb: to bend or collapse from pressure or heat
Cabinet	noun: a piece of furniture used for storing things	noun: a group of people who give advice to a government leader	-
Channel	noun: a radio or television station	noun: a system used for sending something	noun: a long, narrow place where water flows
Doctor	noun: a person skilled in the science of medicine, dentistry, or one holding a PhD	verb: to change something in a way to trick or deceive	verb: to give medical treatment
Grave	noun: a hole in the ground for burying a dead body	adj: very serious	-
Hamper	noun: a large basket used for holding dirty clothes	verb: to slow the movement, action, or progress of	-
Plane	noun: a mode of transportation that has wings and an engine and can carry people and things in the air	noun: a flat or level surface that extends outward	noun: a level of though, development, or existence
Reservation	noun: an agreement to have something (such as a table, room, or seat) held for use at a later time	noun: a feeling of uncertainty or doubt	noun: an area of land kept separate for Native Americans to live an area of land set aside for animals to live for protection
Season	noun: one of the four periods in which a year is divided (winter, spring, summer, and fall)	noun: a particular period of time during the year	verb: to add spices to something to give it more flavor
Sentence	noun: a group words that expresses a statement, question, command, or wish	noun: the punishment given to someone by a court of law	verb: to officially state the punishment given by a court of law

From this chart you will notice that words with multiple meanings may have different **parts of speech**. A part of speech is a category of words that have the same grammatical properties. Some of the main parts of speech for words in the English language are: nouns, adjectives, verbs, and adverbs.

Part of Speech	Definition	Example
Noun	a person, place, thing, or idea	*Linda, New York City, toaster, happiness*
Adjective	a word that describes a noun or pronoun	*adventurous, young, red, intelligent*
Verb	an action or state of being	*run, is, sleep, become*
Adverb	a word that describes a verb, adjective, or other adverb	*quietly, extremely, carefully, well*

For example, in the chart above, *season* is can be a **noun** or a **verb**.

Using Multiple Meaning Words Properly in Context

When you come across a **multiple meaning word** in a text, it is important to discern which meaning of the word is being used so you do not get confused.

You can once again turn to the **context clues** to clarify which meaning of the word is being used.

Let's take a look at the word *coach*. This word has several definitions:

COACH:
1. noun: a person who teaches and trains an athlete or performer
2. noun: a large bus with comfortable seating used for long trips
3. noun: the section on an airplane with the least expensive seats
4. verb: to teach or train someone in a specific area
5. verb: to give someone instructions on what to do or say in a certain situation

Since *coach* has so many definitions, you need to look at the **context clues** to figure out which definition of the word is being used:

The man was not happy that he had to sit in <u>*coach*</u> *on the 24-hour flight to Australia.*

In this sentence, the context clues **sit in** and **24-hour flight** help you see that *coach* means the least expensive seat on an airplane.

Let's look at another sentence using the word *coach*:

The lawyer needed to <u>*coach*</u> *her witness so he would answer all the questions properly.*

In this sentence, the context clues **so he would answer all the questions properly** help you see that the lawyer was giving the witness instructions on what to say.

Let's Review!
- When you come across an unfamiliar word in a text you can use context clues to help you define it.
- Context clues can also help you determine which definition of a multiple meaning word to use.

SYNONYMS, ANTONYMS, AND ANALOGIES

In order to utilize language to the best of your ability while reading, writing, or speaking, you must know how to interpret and use new vocabulary words, and also understand how these words relate to one another. Sometimes words have the same meaning. Sometimes words are complete opposites of each other. Understanding how the words you read, write, and speak with relate to each other will deepen your understanding of how language works. This lesson will cover (1) synonyms, (2) antonyms, and (3) analogies.

Synonyms

A **synonym** is a word that has the same meaning or close to the same meaning as another word. For example, if you look up the words *irritated* and *annoyed* in a dictionary, you will discover that they both mean "showing or feeling slight anger." Similarly, if you were to look up *blissful* and *joyful*, you will see that they both mean "extremely happy." The dictionary definition of a word is called its **denotation**. This is a word's literal or direct meaning.

When you understand that there are multiple words that have the same **denotation**, it will broaden your vocabulary.

It is also important to know that words with similar meanings have **nuances**, or subtle differences.

One way that words have nuances is in their **shades of meanings.** This means that although they have a similar definition, if you look closely, you will see that they have slight differences.

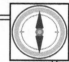

> **FOR EXAMPLE**
> If you quickly glance at the following words, you will see that they all have a similar meaning. However, if you look closely, you will see that their meanings have subtle differences. You can see their differences by looking at their various **levels** or **degrees**:
>
> LEAST ⟶ MOST

nibble	bite	eat	devour
upset	angry	furious	irate
wet	soggy	soaked	drenched
good	great	amazing	phenomenal

Another way that words have nuance are in their **connotations.** A word's connotation is its **positive** or **negative** association. This can be the case even when two words have the same **denotations**, or dictionary definitions.

For example, the words *aroma* and *stench* both have a similar dictionary definition or **denotation**: "a smell." However, their **connotations** are quite different. *Aroma* has a **positive**

58

connotation because it describes a *pleasant* smell. But *stench* has a **negative connotation** because it describes an unpleasant smell.

FOR EXAMPLE

Look at the following words. Although they have the same denotation, their connotations are very different:

Denotation	Positive Connotation	Negative Connotation
CLIQUE and *CLUB* both mean "a group of people."	*CLUB* has a positive connotation because it describes a group of people coming together to accomplish something.	*CLIQUE* has a negative connotation because it describes a group of people who exclude others.
INTERESTED and *NOSY* both mean "showing curiosity."	*INTERESTED* has a positive connotation because it means having a genuine curiosity about someone or something.	*NOSY* has a negative connotation because it describes who tries to pry information out of someone else to gossip or judge.
EMPLOY and *EXPLOIT* both mean "to use someone."	*EMPLOY* has a positive connotation because it means to use someone for a job.	*EXPLOIT* has a negative connotation because it means to use someone for one's own advantage.

Seeing that synonymous words have different **shades of meaning** and **connotations** will allow you to more precisely interpret and understand the nuances of language.

Antonyms

An **antonym** is a word that means the opposite or close to the opposite of another word. Think of an antonym as the direct opposite of a **synonym**. For example, *caring* and *apathetic* are antonyms because *caring* means "displaying concern and kindness for others" whereas *apathetic* means "showing no interest or concern."

Antonyms can fall under three categories:

GRADED ANTONYMS:	Word pairs whose meanings are opposite and lie on a spectrum or continuum; there are many other words that fall between the two words. If you look at *hot* and *cold*, there are other words on this spectrum:
	scalding, **hot***, warm, tepid, cool,* **cold**
RELATIONAL ANTONYMS:	Word pairs whose opposites make sense only in the context of the relationship between the two meanings. These two words could not exist without the other: **open - close**
COMPLEMENTARY ANTONYMS:	Word pairs that have no degree of meaning at all; there are only two possibilities, one or the other:
	dead - alive

Here are some more examples of the three types of antonyms:

Graded Antonyms	Relational Antonyms	Complementary Antonyms
hard - soft	front - back	day - night
fast - slow	predator - prey	sink - float
bad - good	top - bottom	input - output
wet - dry	capture - release	interior - exterior
big - small	on - off	occupied - vacant

There are also common **prefixes** that help make antonyms. The most common prefixes for antonyms of words are: **UN**, **NON**, and **IN**. All these prefixes mean "not" or "without."

FOR EXAMPLE

UN:

likely – **un**likely
fortunate – **un**fortunate

IN:

tolerant – **in**tolerant
excusable – **in**excusable

NON:

conformist – **non**conformist
payment – **non**payment

Analogies

An **analogy** is a simple comparison between two things. Analogies help us understand the world around us by seeing how different things relate to one another.

In looking closely at words, analogies help us understand how they are connected.

In word analogies, they are usually set up using colons in the following way:

Pleasure: Smile :: Pain: _____

This can be read as: Pleasure **IS TO** Smile **AS** Pain **IS TO** _____

The answer: "grimace"

Sometimes you see analogies written out like this:

Pleasure is to Smile as Pain is to _____

These are the common types of word analogies that illustrate how different words relate to one another:

Type of Analogy	Relationship	Example
Synonyms	Two words with the same meaning	Beginner : Novice:: Expert : Pro
Antonyms	Two words with the opposite meaning	Hot : Cold :: Up : Down
Part/Whole	One word is a part of another word	Stars : Galaxy :: Pages : Book
Cause/Effect	One word describes a condition or action, and the other describes an outcome	Tornado : Damage :: Joke : Laughter
Object/Function	One word describes something, and the other word describes what it's used for	Needle : Sew :: Saw : Cut

Category/Type	One word is a general category, and the other is something that falls in that category	Music : Folk :: Dance : Ballet
Performer/Related Action	One word is a person or object, and the other words is the action he/she/it commonly performs	Thief : Steal :: Surgeon : Operate
Degree of Intensity	These words have similar meanings, but one word is stronger or more intense than the other	Glad : Elated :: Angry : Furious

By recognizing the type of analogy two words have, you then can explore how they are connected.

Let's Review!

- Synonyms are words that have the same meaning. Synonyms also have nuances.
- Analogies are words that have an opposite meaning. There are three types of antonyms.
- Analogies show how words relate to each other. There are different types of analogy relationships to look for.
- Understanding how words relate to each other will help you better understand language, pull meaning from texts, and write and speak with a wider vocabulary.

CHAPTER 4 VOCABULARY ACQUISITION PRACTICE QUIZ

1. Select the word from the following sentence that has more than one meaning.

   Cassandra's voice has a much different pitch than her brother's, so they sound great when they sing together.

   A. Voice   C. Pitch

   B. Different   D. Sing

2. Select the correct definition of the underlined word that has multiple meanings in the sentence.

   When the young boy saw his angry mother coming toward him, he made a <u>bolt</u> for the door.

   A. A large roll of cloth

   B. A quick movement in a particular direction

   C. A sliding bar that is used to lock a window or door

   D. A bright line of light appearing in the sky during a storm

3. Select the meaning of the underlined word in the sentence based on the context clues.

   When visiting the desert, the temperature tends to <u>fluctuate</u>, so you need to bring a variety of clothing.

   A. Rise   C. Change

   B. Drop   D. Stabilize

4. The use of the suffix -*ous* in the word <u>parsimonious</u> indicates what about a person?

   A. He/she is full of stinginess.

   B. He/she is against stinginess.

   C. He/she is supportive of stinginess.

   D. He/she is a person who studies stinginess.

5. Which of the following prefixes means <u>incorrect</u>?

   A. un-   C. mis-

   B. non-   D. over-

6. What is the best definition of the word <u>pugnacious</u>?

   A. Rude   C. Deceiving

   B. Harmful   D. Combative

7. The following words have the same denotation. Which word has a negative connotation?

   A. Poised   C. Arrogant

   B. Assured   D. Confident

8. Whisk : Mix :: Flashlight : _____

   A. Hike   C. Camp

   B. Light   D. Travel

9. Which word in the list of synonyms shows the strongest degree of the word?

   A. Amusing   C. Uproarious

   B. Comical   D. Entertaining

CHAPTER 4 VOCABULARY ACQUISITION PRACTICE QUIZ — ANSWER KEY

1. C. The word "pitch" has more than one meaning. **See Lesson: Context Clues and Multiple Meaning Words.**

2. B. The meaning of <u>bolt</u> in the context of this sentence is "a quick movement in a particular direction." **See Lesson: Context Clues and Multiple Meaning Words.**

3. C. The meaning of <u>fluctuate</u> in the context of this sentence is "change." **See Lesson: Context Clues and Multiple Meaning Words.**

4. A. The suffix *-ous* means "full of or possessing," so a parsimonious person is one who is full of stinginess. **See Lesson: Root Words, Prefixes, and Suffixes.**

5. C. The prefix that means "incorrect" is *mis*. **See Lesson: Root Words, Prefixes, and Suffixes.**

6. D. The root *pug* means "war" or "fight," so pugnacious means combative. **See Lesson: Root Words, Prefixes, and Suffixes.**

7. C. Arrogant has a negative connotation. **See Lesson: Synonyms, Antonyms, and Analogies.**

8. B. A whisk is a tool used to mix in the same way that a flashlight is a tool used to light. **See Lesson: Synonyms, Antonyms, and Analogies.**

9. C. Uproarious is the word that shows the strongest degree in the list of synonyms. **See Lesson: Synonyms, Antonyms, and Analogies.**

SECTION II. MATHEMATICS

CHAPTER 5 NUMBER AND QUANTITY

BASIC ADDITION AND SUBTRACTION

This lesson introduces the concept of numbers and their symbolic and graphical representations. It also describes how to add and subtract whole numbers.

Numbers

A **number** is a way to quantify a set of entities that share some characteristic. For example, a fruit basket might contain nine pieces of fruit. More specifically, it might contain three apples, two oranges, and four bananas. Note that a number is a quantity, but a **numeral** is the symbol that represents the number: 8 means the number eight, for instance.

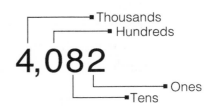

Although number representations vary, the most common is **base 10.** In base-10 format, each **digit** (or individual numeral) in a number is a quantity based on a multiple of 10. The base-10 system designates 0 through 9 as the numerals for zero through nine, respectively, and combines them to represent larger numbers. Thus, after counting from 1 to 9, the next number uses an additional digit: 10. That number means 1 group of 10 ones plus 0 additional ones. After 99, another digit is necessary, this time representing a hundred (10 sets of 10). This process of adding digits can go on indefinitely to express increasingly large numbers. For whole numbers, the rightmost digit is the ones place, the next digit to its left is the tens place, the next is the hundreds place, then the thousands place, and so on.

Classifying numbers can be convenient. The chart below lists a few common number sets.

Sets of Numbers	Members	Remarks
Natural numbers	1, 2, 3, 4, 5,...	The "counting" numbers
Whole numbers	0, 1, 2, 3, 4,...	The natural numbers plus 0
Integers	..., −3, −2, −1, 0, 1, 2, 3,...	The whole numbers plus all negative whole numbers
Real numbers	All numbers	The integers plus all fraction/decimal numbers in between
Rational numbers	All real numbers that can be expressed as p/q, where p and q are integers and q is nonzero	The natural numbers, whole numbers, and integers are all rational numbers
Irrational numbers	All real numbers that are not rational	The rational and irrational numbers together constitute the entire set of real numbers

Example

Jane has 4 pennies, 3 dimes, and 7 dollars. How many cents does she have?

    A. 347   B. 437   C. 734   D. 743

The correct answer is **C**. The correct solution is 734. A penny is 1 cent. A dime (10 pennies) is 10 cents, and a dollar (100 pennies) is 100 cents. Place the digits in base-10 format: 7 hundreds, 3 tens, 4 ones, or 734.

The Number Line

The **number line** is a model that illustrates the relationships among numbers. The complete number line is infinite and includes every real number—both positive and negative. A ruler, for example, is a portion of a number line that assigns a **unit** (such as inches or centimeters) to each number. Typically, number lines depict smaller numbers to the left and larger numbers to the right. For example, a portion of the number line centered on 0 might look like the following:

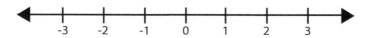

Because people learn about numbers in part through counting, they have a basic sense of how to order them. The number line builds on this sense by placing all the numbers (at least conceptually) from least to greatest. Whether a particular number is greater than or less than another is determined by comparing their relative positions. One number is greater than another if it is farther right on the number line. Likewise, a number is less than another if it is farther left on the number line. Symbolically, < means "is less than" and > means "is greater than." For example, 5 > 1 and 9 < 25.

Example

Place the following numbers in order from greatest to least: 5, –12, 0.

    A. 0, 5, –12   C. 5, 0, –12

    B. –12, 5, 0   D. –12, 0, 5

> **BE CAREFUL!**
>
> When ordering negative numbers, think of the number line. Although –10 > –2 may seem correct, it is incorrect. Because –10 is to the left of –2 on the number line, –10 < –2.

The correct answer is **C**. The correct solution is 5, 0, –12. Use the number line to order the numbers. Note that the question says *from greatest to least*.

Addition

Addition is the process of combining two or more numbers. For example, one set has 4 members and another set has 5 members. To combine the sets and find out how many members are in the new set, add 4 and 5 to get the **sum**. Symbolically, the expression is 4 + 5, where + is the **plus sign**. Pictorially, it might look like the following:

$$\underset{\circ\ \circ}{\circ\ \circ} \quad + \quad \underset{\circ\ \circ\ \circ}{\circ\ \circ} \quad = \quad \underset{\circ\ \circ\ \circ\ \circ\ \circ}{\circ\ \circ\ \circ\ \circ}$$

To get the sum, combine the two sets of circles and then count them. The result is 9.

> **KEY POINT**
> The order of the numbers is irrelevant when adding.

Another way to look at addition involves the number line. When adding 4 + 5, for example, start at 4 on the number line and take 5 steps to the right. The stopping point will be 9, which is the sum.

Counting little pictures or using the number line works for small numbers, but it becomes unwieldy for large ones—even numbers such as 24 and 37 would be difficult to add quickly and accurately. A simple algorithm enables much faster addition of large numbers. It works with two or more numbers.

STEP BY STEP

Step 1. Stack the numbers, vertically aligning the digits for each place.

Step 2. Draw a plus sign (+) to the left of the bottom number and draw a horizontal line below the last number.

Step 3. Add the digits in the ones place.

Step 4. If the sum from Step 3 is less than 10, write it in the same column below the horizontal line. Otherwise, write the first (ones) digit below the line, then **carry** the second (tens) digit to the top of the next column.

Step 5. Going from right to left, repeat Steps 3–4 for the other places.

Step 6. If applicable, write the remaining carry digit as the leftmost digit in the sum.

Example

Evaluate the expression 154 + 98.

A. 250   B. 252   C. 352   D. 15,498

The correct answer is **B**. The correct solution is 252. Carefully follow the addition algorithm (see below). The process involves carrying a digit twice.

$$
\begin{array}{r} 154 \\ +\ 98 \\ \hline \end{array}
\rightarrow
\begin{array}{r} {}^{1} \\ 154 \\ +\ 98 \\ \hline 2 \end{array}
\rightarrow
\begin{array}{r} {}^{11} \\ 154 \\ +\ 98 \\ \hline 52 \end{array}
\rightarrow
\begin{array}{r} {}^{11} \\ 154 \\ +\ 98 \\ \hline 252 \end{array}
$$

Subtraction

Subtraction is the inverse (opposite) of addition. Instead of representing the sum of numbers, it represents the difference between them. For example, given a set containing 15 members, subtracting 3 of those members yields a **difference** of 12. Using the **minus sign,** the expression for this operation is 15 − 3 = 12. As with addition, two approaches are counting pictures and using the number line. The first case might involve drawing 15 circles and then crossing off 3 of them; the difference is the number of remaining circles (12). To use the number line, begin at 15 and move left 3 steps to reach 12.

Again, these approaches are unwieldy for large numbers, but the subtraction algorithm eases evaluation by hand. This algorithm is only practical for two numbers at a time.

STEP BY STEP

Step 1. Stack the numbers, vertically aligning the digits in each place. Put the number you are subtracting *from* on top.

Step 2. Draw a minus sign (−) to the left of the bottom number and draw a horizontal line below the stack of numbers.

Step 3. Start at the ones place. If the digit at the top is larger than the digit below it, write the difference under the line. Otherwise, **borrow** from the top digit in the next-higher place by crossing it off, subtracting 1 from it, and writing the difference above it. Then add 10 to the digit in the ones place and perform the subtraction as normal.

Step 4. Going from right to left, repeat Step 3 for the rest of the places. If borrowing was necessary, make sure to use the new digit in each place, not the original one.

When adding or subtracting with negative numbers, the following rules are helpful. Note that x and y are used as placeholders for any real number.

$x + (-y) = x - y$

$-x - y = -(x + y)$

$(-x) + (-y) = -(x + y)$

$x - y = -(y - x)$

BE CAREFUL!

When dealing with numbers that have units (such as weights, currencies, or volumes), addition and subtraction are only possible when the numbers have the same unit. If necessary, convert one or more of them to equivalent numbers with the same unit.

Example

Kevin has 120 minutes to complete an exam. If he has already used 43, how many minutes does he have left?

   A. 43   B. 77   C. 87   D. 163

The correct answer is **B**. The correct solution is 77. The first step is to convert this problem to a math expression. The goal is to find the difference between how many minutes Kevin has for the exam and how many he has left after 43 minutes have elapsed. The expression would be 120 − 43. Carefully follow the subtraction algorithm (see below). The process will involve borrowing a digit twice.

$$
\begin{array}{c}
120 \\
-\ 43 \\
\hline
\end{array}
\longrightarrow
\begin{array}{c}
\overset{1\,10}{1\cancel{2}0} \\
-\ 43 \\
\hline
7 \\
\end{array}
\longrightarrow
\begin{array}{c}
\overset{0\ 11\,10}{\cancel{1}\cancel{2}0} \\
-\ 43 \\
\hline
77 \\
\end{array}
$$

Let's Review!

- Numbers are positive and negative quantities and often appear in base-10 format.
- The number line illustrates the ordering of numbers.
- Addition is the combination of numbers. It can be performed by counting objects or pictures, moving on the number line, or using the addition algorithm.
- Subtraction is finding the difference between numbers. Like addition, it can be performed by counting, moving on the number line, or using the subtraction algorithm.

BASIC MULTIPLICATION AND DIVISION

This lesson describes the process of multiplying and dividing numbers and introduces the order of operations, which governs how to evaluate expressions containing multiple arithmetic operations.

Multiplication

Addition can be tedious if it involves multiple instances of the same numbers. For example, evaluating 29 + 29 is easy, but evaluating 29 + 29 + 29 + 29 + 29 is laborious. Note that this example contains five instances—or multiples—of 29. **Multiplication** replaces the repeated addition of the same number with a single, more concise operation. Using the **multiplication (or times) symbol** (×), the expression is

$$29 + 29 + 29 + 29 + 29 = 5 \times 29$$

The expression contains 5 multiples of 29. These numbers are the **factors** of multiplication. The result is called the **product**. In this case, addition shows that the product is 145. As with the other arithmetic operations, multiplication is easy for small numbers. Below is the multiplication table for whole numbers up to 12.

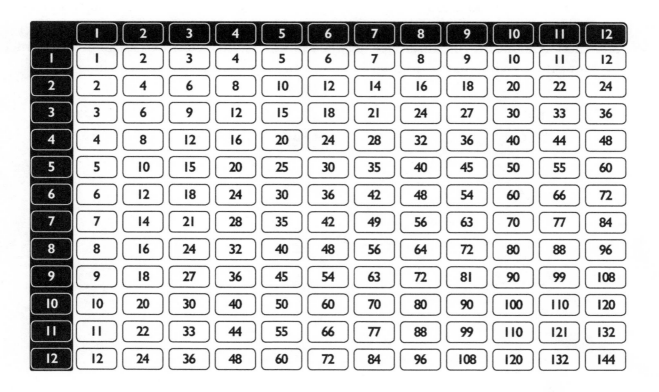

	1	2	3	4	5	6	7	8	9	10	11	12
1	1	2	3	4	5	6	7	8	9	10	11	12
2	2	4	6	8	10	12	14	16	18	20	22	24
3	3	6	9	12	15	18	21	24	27	30	33	36
4	4	8	12	16	20	24	28	32	36	40	44	48
5	5	10	15	20	25	30	35	40	45	50	55	60
6	6	12	18	24	30	36	42	48	54	60	66	72
7	7	14	21	28	35	42	49	56	63	70	77	84
8	8	16	24	32	40	48	56	64	72	80	88	96
9	9	18	27	36	45	54	63	72	81	90	99	108
10	10	20	30	40	50	60	70	80	90	100	110	120
11	11	22	33	44	55	66	77	88	99	110	121	132
12	12	24	36	48	60	72	84	96	108	120	132	144

When dealing with large numbers, the multiplication algorithm is more practical than memorization. The ability to quickly recall the products in the multiplication table is nevertheless crucial to using this algorithm.

STEP BY STEP

Step 1. Stack the two factors, vertically aligning the digits in each place.

Step 2. Draw a multiplication symbol (×) to the left of the bottom number and draw a horizontal line below the stack.

Step 3. Begin with the ones digit in the lower factor. Multiply it with the ones digit from the top factor.

Step 4. If the product from Step 3 is less than 10, write it in the same column below the horizontal line. Otherwise, write the first (ones) digit below the line and carry the second (tens) digit to the top of the next column.

Step 5. Perform Step 4 for each digit in the top factor, adding any carry digit to the result. If an extra carry digit appears at the end, write it as the leftmost digit in the product.

Step 6. Going right to left, repeat Steps 3–4 for the other places in the bottom factor, starting a new line in each case.

Step 7. Add the numbers below the line to get the product.

Example

A certain type of screw comes in packs of 35. If a contractor orders 52 packs, how many screws does he receive?

A. 2   B. 57   C. 245   D. 1,820

The correct answer is **D**. The first step is to convert this problem to a math expression. The goal is to find how many screws the contractor receives if he orders 52 packs of 35 each. The expression would be 52×35 (or 35×52). Carefully follow the multiplication algorithm (see below).

$$
\begin{array}{c}
52 \\
\times\, 35 \\
\hline
\end{array}
\rightarrow
\begin{array}{c}
\overset{1}{}52 \\
\times\, 35 \\
\hline
0 \\
\end{array}
\rightarrow
\begin{array}{c}
\overset{1}{}52 \\
\times\, 35 \\
\hline
260 \\
\end{array}
\rightarrow
\begin{array}{c}
\overset{1}{}52 \\
\times\, 35 \\
\hline
260 \\
6 \\
\end{array}
\rightarrow
\begin{array}{c}
\overset{11}{}52 \\
\times\, 35 \\
\hline
260 \\
56 \\
\end{array}
\rightarrow
\begin{array}{c}
\overset{11}{}52 \\
\times\, 35 \\
\hline
260 \\
156 \\
\end{array}
\rightarrow
\begin{array}{c}
\overset{11}{}52 \\
\times\, 35 \\
\hline
260 \\
+\,156 \\
\hline
1,820 \\
\end{array}
$$

KEY POINT

As with addition, the order of numbers in a multiplication expression is irrelevant to the product. For example, $6 \times 9 = 9 \times 6$.

Division

Division is the inverse of multiplication, like subtraction is the inverse of addition. Whereas multiplication asks how many individuals are in 8 groups of 9 ($8 \times 9 = 72$), for example, division asks how many groups of 8 (or 9) are in 72. Division expressions use either the / or ÷ symbol. Therefore, $72 \div 9$ means: How many groups of 9 are in 72, or how many times does 9 go into 72? Thinking about the meaning of multiplication shows that $72 \div 9 = 8$ and $72 \div 8 = 9$. In the expression $72 \div 8 = 9$, 72 is the **dividend,** 8 is the **divisor,** and 9 is the **quotient.**

When the dividend is unevenly divisible by the divisor (e.g., $5 \div 2$), calculating the quotient with a **remainder** can be convenient. The quotient in this case is the maximum number of times the divisor goes into the dividend plus how much of the dividend is left over. To express the remainder, use an R. For example, the quotient of $5 \div 2$ is 2R1 because 2 goes into 5 twice with 1 left over.

Knowing the multiplication table allows quick evaluation of simple whole-number division. For larger numbers, the division algorithm enables evaluation by hand.

Unlike multiplication—but like subtraction—the order of the numbers in a division expression is important. Generally, changing the order changes the quotient.

STEP BY STEP

Step 1. Write the divisor and then the dividend on a single line.

Step 2. Draw a vertical line between them, connecting to a horizontal line over the dividend.

Step 3. If the divisor is smaller than the leftmost digit of the dividend, perform the remainder division and write the quotient (without the remainder) above that digit. If the divisor is larger than the leftmost digit, use the first two digits (or however many are necessary) until the number is greater than the divisor. Write the quotient over the rightmost digit in that number.

Step 4. Multiply the quotient digit by the divisor and write it under the dividend, vertically aligning the ones digit of the product with the quotient digit.

Step 5. Subtract the product from the digits above it.

Step 6. Bring down the next digit from the quotient.

Step 7. Perform Steps 3–6, using the most recent difference as the quotient.

Step 8. Write the remainder next to the quotient.

Example

Evaluate the expression 468 ÷ 26.

    A. 18   B. 18R2   C. 494   D. 12,168

The correct answer is **A.** Carefully follow the division algorithm. In this case, the answer has no remainder.

$$
26\overline{)468} \rightarrow 26\overline{)468} \atop 26 \rightarrow 26\overline{)468} \atop -26 \atop 20 \rightarrow 26\overline{)468} \atop -26\downarrow \atop 208 \rightarrow 26\overline{)468} \atop -26\downarrow \atop 208 \atop -208 \atop 0
$$

> **KEY POINT**
> Division by 0 is undefined. If it appears in an expression, something is wrong.

Signed Multiplication and Division

Multiplying and dividing signed numbers is simpler than adding and subtracting them because it only requires remembering two simple rules. First, if the two numbers have the same sign, their product or quotient is positive. Second, if they have different signs, their product or quotient is negative.

As a result, negative numbers can be multiplied or divided as if they are positive. Just keep track of the sign separately for the product or quotient. Note that negative numbers are sometimes written in parentheses to avoid the appearance of subtraction.

For Example:

$$5 \times (-3) = -15$$

$$(-8) \times (-8) = 64$$

$$(-12) \div 3 = -4$$

$$(-100) \div (-25) = 4$$

Example

Evaluate the expression (–7) × (–9).

    A. −63   B. −16   C. 16   D. 63

The correct answer is **D.** Because both factors are negative, the product will be positive. Because the product of 7 and 9 is 63, the product of −7 and −9 is also 63.

Order of Operations

By default, math expressions work like most Western languages: they should be read and evaluated from left to right. However, some operations take precedence over others, which can change this default evaluation. Following this **order of operations** is critical. The mnemonic **PEMDAS** (Please Excuse My Dear Aunt Sally) helps in remembering how to evaluate an expression with multiple operations.

STEP BY STEP

P.	Evaluate operations in parentheses (or braces/brackets). If the expression has parentheses within parentheses, begin with the innermost ones.
E.	Evaluate exponential operations. (For expressions without exponents, ignore this step.)
MD.	Perform all multiplication and division operations, going through the expression from left to right.
AS.	Perform all addition and subtraction operations, going through the expression from left to right.

Because the order of numbers in multiplication and addition does not affect the result, the PEMDAS procedure only requires going from left to right when dividing or subtracting. At those points, going in the correct direction is critical to getting the right answer.

Calculators that can handle a series of numbers at once automatically evaluate an expression according to the order of operations. When available, calculators are a good way to check the results.

BE CAREFUL!

When evaluating an expression like $4 - 3 + 2 \times 5$, remember to go from left to right when adding and subtracting or when multiplying and dividing. The first step in this case (MD) yields $4 - 3 + 10$. Avoid the temptation to add first in the next step; instead, go from left to right. The result is $1 + 10 = 11$, *not* $4 - 13 = -9$.

Example

Evaluate the expression 8 × (3 + 6) ÷ 3–2 + 5.

A. 13   B. 17   C. 27   D. 77

The correct answer is **C**. Use the PEMDAS mnemonic. Start with parentheses. Then, do multiplication/division from left to right. Finally, do addition/subtraction from left to right.

8 × (3 + 6) ÷ 3–2 + 5

8 × 9 ÷ 3–2 + 5

72 ÷ 3–2 + 5

24–2 + 5

22 + 5

27

Let's Review!

- The multiplication table is important to memorize for both multiplying and dividing small whole numbers (up to about 12).
- Multiplication and division of large numbers by hand typically requires the multiplication and division algorithms.
- Multiplying and dividing signed numbers follows two simple rules: If the numbers have the same sign, the product or quotient is positive. If they have different signs, the product or quotient is negative.
- When evaluating expressions with several operations, carefully follow the order of operations; PEMDAS is a helpful mnemonic.

FACTORS AND MULTIPLES

This lesson shows the relationship between factors and multiples of a number. In addition, it introduces prime and composite numbers and demonstrates how to use prime factorization to determine all the factors of a number.

Factors of a Number

Multiplication converts two or more factors into a product. A given number, however, may be the product of more than one combination of factors; for example, 12 is the product of 3 and 4 and the product of 2 and 6. Limiting consideration to the set of whole numbers, a **factor of a number** (call it x) is a whole number whose product with any other whole number is equal to x. For instance, 2 is a factor of 12 because $12 \div 2$ is a whole number (6). Another way of expressing it is that 2 is a factor of 12 because 12 is **divisible** by 2.

> **BE CAREFUL!**
>
> The term *factor* can mean any number being multiplied by another number, or it can mean a number by which another number is divisible. The two uses are related but slightly different. The context will generally clarify which meaning applies.

A whole number always has at least two factors: 1 and itself. That is, for any whole number y, $1 \times y = y$. To test whether one number is a factor of a second number, divide the second by the first. If the quotient is whole, it is a factor. If the quotient is not whole (or it has a remainder), it is not a factor.

Example

Which number is not a factor of 54?

   A. 1   B. 2   C. 4   D. 6

The correct answer is **C**. A number is a factor of another number if the latter is divisible by the former. The number 54 is divisible by 1 because $54 \times 1 = 54$, and it is divisible by 2 because $27 \times 2 = 54$. Also, $6 \times 9 = 54$. But $54 \div 4 = 13.5$ (or 13R2). Therefore, 4 is not a factor.

Multiples of a Number

Multiples of a number are related to factors of a number. A **multiple of a number** is that number's product with some integer. For example, if a hardware store sells a type of screw that only comes in packs of 20, customers must buy these screws in *multiples* of 20: that is, 20, 40, 60, 80, and so on. (Technically, 0 is also a multiple.) These numbers are equal to 20×1, 20×2, 20×3, 20×4, and so on. Similarly, measurements in feet represent multiples of 12 inches. A (whole-number) measurement in feet would be equivalent to 12 inches, 24 inches, 36 inches, and so on.

When counting by twos or threes, multiples are used. But because the multiples of a number are the product of that number with the integers, multiples can also be negative. For the number 2, the multiples are the set {..., −6, −4, −2, 0, 2, 4, 6,...}, where the ellipsis dots indicate that the set continues the pattern indefinitely in both directions. Also, the number can be any real number: the multiples of π (approximately 3.14) are {..., −3π, −2π, −1π, 0, 1π, 2π, 3π,...}. Note that the notation 2π, for example, means $2 \times \pi$.

The positive multiples (along with 0) of a whole number are all numbers for which that whole number is a factor. For instance, the positive multiples of 5 are 0, 5, 10, 15, 20, 25, 30, and so on. That full set contains all (whole) numbers for which 5 is a factor. Thus, one number is a multiple of a second number if the second number is a factor of the first.

Example

If a landowner subdivides a parcel of property into multiples of 7 acres, how many acres can a buyer purchase?

   A. 1   B. 15   C. 29   D. 42

The correct answer is **D**. Because the landowner subdivides the property into multiples of 7 acres, a buyer must choose an acreage from the list 7 acres, 14 acres, 21 acres, and so on. That list includes 42 acres. Another way to solve the problem is to find which answer is divisible by 7 (that is, which number has 7 as a factor).

Prime and Composite Numbers

For some real-world applications, such as cryptography, factors and multiples play an important role. One important way to classify whole numbers is by whether they are prime or composite. A **prime** number is any whole (or natural) number greater than 1 that has only itself and 1 as factors. The smallest example is 2: because 2 only has 1 and 2 as factors, it is prime. **Composite** numbers have at least one factor other than 1 and themselves. The smallest composite number is 4: in addition to 1 and 4, it has 2 as a factor.

Determining whether a number is prime can be extremely difficult—hence its value in cryptography. One simple test that works for some numbers is to check whether the number is even or odd. An **even number** is divisible by 2; an **odd number** is not. To determine whether a number is even or odd, look at the last (rightmost) digit.

> **BE CAREFUL!**
>
> Avoid the temptation to call 1 a prime number. Although it only has itself and 1 as factors, those factors are the same number. Hence, 1 is fundamentally different from the prime numbers, which start at 2.

If that digit is even (0, 2, 4, 6, or 8), the number is even. Otherwise, it is odd. Another simple test works for multiples of 3. Add all the digits in the number. If the sum is divisible by 3, the original number is also divisible by 3. This rule can be successively applied multiple times until the sum of digits is manageable. That number is then composite.

Example

Which number is prime?

A. 6　　　　　　　B. 16　　　　　　　C. 61　　　　　　　D. 116

The correct answer is **C**. When applicable, the easiest way to identify a number greater than 2 as composite rather than prime is to check whether it is even. All even numbers greater than 2 are composite. By elimination, 61 is prime.

Prime Factorization

Determining whether a number is prime, even for relatively small numbers (less than 100), can be difficult. One tool that can help both solve this problem and identify all factors of a number is **prime factorization.** One way to do prime factorization is to make a **factor tree.**

The procedure below demonstrates the process.

> **STEP BY STEP**
> **Step 1.**　Write the number you want to factor.
> **Step 2.**　If the number is prime, stop. Otherwise, go to Step 3.
> **Step 3.**　Find any two factors of the number and write them on the line below the number.
> **Step 4.**　"Connect" the factors and the number using line segments. The result will look somewhat like an inverted tree, particularly as the process continues.
> **Step 5.**　Repeat Steps 2–4 for all composite factors in the tree.

The numbers in the factor tree are either "branches" (if they are connected downward to other numbers) or "leaves" (if they have no further downward connections). The leaves constitute all the prime factors of the original number: when multiplied together, their product is that number. Moreover, any product of two or more of the leaves is a factor of the original number. Thus, using prime factorization helps find any and all factors of a number, although the process can be tedious when performed by hand (particularly for large numbers). Below is a factor tree for the number 96. All the leaves are circled for emphasis.

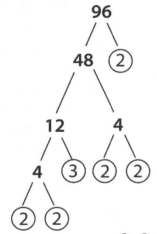

$$2 \times 2 \times 3 \times 2 \times 2 \times 2 = 96$$

Example

Which list includes all the unique prime factors of 84?

A. 2, 3, 7   B. 3, 4, 7   C. 3, 5, 7   D. 1, 2, 3, 7

The correct answer is **A**. One approach is to find the prime factorization of 84. The factor tree shows that $84 = 2 \times 2 \times 3 \times 7$. Alternatively, note that answer D includes 1, which is not prime. Answer B includes 4, which is a composite number. Since answer C includes 5, which is not a factor of 84, the only possible answer is A.

Let's Review!

- A whole number is divisible by all of its factors, which are also whole numbers by definition.
- Multiples of a number are all possible products of that number and the integers.
- A prime number is a whole number greater than 1 that has no factors other than itself and 1.
- A composite number is a whole number greater than 1 that is not prime (that is, it has factors other than itself and 1).
- Even numbers are divisible by 2; odd numbers are not.
- Prime factorization yields all the prime factors of a number. The factor-tree method is one way to determine prime factorization.

STANDARDS OF MEASURE

This lesson discusses the conversion within and between the standard system and the metric system and between 12-hour clock time and military time.

Length Conversions

The basic units of measure of length in the standard measurement system are inches, feet, yards, and miles. There are 12 inches (in.) in 1 foot (ft.), 3 feet (ft.) in 1 yard (yd.), and 5,280 feet (ft.) in 1 mile (mi.).

The basic unit of measure of metric length is meters. There are 1,000 millimeters (mm), 100 centimeters (cm), and 10 decimeters (dm) in 1 meter (m). There are 10 meters (m) in 1 dekameter (dam), 100 meters (m) in 1 hectometer (hm), and 1,000 meters (m) in 1 kilometer (km).

BE CAREFUL!

There are some cases where multiple conversions must be performed to determine the correct units.

To convert from one unit to the other, multiply by the appropriate factor.

Examples

1. **Convert 27 inches to feet.**

   A. 2 feet   B. 2.25 feet   C. 3 feet   D. 3.25 feet

   The correct answer is **B**. The correct solution is 2.25 feet. $27 \text{ in} \times \frac{1 \text{ ft}}{12 \text{ in}} = \frac{27}{12} = 2.25$ ft.

2. **Convert 67 millimeters to centimeters.**

   A. 0.0067 centimeters   C. 0.67 centimeters

   B. 0.067 centimeters   D. 6.7 centimeters

   The correct answer is **D**. The correct solution is 6.7 centimeters. $67 \text{ mm} \times \frac{1 \text{ cm}}{10 \text{ mm}} = \frac{67}{10} = 6.7$ cm.

Volume and Weight Conversions

There are volume conversion factors for standard and metric volumes.

The volume conversions for standard volume are shown in the table.

Measurement	Conversion
Pints (pt.) and fluid ounces (fl. oz.)	1 pint equals 16 fluid ounces
Quarts (qt.) and pints (pt.)	1 quart equals 2 pints
Quarts (qt.) and gallons (gal.)	1 gallon equals 4 quarts

The basic unit of volume for the metric system is liters. There are 1,000 milliliters (mL) in 1 liter (L) and 1,000 liters (L) in 1 kiloliter (kL).

There are weight conversion factors for standard and metric weights.

The basic unit of weight for the standard measurement system is pounds. There are

16 ounces (oz.) in 1 pound (lb.) and

2,000 pounds (lb.) in 1 ton (T).

The basic unit of weight for the metric system is grams.

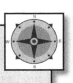

KEEP IN MIND
The conversions within the metric system are multiples of 10.

Measurement	Conversion
Milligrams (mg) and grams (g)	1,000 milligrams equals 1 gram
Centigrams (cg) and grams (g)	100 centigrams equals 1 gram
Kilograms (kg) and grams (g)	1 kilogram equals 1,000 grams
Metric tons (t) and kilograms (kg)	1 metric ton equals 1,000 kilograms

Examples

1. **Convert 8 gallons to pints.**

   A. 1 pint   B. 4 pints   C. 16 pints   D. 64 pints

   The correct answer is **D**. The correct solution is 64 pints. $8 \text{ gal} \times \frac{4 \text{ qt}}{1 \text{ gal}} \times \frac{2 \text{ pt}}{1 \text{ qt}} = 64 \text{ pt}$.

2. **Convert 7.5 liters to milliliters.**

   A. 75 milliliters   B. 750 milliliters   C. 7,500 milliliters   D. 75,000 milliliters

   The correct answer is **C**. The correct solution is 7,500 milliliters. $7.5 \text{ L} \times \frac{1,000 \text{ mL}}{1 \text{ L}} = 7,500 \text{ mL}$.

3. **Convert 12.5 pounds to ounces.**

   A. 142 ounces   B. 150 ounces   C. 192 ounces   D. 200 ounces

   The correct answer is **D**. The correct solution is 200 ounces. $12.5 \text{ lb} \times \frac{16 \text{ oz}}{1 \text{ lb}} = 200 \text{ oz}$.

4. **Convert 84 grams to centigrams.**

   A. 0.84 centigrams   B. 8.4 centigrams   C. 840 centigrams   D. 8,400 centigrams

   The correct answer is **D**. The correct solution is 8,400 centigrams. $84 \text{ g} \times \frac{100 \text{ cg}}{1 \text{ g}} = 8,400 \text{ cg}$.

Conversions between Standard and Metric Systems

The table shows the common conversions of length, volume, and weight between the standard and metric systems.

Measurement	Conversion
Centimeters (cm) and inches (in.)	2.54 centimeters equals 1 inch
Meters (m) and feet (ft.)	1 meter equals 3.28 feet
Kilometers (km) and miles (mi.)	1.61 kilometers equals 1 mile
Quarts (qt.) and liters (L)	1.06 quarts equals 1 liter
Liters (L) and gallons (gal.)	3.79 liters equals 1 gallon
Grams (g) and ounces (oz.)	28.3 grams equals 1 ounce
Kilograms (kg) and pounds (lb.)	1 kilogram equals 2.2 pounds

There are many additional conversion factors, but this lesson uses only the common ones. Most factors have been rounded to the nearest hundredth for accuracy.

STEP BY STEP

Step 1. Choose the appropriate conversion factor within each system, if necessary.

Step 2. Choose the appropriate conversion factor from the standard and metric conversion.

Step 3. Multiply and simplify to the nearest hundredth.

Examples

1. **Convert 12 inches to centimeters.**

    A. 4.72 centimeters   B. 14.54 centimeters   C. 28.36 centimeters   D. 30.48 centimeters

    The correct answer is **D**. The correct solution is 30.48 centimeters. $12 \text{ in} \times \frac{2.54 \text{ cm}}{1 \text{ in}} = 30.48$ cm.

2. **Convert 8 kilometers to feet.**

    A. 13,118.01 feet   B. 26,236.02 feet   C. 34,003.20 feet   D. 68,006.40 feet

    The correct answer is **B**. The correct solution is 26,236.02 feet. $8 \text{ km} \times \frac{1 \text{ mi}}{1.61 \text{ km}} \times \frac{5{,}280 \text{ ft}}{1 \text{ mi}} = \frac{42{,}240}{1.61} = 26{,}236.02$ ft.

3. **Convert 2 gallons to milliliters.**

    A. 527 milliliters   B. 758 milliliters   C. 5,270 milliliters   D. 7,580 milliliters

    The correct answer is **D**. The correct solution is 7,580 milliliters.
    $2 \text{ gal} \times \frac{3.79 \text{ L}}{1 \text{ gal}} \times \frac{1{,}000 \text{ mL}}{1 \text{ L}} = 7{,}580$ mL.

4. **Convert 16 kilograms to pounds.**

   A. 7.27 pounds   B. 18.2 pounds   C. 19.27 pounds   D. 35.2 pounds

   The correct answer is **D**. The correct solution is 35.2 pounds. $16 \text{ kg} \times \frac{2.2 \text{ lb}}{1 \text{ kg}} = 35.2 \text{ lb}$.

Time Conversions

Two ways to keep time are 12-hour clock time using a.m. and p.m. and military time based on a 24-hour clock. Keep these three key points in mind:

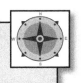

KEEP IN MIND
Midnight (12:00 a.m.) is 2400 or 0000 in military time.

- The hours from 1:00 a.m. to 12:59 p.m. are the same in both methods. For example, 9:15 a.m. in 12-hour clock time is 0915 in military time.
- From 1:00 p.m. to 11:59 p.m., add 12 hours to obtain military time. For example, 4:07 p.m. in 12-hour clock time is 1607 in military time.
- From 12:01 a.m. to 12:59 a.m. in 12-hour clock time, military time is from 0001 to 0059.

Example

Identify 9:27 p.m. in military time.

   A. 0927   B. 1927   C. 2127   D. 2427

   The correct answer is **C**. The correct solution is 2127. Add 1200 to the time, 1200 + 927 = 2127.

Let's Review!

- To convert from one unit to another, choose the appropriate conversion factors.
- In many cases, it is necessary to use multiple conversion factors.

CHAPTER 5 NUMBER AND QUANTITY PRACTICE QUIZ

1. Evaluate the expression 8 − 27.

    A. −35   C. 0

    B. −19   D. 19

2. Evaluate the expression 102 + 3 + 84 + 27.

    A. 105   C. 250

    B. 216   D. 513

3. How much change should a customer expect if she is buying a $53 item and hands the cashier two $50 bills?

    A. $3   C. $57

    B. $47   D. $100

4. When dealing with a series of multiplication and division operations, which is the correct approach to evaluating them?

    A. Evaluate all division operations first.

    B. Evaluate the expression from left to right.

    C. Evaluate all multiplication operations first.

    D. None of the above.

5. Evaluate the expression 28 × 43.

    A. 71   C. 1,204

    B. 196   D. 1,960

6. Evaluate the expression 3 + 1 − 5 + 2 − 6.

    A. −9   C. 0

    B. −5   D. 17

7. Which number is a factor of 128?

    A. 3   C. 12

    B. 6   D. 16

8. How many prime factors does 42 have?

    A. 1   C. 3

    B. 2   D. 4

9. If a factor tree for a prime factorization has four leaves—3, 2, 5, and 7—what is the number being factored?

    A. 7   C. 210

    B. 5   D. Not enough information

10. Convert 16,000 ounces to tons.

    A. 0.5 ton   C. 1.5 tons

    B. 1 ton   D. 2 tons

11. Convert 99 meters to kilometers.

    A. 0.0099 kilometers

    B. 0.099 kilometers

    C. 0.9 centimeters

    D. 9.9 centimeters

12. Identify 12:45 a.m. in military time.

    A. 0045   C. 1245

    B. 0145   D. 1345

CHAPTER 5 NUMBER AND QUANTITY PRACTICE QUIZ — ANSWER KEY

1. B. The correct solution is –19. Because the subtraction algorithm does not apply directly in this case (the first number is smaller than the second), first use the rule that $x - y = -(y - x)$. So, $8 - 27 = -(27 - 8)$. Applying the algorithm to $27 - 8$ yields 19, then $-(27 - 8) = -19$. **See Lesson: Basic Addition and Subtraction.**

2. B. The correct solution is 216. Use the addition algorithm. Add the numbers two at a time or all at once. The latter approach will involve two carry digits. **See Lesson: Basic Addition and Subtraction.**

3. B. The correct solution is $47. The customer gives the cashier $100, which is the sum of $50 and $50. To find out how much change she receives, calculate the difference between $100 and $53, which is $47. **See Lesson: Basic Addition and Subtraction.**

4. B. Multiplication and division have equivalent priority in the order of operations. In this case, the expression must be evaluated from left to right. **See Lesson: Basic Multiplication and Division.**

5. C. Use the multiplication algorithm. It involves adding 84 and 1,120 to get the product of 1,204. **See Lesson: Basic Multiplication and Division.**

6. B. This expression only involves addition and subtraction, but its evaluation must go from left to right. **See Lesson: Basic Multiplication and Division.**

$$3 + 1 - 5 + 2 - 6$$
$$4 - 5 + 2 - 6$$
$$(-1) + 2 - 6$$
$$1 - 6$$
$$-5$$

7. D. To determine whether a number is a factor of another number, divide the second number by the first number. If the quotient is whole, the first number is a factor. In this case, 128 is only divisible by 16. **See Lesson: Factors and Multiples.**

8. C. The prime factorization—for example, using a factor tree—shows that 42 has the prime factors 2, 3, and 7 because $2 \times 3 \times 7 = 42$. **See Lesson: Factors and Multiples.**

9. C. The number being factored in a prime factorization is the product of all its prime factors. The leaves in a factor tree are these prime factors. Therefore, the number is their product. In this case, it is $3 \times 2 \times 5 \times 7 = 210$. **See Lesson: Factors and Multiples.**

10. A. The correct solution is 0.5 ton.
$16,000 \text{ oz} \times \frac{1 \text{ lb}}{16 \text{ oz}} \times \frac{1\text{T}}{2,000 \text{ lb}} = \frac{16,000}{32,000} = 0.5$ T. **See Lesson: Standards of Measure.**

11. B. The correct solution is 0.099 kilometers. $99 \text{ m} \times \frac{1 \text{ km}}{1,000 \text{ m}} = \frac{99}{1,000} = 0.099$ km. **See Lesson: Standards of Measure.**

12. A. The correct solution is 0045. Subtract 1200 from the time, $1245 - 1200 = 0045$. **See Lesson: Standards of Measure.**

CHAPTER 6 ALGEBRA

DECIMALS AND FRACTIONS

This lesson introduces the basics of decimals and fractions. It also demonstrates changing decimals to fractions, changing fractions to decimals, and converting between fractions, decimals, and percentages.

Introduction to Fractions

A fraction represents part of a whole number. The top number of a fraction is the **numerator**, and the bottom number of a fraction is the **denominator**. The numerator is smaller than the denominator for a **proper fraction**. The numerator is larger than the denominator for an **improper fraction**.

Proper Fractions	Improper Fractions
$\frac{2}{5}$	$\frac{5}{2}$
$\frac{7}{12}$	$\frac{12}{7}$
$\frac{19}{20}$	$\frac{20}{19}$

An improper fraction can be changed to a **mixed number**. A mixed number is a whole number and a proper fraction. To write an improper fraction as a mixed number, divide the denominator into the numerator. The result is the whole number.

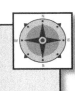

KEEP IN MIND

When comparing fractions, the denominators of the fractions must be the same.

The remainder is the numerator of the proper fraction, and the value of the denominator does not change. For example, $\frac{5}{2}$ is $2\frac{1}{2}$ because 2 goes into 5 twice with a remainder of 1. To write an improper fraction as a mixed number, multiply the whole number by the denominator and add the result to the numerator. The results become the new numerator. For example, $2\frac{1}{2}$ is $\frac{5}{2}$ because 2 times 2 plus 1 is 5 for the new numerator.

When comparing fractions, the denominators must be the same. Then, look at the numerator to determine which fraction is larger. If the fractions have different denominators, then a **least common denominator** must be found. This number is the smallest number that can be divided evenly into the denominators of all fractions being compared.

To determine the largest fraction from the group $\frac{1}{3}, \frac{3}{5}, \frac{2}{3}, \frac{2}{5}$, the first step is to find a common denominator. In this case, the least common denominator is 15 because 3 times 5 and 5 times 3 is 15. The second step is to convert the fractions to a denominator of 15.

The fractions with a denominator of 3 have the numerator and denominator multiplied by 5, and the fractions with a denominator of 5 have the numerator and denominator multiplied by 3, as shown below:

$$\frac{1}{3} \times \frac{5}{5} = \frac{5}{15}, \; \frac{3}{5} \times \frac{3}{3} = \frac{9}{15}, \; \frac{2}{3} \times \frac{5}{5} = \frac{10}{15}, \; \frac{2}{5} \times \frac{3}{3} = \frac{6}{15}$$

Now, the numerators can be compared. The largest fraction is $\frac{2}{3}$ because it has a numerator of 10 after finding the common denominator.

Examples

1. **Which fraction is the least?**

   A. $\frac{3}{5}$ B. $\frac{3}{4}$ C. $\frac{1}{5}$ D. $\frac{1}{4}$

   The correct answer is **C**. The correct solution is $\frac{1}{5}$ because it has the smallest numerator compared to the other fractions with the same denominator. The fractions with a common denominator of 20 are $\frac{3}{5} = \frac{12}{20}, \frac{3}{4} = \frac{15}{20}, \frac{1}{5} = \frac{4}{20}, \frac{1}{4} = \frac{5}{20}$.

2. **Which fraction is the greatest?**

   A. $\frac{5}{6}$ B. $\frac{1}{2}$ C. $\frac{2}{3}$ D. $\frac{1}{6}$

   The correct answer is **A**. The correct solution is $\frac{5}{6}$ because it has the largest numerator compared to the other fractions with the same denominator. The fractions with a common denominator of 6 are $\frac{5}{6} = \frac{5}{6}, \frac{1}{2} = \frac{3}{6}, \frac{2}{3} = \frac{4}{6}, \frac{1}{6} = \frac{1}{6}$.

Introduction to Decimals

A **decimal** is a number that expresses part of a whole. Decimals show a portion of a number after a decimal point. Each number to the left and right of the decimal point has a specific place value. Identify the place values for 645.3207.

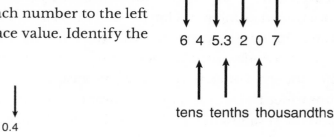

When comparing decimals, compare the numbers in the same place value. For example, determine the greatest decimal from the group 0.4, 0.41, 0.39, and 0.37. In these numbers, there is a value to the right of the decimal point. Comparing the tenths places, the numbers with 4 tenths (0.4 and 0.41) are greater than the numbers with three tenths (0.39 and 0.37).

0.4

0.41

0.39

0.37

KEEP IN MIND

When comparing decimals, compare the place value where the numbers are different.

Then, compare the hundredths in the 4 tenths numbers. The value of 0.41 is greater because there is a 1 in the hundredths place versus a 0 in the hundredths place.

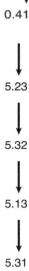

0.4

0.41

Here is another example: determine the least decimal of the group 5.23, 5.32, 5.13, and 5.31. In this group, the ones value is 5 for all numbers. Then, comparing the tenths values, 5.13 is the smallest number because it is the only value with 1 tenth.

5.23

5.32

5.13

5.31

Examples

1. **Which decimal is the greatest?**

   A. 0.07   B. 0.007   C. 0.7   D. 0.0007

   The correct answer is **C**. The solution is 0.7 because it has the largest place value in the tenths.

2. **Which decimal is the least?**

   A. 0.0413   B. 0.0713   C. 0.0513   D. 0.0613

   The correct answer is **A**. The correct solution is 0.0413 because it has the smallest place value in the hundredths place.

Changing Decimals and Fractions

Three steps change a decimal to a fraction.

> **STEP BY STEP**
> **Step 1.** Write the decimal divided by 1 with the decimal as the numerator and 1 as the denominator.
> **Step 2.** Multiply the numerator and denominator by 10 for every number after the decimal point. (For example, if there is 1 decimal place, multiply by 10. If there are 2 decimal places, multiply by 100).
> **Step 3.** Reduce the fraction completely.

To change the decimal 0.37 to a fraction, start by writing the decimal as a fraction with a denominator of one, $\frac{0.37}{1}$. Because there are two decimal places, multiply the numerator and denominator by 100, $\frac{0.37 \times 100}{1 \times 100} = \frac{37}{100}$. The fraction does not reduce, so $\frac{37}{100}$ is 0.37 in fraction form.

Similarly, to change the decimal 2.4 to a fraction start by writing the decimal as a fraction with a denominator of one, $\frac{0.4}{1}$, and ignore the whole number. Because there is one decimal place, multiply the numerator and denominator by 10, $\frac{0.4 \times 10}{1 \times 10} = \frac{4}{10}$. The fraction does reduce: $2\frac{4}{10} = 2\frac{2}{5}$ is 2.4 in fraction form.

The decimal $0.\overline{3}$ as a fraction is $\frac{0.\overline{3}}{1}$. In the case of a repeating decimal, let $n = 0.\overline{3}$ *and* $10 = 3.\overline{3}$. Then, $10n - n = 3.\overline{3} - 0.\overline{3}$, resulting in $9n = 3$ and solution of $n = \frac{3}{9} = \frac{1}{3}$. The decimal $0.\overline{3}$ is $\frac{1}{3}$ as a fraction.

Examples

1. **Change 0.38 to a fraction. Simplify completely.**

   A. $\frac{3}{10}$ 　　　　 B. $\frac{9}{25}$ 　　　　 C. $\frac{19}{50}$ 　　　　 D. $\frac{2}{5}$

   The correct answer is **C**. The correct solution is $\frac{19}{50}$ because $\frac{0.38}{1} = \frac{38}{100} = \frac{19}{50}$.

2. **Change $1.\overline{1}$ to a fraction. Simplify completely.**

   A. $1\frac{1}{11}$ 　　　　 B. $1\frac{1}{9}$ 　　　　 C. $1\frac{1}{6}$ 　　　　 D. $1\frac{1}{3}$

   The correct answer is **B**. The correct solution is $1\frac{1}{9}$. Let $n = 1.\overline{1}$ and $10n = 11.\overline{1}$. Then, $10n - n = 11.\overline{1} - 1.\overline{1}$, resulting in $9n = 10$ and solution of $n = \frac{10}{9} = 1\frac{1}{9}$.

Two steps change a fraction to a decimal.

STEP BY STEP

Step 1. Divide the denominator by the numerator. Add zeros after the decimal point as needed.

Step 2. Complete the process when there is no remainder or the decimal is repeating.

To convert $\frac{1}{5}$ to a decimal, rewrite $\frac{1}{5}$ as a long division problem and add zeros after the decimal point, $1.0 \div 5$. Complete the long division and $\frac{1}{5}$ as a decimal is 0.2. The division is complete because there is no remainder.

To convert $\frac{8}{9}$ to a decimal, rewrite $\frac{8}{9}$ as a long division problem and add zeros after the decimal point, $8.00 \div 9$. Complete the long division, and $\frac{8}{9}$ as a decimal is $0.\overline{8}$. The process is complete because the decimal is complete.

To rewrite the mixed number $2\frac{3}{4}$ as a decimal, the fraction needs changed to a decimal. Rewrite $\frac{3}{4}$ as a long division problem and add zeros after the decimal point, $3.00 \div 4$. The whole number is needed for the answer and is not included in the long division. Complete the long division, and $2\frac{3}{4}$ as a decimal is 2.75.

Examples

1. **Change $\frac{9}{10}$ to a decimal. Simplify completely.**

   A. 0.75   B. 0.8   C. 0.85   D. 0.9

   The correct answer is **D**. The correct answer is 0.9 because $\frac{9}{10} = 9.0 \div 10 = 0.9$.

2. **Change $\frac{5}{6}$ to a decimal. Simplify completely.**

   A. 0.73   B. $0.7\overline{6}$ C. $0.8\overline{3}$ D. 0.86

   The correct answer is **C**. The correct answer is $0.8\overline{3}$ because $\frac{5}{6} = 5.000 \div 6 = 0.8\overline{3}$.

Convert among Fractions, Decimals, and Percentages

Fractions, decimals, and percentages can change forms, but they are equivalent values.

There are two ways to change a decimal to a percent. One way is to multiply the decimal by 100 and add a percent sign. 0.24 as a percent is 24%.

Another way is to move the decimal point two places to the right. The decimal 0.635 is 63.5% as a percent when moving the decimal point two places to the right.

Any decimal, including repeating decimals, can change to a percent. $0.\overline{3}$ as a percent is $0.\overline{3} \times 100 = 33.\overline{3}\%$.

Example

Write 0.345 as a percent.

A. 3.45%   B. 34.5%   C. 345%   D. 3450%

The correct answer is **B.** The correct answer is 34.5% because 0.345 as a percent is 34.5%.

There are two ways to change a percent to a decimal. One way is to remove the percent sign and divide the decimal by 100. For example, 73% as a decimal is 0.73.

Another way is to move the decimal point two places to the left. For example, 27.8% is 0.278 as a decimal when moving the decimal point two places to the left.

Any percent, including repeating percents, can change to a decimal. For example, $44.\overline{4}\%$ as a decimal is $44.\overline{4} \div 100 = 0.\overline{4}$.

Example

Write 131% as a decimal.

A. 0.131   B. 1.31   C. 13.1   D. 131

The correct answer is **B.** The correct answer is 1.31 because 131% as a decimal is 131 ÷ 100 = 1.31.

Two steps change a fraction to a percent.

STEP BY STEP
Step 1.   Divide the numerator and denominator.
Step 2.   Multiply by 100 and add a percent sign.

To change the fraction $\frac{3}{5}$ to a decimal, perform long division to get 0.6. Then, multiply 0.6 by 100 and $\frac{3}{5}$ is the same as 60%.

To change the fraction $\frac{7}{8}$ to a decimal, perform long division to get 0.875. Then, multiply 0.875 by 100 and $\frac{7}{8}$ is the same as 87.5%.

Fractions that are repeating decimals can also be converted to a percent. To change the fraction $\frac{2}{3}$ to a decimal, perform long division to get $0.\overline{6}$. Then, multiply $0.\overline{6}$ by 100 and the percent is $66.\overline{6}\%$.

Example

Write $2\frac{1}{8}$ as a percent.

A. 21.2%   B. 21.25%   C. 212%   D. 212.5%

The correct answer is **D.** The correct answer is 212.5% because $2\frac{1}{8}$ as a percent is 2.125 x 100 = 212.5%.

Two steps change a percent to a fraction.

> **STEP BY STEP**
>
> **Step 1.** Remove the percent sign and write the value as the numerator with a denominator of 100.
>
> **Step 2.** Simplify the fraction.

Remove the percent sign from 45% and write as a fraction with a denominator of 100, $\frac{45}{100}$. The fraction reduces to $\frac{9}{20}$.

Remove the percent sign from 22.8% and write as a fraction with a denominator of 100, $\frac{22.8}{100}$. The fraction reduces to $\frac{228}{1000} = \frac{57}{250}$.

Repeating percentages can change to a fraction. Remove the percent sign from $16.\overline{6}\%$ and write as a fraction with a denominator of 100, $\frac{16.\overline{6}}{100}$. The fraction simplifies to $\frac{0.1\overline{6}}{1} = \frac{1}{6}$.

Example

Write 72% as a fraction.

A. $\frac{27}{50}$ B. $\frac{7}{10}$ C. $\frac{18}{25}$ D. $\frac{3}{4}$

The correct answer is **C**. The correct answer is $\frac{18}{25}$ because 72% as a fraction is $\frac{72}{100} = \frac{18}{25}$.

Let's Review!

- A fraction is a number with a numerator and a denominator. A fraction can be written as a proper fraction, an improper fraction, or a mixed number. Changing fractions to a common denominator enables you to determine the least or greatest fraction in a group of fractions.
- A decimal is a number that expresses part of a whole. By comparing the same place values, you can find the least or greatest decimal in a group of decimals.
- A number can be written as a fraction, a decimal, and a percent. These are equivalent values. Numbers can be converted between fractions, decimals, and percents by following a series of steps.

MULTIPLICATION AND DIVISION OF FRACTIONS

This lesson introduces how to multiply and divide fractions.

Multiplying a Fraction by a Fraction

The multiplication of fractions does not require changing any denominators like adding and subtracting fractions do. To multiply a fraction by a fraction, multiply the numerators together and multiply the denominators together. For example, $\frac{2}{3} \times \frac{4}{5}$ is $\frac{2 \times 4}{3 \times 5}$, which is $\frac{8}{15}$.

Sometimes, the final solution reduces. For example, $\frac{3}{5} \times \frac{1}{9} = \frac{3 \times 1}{5 \times 9} = \frac{3}{45}$. The fraction $\frac{3}{45}$ reduces to $\frac{1}{15}$.

Simplifying fractions can occur before completing the multiplication. In the previous problem, the numerator of 3 can be simplified with the denominator of 9: $\frac{1\cancel{3}}{5} \times \frac{1}{\cancel{9}3} = \frac{1}{15}$. This method of simplifying only occurs with the multiplication of fractions.

KEEP IN MIND
The product of multiplying a fraction by a fraction is always less than 1.

Examples

1. **Multiply $\frac{1}{2} \times \frac{3}{4}$.**

   A. $\frac{1}{4}$ B. $\frac{1}{2}$ C. $\frac{3}{8}$ D. $\frac{2}{3}$

   The correct answer is **C.** The correct solution is $\frac{3}{8}$ because $\frac{1}{2} \times \frac{3}{4} = \frac{3}{8}$.

2. **Multiply $\frac{2}{3} \times \frac{5}{6}$.**

   A. $\frac{1}{9}$ B. $\frac{5}{18}$ C. $\frac{5}{9}$ D. $\frac{7}{18}$

   The correct answer is **C.** The correct solution is $\frac{5}{9}$ because $\frac{2}{3} \times \frac{5}{6} = \frac{10}{18} = \frac{5}{9}$.

Multiply a Fraction by a Whole or Mixed Number

Multiplying a fraction by a whole or mixed number is similar to multiplying two fractions. When multiplying by a whole number, change the whole number to a fraction with a denominator of 1. Next, multiply the numerators together and the denominators together. Rewrite the final answer as a mixed number. For example: $\frac{9}{10} \times 3 = \frac{9}{10} \times \frac{3}{1} = \frac{27}{10} = 2\frac{7}{10}$.

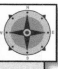

When multiplying a fraction by a mixed number or multiplying two mixed numbers, the process is similar.

KEEP IN MIND
Always change a mixed number to an improper fraction when multiplying by a mixed number.

For example, multiply $\frac{10}{11} \times 3\frac{1}{2}$. Change the mixed number to an improper fraction, $\frac{10}{11} \times \frac{7}{2}$. Multiply the numerators together and multiply the denominators together, $\frac{70}{22}$. Write the improper fraction as a mixed number, $3\frac{4}{22}$. Reduce if necessary, $3\frac{2}{11}$.

This process can also be used when multiplying a whole number by a mixed number or multiplying two mixed numbers.

Examples

1. **Multiply** $4 \times \frac{5}{6}$.

    A. $\frac{5}{24}$ 　　　　 B. $2\frac{3}{4}$ 　　　　 C. $3\frac{1}{3}$ 　　　　 D. $4\frac{5}{6}$

    The correct answer is **C**. The correct solution is $3\frac{1}{3}$ because $\frac{4}{1} \times \frac{5}{6} = \frac{20}{6} = 3\frac{2}{6} = 3\frac{1}{3}$.

2. **Multiply** $1\frac{1}{2} \times 1\frac{1}{6}$.

    A. $1\frac{1}{12}$ 　　　　 B. $1\frac{1}{4}$ 　　　　 C. $1\frac{3}{8}$ 　　　　 D. $1\frac{3}{4}$

    The correct answer is **D**. The correct solution is $1\frac{3}{4}$ because $\frac{3}{2} \times \frac{7}{6} = \frac{21}{12} = 1\frac{9}{12} = 1\frac{3}{4}$.

Dividing a Fraction by a Fraction

Some basic steps apply when dividing a fraction by a fraction. The information from the previous two sections is applicable to dividing fractions.

STEP BY STEP

Step 1. Leave the first fraction alone.

Step 2. Find the reciprocal of the second fraction.

Step 3. Multiply the first fraction by the reciprocal of the second fraction.

Step 4. Rewrite the fraction as a mixed number and reduce the fraction completely.

Divide, $\frac{3}{10} \div \frac{1}{2}$. Find the reciprocal of the second fraction, which is $\frac{2}{1}$.

Now, multiply the fractions, $\frac{3}{10} \times \frac{2}{1} = \frac{6}{10}$. Reduce $\frac{6}{10}$ to $\frac{3}{5}$.

Divide, $\frac{4}{5} \div \frac{3}{8}$. Find the reciprocal of the second fraction, which is $\frac{8}{3}$.

Now, multiply the fractions, $\frac{4}{5} \times \frac{8}{3} = \frac{32}{15}$. Rewrite the fraction as a mixed number, $\frac{32}{15} = 2\frac{2}{15}$.

Examples

1. **Divide** $\frac{1}{2} \div \frac{5}{6}$.

    A. $\frac{5}{12}$ 　　　　 B. $\frac{3}{5}$ 　　　　 C. $\frac{5}{6}$ 　　　　 D. $1\frac{2}{3}$

    The correct answer is **B**. The correct solution is $\frac{3}{5}$ because $\frac{1}{2} \times \frac{6}{5} = \frac{6}{10} = \frac{3}{5}$.

2. **Divide $\frac{2}{3} \div \frac{3}{5}$.**

   A. $\frac{2}{15}$ B. $\frac{2}{5}$ C. $1\frac{1}{15}$ D. $1\frac{1}{9}$

The correct answer is **D**. The correct solution is $1\frac{1}{9}$ because $\frac{2}{3} \times \frac{5}{3} = \frac{10}{9} = 1\frac{1}{9}$.

Dividing a Fraction and a Whole or Mixed Number

Some basic steps apply when dividing a fraction by a whole number or a mixed number.

STEP BY STEP	
Step 1.	Write any whole number as a fraction with a denominator of 1. Write any mixed numbers as improper fractions.
Step 2.	Leave the first fraction (improper fraction) alone.
Step 3.	Find the reciprocal of the second fraction.
Step 4.	Multiply the first fraction by the reciprocal of the second fraction.
Step 5.	Rewrite the fraction as a mixed number and reduce the fraction completely.

Divide, $\frac{3}{10} \div 3$. Rewrite the expression as $\frac{3}{10} \div \frac{3}{1}$. Find the reciprocal of the second fraction, which is $\frac{1}{3}$. Multiply the fractions, $\frac{3}{10} \times \frac{1}{3} = \frac{3}{30} = \frac{1}{10}$. Reduce $\frac{3}{30}$ to $\frac{1}{10}$.

Divide, $2\frac{4}{5} \div 1\frac{3}{8}$. Rewrite the expression as $\frac{14}{5} \div \frac{11}{8}$. Find the reciprocal of the second fraction, which is $\frac{8}{11}$.

Multiply the fractions, $\frac{14}{5} \times \frac{8}{11} = \frac{112}{55} = 2\frac{2}{55}$. Reduce $\frac{112}{55}$ to $2\frac{2}{55}$.

Examples

1. **Divide $\frac{2}{3} \div 4$.**

   A. $\frac{1}{12}$ B. $\frac{1}{10}$ C. $\frac{1}{8}$ D. $\frac{1}{6}$

The correct answer is **D**. The correct answer is $\frac{1}{6}$ because $\frac{2}{3} \times \frac{1}{4} = \frac{2}{12} = \frac{1}{6}$.

2. **Divide $1\frac{5}{12} \div 1\frac{1}{2}$.**

   A. $\frac{17}{18}$ B. $1\frac{5}{24}$ C. $1\frac{5}{6}$ D. $2\frac{1}{8}$

The correct answer is **A**. The correct answer is $\frac{17}{18}$ because $\frac{17}{12} \div \frac{3}{2} = \frac{17}{12} \times \frac{2}{3} = \frac{34}{36} = \frac{17}{18}$.

Let's Review!

- The process to multiply fractions is to multiply the numerators together and multiply the denominators together. When there is a mixed number, change the mixed number to an improper fraction before multiplying.
- The process to divide fractions is to find the reciprocal of the second fraction and multiply the fractions. As with multiplying, change any mixed numbers to improper fractions before dividing.

EQUATIONS WITH ONE VARIABLE

This lesson introduces how to solve linear equations and linear inequalities.

One-Step Linear Equations

A **linear equation** is an equation where two expressions are set equal to each other. The equation is in the form $ax + b = c$, where a is a non-zero constant and b and c are constants. The exponent on a linear equation is always 1, and there is no more than one solution to a linear equation.

There are four properties to help solve a linear equation.

Property	Definition	Example with Numbers	Example with Variables
Addition Property of Equality	Add the same number to both sides of the equation.	$x-3 = 9$ $x-3+3 = 9+3$ $x = 12$	$x-a = b$ $x-a+a = b+a$ $x = a+b$
Subtraction Property of Equality	Subtract the same number from both sides of the equation.	$x+3 = 9$ $x+3-3 = 9-3$ $x = 6$	$x+a = b$ $x+a-a = b-a$ $x = b-a$
Multiplication Property of Equality	Multiply both sides of the equation by the same number.	$\frac{x}{3} = 9$ $\frac{x}{3} \times 3 = 9 \times 3$ $x = 27$	$\frac{x}{a} = b$ $\frac{x}{a} \times a = b \times a$ $x = ab$
Division Property of Equality	Divide both sides of the equation by the same number.	$3x = 9$ $\frac{3x}{3} = \frac{9}{3}$ $x = 3$	$ax = b$ $\frac{ax}{a} = \frac{b}{a}$ $x = \frac{b}{a}$

Example

Solve the equation for the unknown, $\frac{w}{2} = -6$.

A. −12　　　　　　B. −8　　　　　　C. −4　　　　　　D. −3

The correct answer is **A**. The correct solution is −12 because both sides of the equation are multiplied by 2.

Two-Step Linear Equations

A two-step linear equation is in the form $ax + b = c$, where a is a non-zero constant and b and c are constants. There are two basic steps in solving this equation.

> **STEP BY STEP**
>
> **Step 1.** Use addition and subtraction properties of an equation to move the variable to one side of the equation and all number terms to the other side of the equation.
>
> **Step 2.** Use multiplication and division properties of an equation to remove the value in front of the variable.

Examples

1. **Solve the equation for the unknown, $\frac{x}{-2} - 3 = 5$.**

   A. -16 B. -8 C. 8 D. 16

   The correct answer is **A**. The correct solution is -16.

$\frac{x}{-2} = 8$	Add 3 to both sides of the equation.
$x = -16$	Multiply both sides of the equation by -2.

2. **Solve the equation for the unknown, $4x + 3 = 8$.**

   A. -2 B. $-\frac{5}{4}$ C. $\frac{5}{4}$ D. 2

   The correct answer is **C**. The correct solution is $\frac{5}{4}$.

$4x = 5$	Subtract 3 from both sides of the equation.
$x = \frac{5}{4}$	Divide both sides of the equation by 4.

3. **Solve the equation for the unknown w, $P = 2l + 2w$.**

   A. $2P - 2l = w$ B. $\frac{P-2l}{2} = w$ C. $2P + 2l = w$ D. $\frac{P+2l}{2} = w$

   The correct answer is **B**. The correct solution is $\frac{P-2l}{2} = w$.

$P - 2l = 2w$	Subtract 2l from both sides of the equation.
$\frac{P-2l}{2} = w$	Divide both sides of the equation by 2.

Multi-Step Linear Equations

In these basic examples of linear equations, the solution may be evident, but these properties demonstrate how to use an opposite operation to solve for a variable. Using these properties, there are three steps in solving a complex linear equation.

> **STEP BY STEP**
>
> **Step 1.** Simplify each side of the equation. This includes removing parentheses, removing fractions, and adding like terms.
>
> **Step 2.** Use addition and subtraction properties of an equation to move the variable to one side of the equation and all number terms to the other side of the equation.
>
> **Step 3.** Use multiplication and division properties of an equation to remove the value in front of the variable.

In Step 2, all of the variables may be placed on the left side or the right side of the equation. The examples in this lesson will place all of the variables on the left side of the equation.

When solving for a variable, apply the same steps as above. In this case, the equation is not being solved for a value, but for a specific variable.

Examples

1. **Solve the equation for the unknown, $2(4x + 1)-5 = 3-(4x-3)$.**

   A. $\frac{1}{4}$ B. $\frac{3}{4}$ C. $\frac{4}{3}$ D. 4

   The correct answer is **B**. The correct solution is $\frac{3}{4}$.

$8x + 2-5 = 3-4x + 3$	Apply the distributive property.
$8x-3 = -4x + 6$	Combine like terms on both sides of the equation.
$12x-3 = 6$	Add $4x$ to both sides of the equation.
$12x = 9$	Add 3 to both sides of the equation.
$x = \frac{3}{4}$	Divide both sides of the equation by 12.

2. **Solve the equation for the unknown, $\frac{2}{3}x + 2 = -\frac{1}{2}x + 2(x + 1)$.**

   A. 0   B. 1   C. 2   D. 3

   The correct answer is **A**. The correct solution is 0.

$\frac{2}{3}x + 2 = -\frac{1}{2}x + 2x + 2$	Apply the distributive property.
$4x + 12 = -3x + 12x + 12$	Multiply all terms by the least common denominator of 6 to eliminate the fractions.
$4x + 12 = 9x + 12$	Combine like terms on the right side of the equation.
$-5x = 12$	Subtract $9x$ from both sides of the equation.
$-5x = 0$	Subtract 12 from both sides of the equation.
$x = 0$	Divide both sides of the equation by -5.

3. Solve the equation for the unknown for x, $y - y_1 = m(x - x_1)$.

A. $y - y_1 + m x_1$ B. $m y - m y_1 + m x_1$ C. $\frac{y - y_1 + x_1}{m}$ D. $\frac{y - y_1 + m x_1}{m}$

The correct answer is **D**. The correct solution is $\frac{y - y_1 + m x_1}{m}$

$$y - y_1 = mx - mx_1$$ Apply the distributive property.

$$y - y_1 + mx_1 = mx$$ Add mx_1 to both sides of the equation.

$$\frac{y - y_1 + mx_1}{m} = x$$ Divide both sides of the equation by m.

Solving Linear Inequalities

A **linear inequality** is similar to a linear equation, but it contains an inequality sign ($<$, $>$, $\leq$, $\geq$). Many of the steps for solving linear inequalities are the same as for solving linear equations. The major difference is that the solution is an infinite number of values. There are four properties to help solve a linear inequality.

Property	Definition	Example
Addition Property of Inequality	Add the same number to both sides of the inequality.	$x - 3 < 9$ $x - 3 + 3 < 9 + 3$ $x < 12$
Subtraction Property of Inequality	Subtract the same number from both sides of the inequality.	$x + 3 > 9$ $x + 3 - 3 > 9 - 3$ $x > 6$
Multiplication Property of Inequality (when multiplying by a positive number)	Multiply both sides of the inequality by the same number.	$\frac{x}{3} \geq 9$ $\frac{x}{3} \times 3 \geq 9 \times 3$ $x \geq 27$
Division Property of Inequality (when multiplying by a positive number)	Divide both sides of the inequality by the same number.	$3x \leq 9$ $\frac{3x}{3} \leq \frac{9}{3}$ $x \leq 3$
Multiplication Property of Inequality (when multiplying by a negative number)	Multiply both sides of the inequality by the same number.	$\frac{x}{-3} \geq 9$ $\frac{x}{-3} \times -3 \geq 9 \times -3$ $x \leq -27$
Division Property of Inequality (when multiplying by a negative number)	Divide both sides of the inequality by the same number.	$-3x \leq 9$ $\frac{-3x}{-3} \leq \frac{9}{-3}$ $x \geq -3$

Multiplying or dividing both sides of the inequality by a negative number reverses the sign of the inequality.

In these basic examples, the solution may be evident, but these properties demonstrate how to use an opposite operation to solve for a variable. Using these properties, there are three steps in solving a complex linear inequality.

> **STEP BY STEP**
>
> **Step 1.** Simplify each side of the inequality. This includes removing parentheses, removing fractions, and adding like terms.
>
> **Step 2.** Use addition and subtraction properties of an inequality to move the variable to one side of the equation and all number terms to the other side of the equation.
>
> **Step 3.** Use multiplication and division properties of an inequality to remove the value in front of the variable. Reverse the inequality sign if multiplying or dividing by a negative number.

In Step 2, all of the variables may be placed on the left side or the right side of the inequality. The examples in this lesson will place all of the variables on the left side of the inequality.

Examples

1. **Solve the inequality for the unknown, $3(2 + x) < 2(3x{-}1)$.**

   A. $x < -\frac{8}{3}$ B. $x > -\frac{8}{3}$ C. $x < \frac{8}{3}$ D. $x > \frac{8}{3}$

   The correct answer is **D**. The correct solution is $x > \frac{8}{3}$.

$6 + 3x < 6x{-}2$	Apply the distributive property.
$6{-}3x < -2$	Subtract $6x$ from both sides of the inequality.
$-3x < -8$	Subtract 6 from both sides of the inequality.
$x > \frac{8}{3}$	Divide both sides of the inequality by 3.

2. **Solve the inequality for the unknown, $\frac{1}{2}(2x{-}3) \geq \frac{1}{4}(2x + 1){-}2$.**

   A. $x > -7$ B. $x > -3$ C. $x \geq -\frac{3}{2}$ D. $x \geq -\frac{1}{2}$

   The correct answer is **D**. The correct solution is $x \geq -\frac{1}{2}$.

$2(2x{-}3) \geq 2x + 1{-}8$	Multiply all terms by the least common denominator of 4 to eliminate the fractions.
$4x{-}6 \geq 2x + 1{-}8$	Apply the distributive property.
$4x{-}6 \geq 2x{-}7$	Combine like terms on the right side of the inequality.
$2x{-}6 \geq -7$	Subtract $2x$ from both sides of the inequality.
$2x \geq -1$	Add 6 to both sides of the inequality.
$x \geq -\frac{1}{2}$	Divide both sides of the inequality by 2.

Let's Review!

- A linear equation is an equation with one solution. Using opposite operations solves a linear equation.
- The process to solve a linear equation or inequality is to eliminate fractions and parentheses and combine like terms on the same side of the sign. Then, solve the equation or inequality by using inverse operations.

EQUATIONS WITH TWO VARIABLES

This lesson discusses solving a system of linear equations by substitution, elimination, and graphing, as well as solving a simple system of a linear and a quadratic equation.

Solving a System of Equations by Substitution

A **system of linear equations** is a set of two or more linear equations in the same variables. A solution to the system is an ordered pair that is a solution in all the equations in the system. The ordered pair (1, -2) is a solution for the system of equations $2x + y = 0$ $-x + 2y = -5$ because $2(1) + (-2) = 0$ $-1 + 2(-2) = -5$ makes both equations true.

One way to solve a system of linear equations is by substitution.

STEP BY STEP	
Step 1.	Solve one equation for one of the variables.
Step 2.	Substitute the expression from Step 1 into the other equation and solve for the other variable.
Step 3.	Substitute the value from Step 2 into one of the original equations and solve.

All systems of equations can be solved by substitution for any one of the four variables in the problem. The most efficient way of solving is locating the $1x$ or $1y$ in the equations because this eliminates the possibility of having fractions in the equations.

Examples

1. **Solve the system of equations,** $\begin{array}{c} x = y + 6 \\ 4x + 5y = 60 \end{array}$.

   A. (10, 12)   B. (6, 12)   C. (6, 4)   D. (10, 4)

   The correct answer is **D**. The correct solution is (10, 4).

   The first equation is already solved for x.

$4(y + 6) + 5y = 60$	Substitute $y + 6$ in for x in the first equation.
$4y + 24 + 5y = 60$	Apply the distributive property.
$9y + 24 = 60$	Combine like terms on the left side of the equation.
$9y = 36$	Subtract 24 from both sides of the equation.
$y = 4$	Divide both sides of the equation by 9.
$x = 4 + 6$	Substitute 4 in the first equation for y.
$x = 10$	Simplify using order of operations.

2. Solve the system of equations, $\begin{array}{l} 3x + 2y = 41 \\ -4x + y = -18 \end{array}$.

  A. (5, 13)   B. (6, 6)   C. (7, 10)   D. (10, 7)

The correct answer is **C**. The correct solution is (7, 10).

$y = 4x-18$	Solve the second equation for y by adding $4x$ to both sides of the equation.
$3x + 2(4x-18) = 41$	Substitute $4x-18$ in for y in the first equation.
$3x + 8x-36 = 41$	Apply the distributive property.
$11x-36 = 41$	Combine like terms on the left side of the equation.
$11x = 77$	Add 36 to both sides of the equation.
$x = 7$	Divide both sides of the equation by 11.
$-4(7) + y = -18$	Substitute 7 in the second equation for x.
$-28 + y = -18$	Simplify using order of operations.
$y = 10$	Add 28 to both sides of the equation.

Solving a System of Equations by Elimination

Another way to solve a system of linear equations is by elimination.

STEP BY STEP

Step 1. Multiply, if necessary, one or both equations by a constant so at least one pair of like terms has opposite coefficients.

Step 2. Add the equations to eliminate one of the variables.

Step 3. Solve the resulting equation.

Step 4. Substitute the value from Step 3 into one of the original equations and solve for the other variable.

All system of equations can be solved by the elimination method for any one of the four variables in the problem. One way of solving is locating the variables with opposite coefficients and adding the equations. Another approach is multiplying one equation to obtain opposite coefficients for the variables.

Examples

1. **Solve the system of equations,** $\begin{array}{l} 3x + 5y = 28 \\ -4x - 5y = -34 \end{array}$.

   A. (12, 6)   B. (6, 12)   C. (6, 2)   D. (2, 6)

   The correct answer is **C**. The correct solution is (6, 2).

$-x = -6$	Add the equations.
$x = 6$	Divide both sides of the equation by -1.
$3(6) + 5y = 28$	Substitute 6 in the first equation for x.
$18 + 5y = 28$	Simplify using order of operations.
$5y = 10$	Subtract 18 from both sides of the equation.
$y = 2$	Divide both sides of the equation by 5.

2. **Solve the system of equations,** $\begin{array}{l} -5x + 5y = 0 \\ 2x - 3y = -3 \end{array}$.

   A. (2, 2)   B. (3, 3)   C. (6, 6)   D. (9, 9)

   The correct answer is **B**. The correct solution is (3, 3).

$-10x + 10y = 0$	Multiply all terms in the first equation by 2.
$10x - 15y = -15$	Multiply all terms in the second equation by 5.
$-5y = -15$	Add the equations.
$y = 3$	Divide both sides of the equation by -5.
$2x - 3(3) = -3$	Substitute 3 in the second equation for y.
$2x - 9 = -3$	Simplify using order of operations.
$2x = 6$	Add 9 to both sides of the equation.
$x = 3$	Divide both sides of the equation by 2.

Solving a System of Equations by Graphing

Graphing is a third method of a solving system of equations. The point of intersection is the solution for the graph. This method is a great way to visualize each graph on a coordinate plane.

> **STEP BY STEP**
> **Step 1.** Graph each equation in the coordinate plane.
> **Step 2.** Estimate the point of intersection.
> **Step 3.** Check the point by substituting for x and y in each equation of the original system.

The best approach to graphing is to obtain each line in slope-intercept form. Then, graph the y-intercept and use the slope to find additional points on the line.

Example

Solve the system of equations by graphing, $\begin{array}{l} y = 3x-2 \\ y = x-4 \end{array}$.

A.

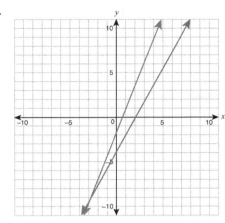

C.

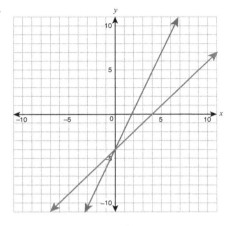

B.

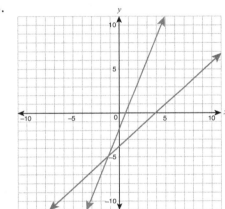

D.

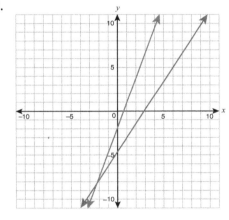

The correct answer is **B**. The correct graph has the two lines intersect at (-1, -5).

Solving a System of a Linear Equation and an Equation of a Circle

There are many other types of systems of equations. One example is the equation of a line $y = mx$ and the equation of a circle $x^2 + y^2 = r^2$ where r is the radius. With this system of equations, there can be two ordered pairs that intersect between the line and the circle. If there is one ordered pair, the line is tangent to the circle.

This system of equations is solved by substituting the expression mx in for y in the equation of a circle. Then, solve the equation for x. The values for x are substituted into the linear equation to find the value for y.

KEEP IN MIND

There will be two solutions in many cases with the system of a linear equation and an equation of a circle.

109

Example

Solve the system of equations, $\begin{array}{l} y = -3x \\ x^2 + y^2 = 10 \end{array}$.

A. (1, 3) and (−1, −3)

C. (−3, 10) and (3, −10)

B. (1, −3) and (−1, 3)

D. (3, 10) and (−3, −10)

The correct answer is **B.** The correct solutions are (1, −3) and (−1, 3).

$x^2 + (-3x)^2 = 10$	Substitute $-3x$ in for y in the second equation.
$x^2 + 9x^2 = 10$	Apply the exponent.
$10x^2 = 10$	Combine like terms on the left side of the equation.
$x^2 = 1$	Divide both sides of the equation by 10.
$x = \pm 1$	Apply the square root to both sides of the equation.
$y = -3(1) = -3$	Substitute 1 in the first equation and multiply.
$y = -3(-1) = 3$	Substitute −1 in the first equation and multiply.

Let's Review!

- There are three ways to solve a system of equations: graphing, substitution, and elimination. Using any method will result in the same solution for the system of equations.
- Solving a system of a linear equation and an equation of a circle uses substitution and usually results in two solutions.

SOLVING REAL-WORLD MATHEMATICAL PROBLEMS

This lesson introduces solving real-world mathematical problems by using estimation and mental computation. This lesson also includes real-world applications involving integers, fractions, and decimals.

Estimating

Estimations are rough calculations of a solution to a problem. The most common use for estimation is completing calculations without a calculator or other tool. There are many estimation techniques, but this lesson focuses on integers, decimals, and fractions.

KEEP IN MIND

An estimation is an educated guess at the solution to a problem.

To round a whole number, round the value to the nearest ten or hundred. The number 142 rounds to 140 for the nearest ten and to 100 for the nearest hundred. The context of the problem determines the place value to which to round.

In most problems with fractions and decimals, the context of the problem requires rounding to the nearest whole number. Rounding these values makes calculation easier and provides an accurate estimation to the solution of the problem.

Other estimation strategies include the following:

- Using friendly or compatible numbers
- Using numbers that are easy to compute
- Adjusting numbers after rounding

Example

There are 168 hours in a week. Carson does the following:

- Sleeps 7.5 hours each day of the week
- Goes to school 6.75 hours five days a week
- Practices martial arts and basketball 1.5 hours each three times a week
- Reads and studies 1.75 hours every day
- Eats 1.5 hours every day

Estimate the remaining number of hours.

A. 30   B. 35   C. 40   D. 45

The correct answer is **C**. The correct solution is 40. He sleeps about 56 hours, goes to school for 35 hours, practices for 9 hours, reads and studies for about 14 hours, and eats for about 14 hours. This is 128 hours. Therefore, Carson has about 40 hours remaining.

Real-World Integer Problems

The following five steps can make solving word problems easier:

1. Read the problem for understanding.
2. Visualize the problem by drawing a picture or diagram.
3. Make a plan by writing an expression to represent the problem.
4. Solve the problem by applying mathematical techniques.
5. Check the answer to make sure it answers the question asked.

BE CAREFUL!
Make sure that you read the problem fully before visualizing and making a plan.

In basic problems, the solution may be evident, but make sure to demonstrate knowledge of writing the expression. In multi-step problems, first make a plan with the correct expression. Then, apply the correct calculation.

Examples

1. **The temperature on Monday was –9°F, and on Tuesday it was 8°F. What is the difference in temperature, in °F?**

   A. –17°   B. –1°   C. 1°   D. 17°

   The correct answer is **D**. The correct solution is 17° because $8-(-9) = 17°F$.

2. **A golfer's last 12 rounds were –2, +4, –3, –1, +5, +3, –4, –5, –2, –6, –1, and 0. What is the average of these rounds?**

   A. –12   B. –1   C. 1   D. 12

   The correct answer is **B**. The correct solution is –1. The total of the scores is –12. The average is –12 divided by 12, which is –1.

Real-World Fraction and Decimal Problems

The five steps in the previous section are applicable to solving real-world fraction and decimal problems. The expressions with one step require only one calculation: addition, subtraction, multiplication, or division. The problems with

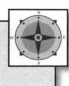

KEEP IN MIND
Estimating the solution first can help determine if a calculation is completed correctly.

multiple steps require writing out the expressions and performing the correct calculations.

Examples

1. **The length of a room is $7\frac{2}{3}$ feet. When the length of the room is doubled, what is the new length in feet?**

   A. $14\frac{2}{3}$ B. $15\frac{1}{3}$ C. $15\frac{2}{3}$ D. $16\frac{1}{3}$

   The correct answer is **B**. The correct solution is $15\frac{1}{3}$. The length is multiplied by 2, $7\frac{2}{3} \times 2 = \frac{23}{3} \times \frac{2}{1} = \frac{46}{3} = 15\frac{1}{3}$ feet.

2. **A fruit salad is a mixture of $1\frac{3}{4}$ pounds of apples, $2\frac{1}{4}$ pounds of grapes, and $1\frac{1}{4}$ pounds of bananas. After the fruit is mixed, $1\frac{1}{2}$ pounds are set aside, and the rest is divided into three containers. What is the weight in pounds of one container?**

   A. $1\frac{1}{5}$ B. $1\frac{1}{4}$ C. $1\frac{1}{3}$ D. $1\frac{1}{2}$

   The correct answer is **B**. The correct solution is $1\frac{1}{4}$. The amount available for the containers is $1\frac{3}{4} + 2\frac{1}{4} + 1\frac{1}{4} - 1\frac{1}{2} = 5\frac{1}{4} - 1\frac{1}{2} = 5\frac{1}{4} - 1\frac{2}{4} = 4\frac{5}{4} - 1\frac{2}{4} = 3\frac{3}{4}$. This amount is divided into three containers, $3\frac{3}{4} \div 3 = \frac{15}{4} \times \frac{15}{12} = 1\frac{3}{12} = 1\frac{1}{4}$ pounds.

3. **In 2016, a town had 17.4 inches of snowfall. In 2017, it had 45.2 inches of snowfall. What is the difference in inches?**

   A. 27.2   B. 27.8   C. 28.2   D. 28.8

   The correct answer is **B**. The correct solution is 27.8 because $45.2 - 17.4 = 27.8$ inches.

4. **Mike bought items that cost $4.78, $3.49, $6.79, $9.78, and $14.05. He had a coupon worth $5.00. If he paid with a $50.00 bill, then how much change does he receive?**

   A. $16.11   B. $18.11   C. $21.11   D. $23.11

   The correct answer is **A**. The correct solution is $16.11. The total bill is $38.89, less the coupon is $33.89. The amount of change is $50.00 - $33.89 = $16.11.

Let's Review!

- Using estimation is beneficial to determine an approximate solution to the problem when the numbers are complex.
- When solving a word problem with integers, fractions, or decimals, first read and visualize the problem. Then, make a plan, solve, and check the answer.

CHAPTER 6 ALGEBRA
PRACTICE QUIZ

1. Which decimal is the greatest?

   A. 1.7805

   B. 1.5807

   C. 1.7085

   D. 1.8057

2. Change $0.\overline{63}$ to a fraction. Simplify completely.

   A. $\frac{5}{9}$

   B. $\frac{7}{11}$

   C. $\frac{2}{3}$

   D. $\frac{5}{6}$

3. Write $0.\overline{1}$ as a percent.

   A. $0.\overline{1}\%$

   B. $1.\overline{1}\%$

   C. $11.\overline{1}\%$

   D. $111.\overline{1}\%$

4. Solve the equation for the unknown, $4x + 3 = 8$.

   A. -2

   B. $-\frac{5}{4}$

   C. $\frac{5}{4}$

   D. 2

5. Solve the inequality for the unknown, $3x + 5 - 2(x + 3) > 4(1-x) + 5$.

   A. $x > 2$

   B. $x > 9$

   C. $x > 10$

   D. $x > 17$

6. Solve the equation for h, $SA = 2\pi rh + 2\pi r^2$.

   A. $2\pi rSA - 2\pi r^2 = h$

   B. $2\pi rSA + 2\pi r^2 = h$

   C. $\frac{SA - 2\pi r^2}{2\pi r} = h$

   D. $\frac{SA + 2\pi r^2}{2\pi r} = h$

7. Solve the system of equations, $y = -2x + 3$ $y + x = 5$.

   A. $(-2, 7)$

   B. $(-2, -7)$

   C. $(2, -7)$

   D. $(2, 7)$

8. Solve the system of equations, $2x - 3y = -1$ $x + 2y = 24$.

   A. $(7, 10)$

   B. $(10, 7)$

   C. $(6, 8)$

   D. $(8, 6)$

9. Divide $1\frac{5}{6} \div 1\frac{1}{3}$.

   A. $1\frac{5}{18}$

   B. $1\frac{3}{8}$

   C. $2\frac{4}{9}$

   D. $3\frac{1}{6}$

10. Multiply $1\frac{1}{4} \times 1\frac{1}{2}$.

   A. $1\frac{1}{8}$

   B. $1\frac{1}{3}$

   C. $1\frac{2}{3}$

   D. $1\frac{7}{8}$

11. Divide $\frac{1}{10} \div \frac{2}{3}$.

   A. $\frac{1}{15}$

   B. $\frac{1}{10}$

   C. $\frac{3}{20}$

   D. $\frac{3}{5}$

12. A store has 75 pounds of bananas. Eight customers buy 3.3 pounds, five customers buy 4.25 pounds, and one customer buys 6.8 pounds. How many pounds are left in stock?

   A. 19.45

   B. 19.55

   C. 20.45

   D. 20.55

13. Solve the system of equations by graphing, $\begin{array}{l} 3x + y = -1 \\ 2x - y = -4 \end{array}$.

A.

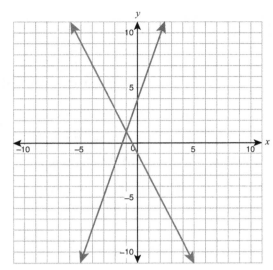

C.

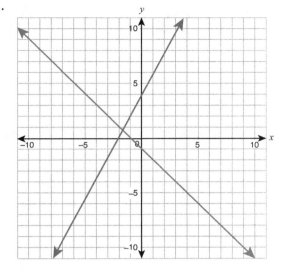

B.

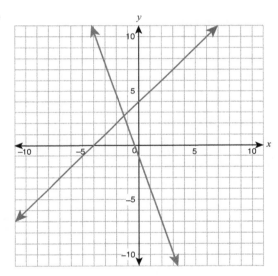

D.

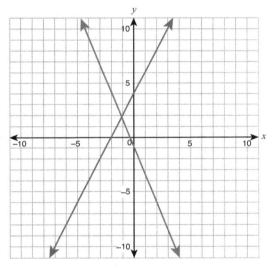

14. A rectangular garden needs a border. The length is $15\frac{3}{5}$ feet, and the width is $3\frac{2}{3}$ feet. What is the perimeter in feet?

A. $18\frac{5}{8}$

C. $37\frac{1}{4}$

B. $19\frac{4}{15}$

D. $38\frac{8}{15}$

15. A historical society has 8 tours daily 5 days a week, with 32 people on each tour. Estimate the number of people who can be on the tour in 50 weeks.

A. 25,000

C. 75,000

B. 50,000

D. 100,000

CHAPTER 6 ALGEBRA
PRACTICE QUIZ – ANSWER KEY

1. D. The correct solution is 1.8057 because 1.8057 contains the largest value in the tenths place. **See Lesson: Decimals and Fractions.**

2. B. The correct solution is $\frac{7}{11}$. Let $n = 0.\overline{63}$ and $100n = 63.\overline{63}$. Then, $100n - n = 63.\overline{63} - 0.\overline{63}$ resulting in $99n = 63$ and solution of $n = \frac{63}{99} = \frac{7}{11}$. **See Lesson: Decimals and Fractions.**

3. C. The correct answer is $11.\overline{1}\%$ because $0.\overline{1}$ as a percent is $0.\overline{1} \times 100 = 11.\overline{1}\%$. **See Lesson: Decimals and Fractions.**

4. C. The correct solution is $\frac{5}{4}$.

$4x = 5$	Subtract 3 from both sides of the equation.
$x = \frac{5}{4}$	Divide both sides of the equation by 4.

See Lesson: Equations with One Variable.

5. A. The correct solution is $x > 2$.

$3x + 5 - 2x - 6 > 4 - 4x + 5$	Apply the distributive property.
$x - 1 > -4x + 9$	Combine like terms on both sides of the inequality.
$5x - 1 > 9$	Add $4x$ to both sides of the inequality.
$5x > 10$	Add 1 to both sides of the inequality.
$x > 2$	Divide both sides of the inequality by 5.

See Lesson: Equations with One Variable.

6. C. The correct solution is $\frac{SA - 2\pi r^2}{2\pi r} = h$.

$SA - 2\pi r^2 = 2\pi rh$	Subtract $2\pi r^2$ from both sides of the equation.
$\frac{SA - 2\pi r^2}{2\pi r} = h$	Divide both sides of the equation by $2\pi r$.

See Lesson: Equations with One Variable.

7. A. The correct solution is (-2, 7).

	The first equation is already solved for y.
$-2x + 3 + x = 5$	Substitute $-2x + 3$ in for y in the second equation.
$-x + 3 = 5$	Combine like terms on the left side of the equation.
$-x = 2$	Subtract 3 from both sides of the equation.
$x = -2$	Divide both sides of the equation by -1.
$y = -2(-2) + 3$	Substitute -2 in the first equation for x.

$y = 4 + 3 = 7$ Simplify using order of operations.

See Lesson: Equations with Two Variables.

8. B. The correct solution is (10, 7).

$-2x - 4y = -48$	Multiply all terms in the second equation by -2.
$-7y = -49$	Add the equations.
$y = 7$	Divide both sides of the equation by -7.
$x + 2(7) = 24$	Substitute 7 in the second equation for y.
$x + 14 = 24$	Simplify using order of operations.
$x = 10$	Subtract 14 from both sides of the equation.

See Lesson: Equations with Two Variables.

9. B. The correct answer is $1\frac{3}{8}$ because $\frac{11}{6} \div \frac{4}{3} = \frac{11}{6} \times \frac{3}{4} = \frac{33}{24} = 1\frac{9}{24} = 1\frac{3}{8}$. **See Lesson: Multiplication and Division of Fractions.**

10. D. The correct solution is $1\frac{7}{8}$ because $\frac{5}{4} \times \frac{3}{2} = \frac{15}{8} = 1\frac{7}{8}$. **See Lesson: Multiplication and Division of Fractions.**

11. C. The correct solution is $\frac{3}{20}$ because $\frac{1}{10} \times \frac{3}{2} = \frac{3}{20}$. **See Lesson: Multiplication and Division of Fractions.**

12. D. The correct solution is 20.55 because the number of pounds purchased is $8(3.3) + 5(4.25) + 6.8 = 26.4 + 21.25 + 6.8 = 54.45$ pounds. The number of pounds remaining is $75 - 54.45 = 20.55$ pounds. **See Lesson: Solving Real-World Mathematical Problems.**

13. D. The correct graph has the two lines intersect at (-1, 2). **See Lesson: Equations with Two Variables.**

14. D. The correct solution is $38\frac{8}{15}$ because $15\frac{3}{5} + 3\frac{2}{3} = 15\frac{9}{15} + 3\frac{10}{15} = 18\frac{19}{15}(2) = \frac{289}{15} \times \frac{2}{1} = \frac{578}{15} = 38\frac{8}{15}$ feet. **See Lesson: Solving Real-World Mathematical Problems.**

15. C. The correct solution is 75,000 because by estimation $10(5)(30)(50) = 75,000$ people can be on the tour in 50 weeks. **See Lesson: Solving Real-World Mathematical Problems.**

CHAPTER 7 FUNCTIONS

SOLVING QUADRATIC EQUATIONS

This lesson introduces solving quadratic equations by the square root method, completing the square, factoring, and using the quadratic formula.

Solving Quadratic Equations by the Square Root Method

A **quadratic equation** is an equation where the highest variable is squared. The equation is in the form $ax^2 + bx + c = 0$, where a is a non-zero constant and b and c are constants. There are at most two solutions to the equation because the highest variable is squared. There are many methods to solve a quadratic equation.

This section will explore solving a quadratic equation by the square root method. The equation must be in the form of $ax^2 = c$, or there is no x term.

> **STEP BY STEP**
>
> **Step 1.** Use multiplication and division properties of an equation to remove the value in front of the variable.
>
> **Step 2.** Apply the square root to both sides of the equation.

Note: The positive and negative square root make the solution true. For the equation $x^2 = 9$, the solutions are –3 and 3 because $3^2 = 9$ and $(-3)^2 = 9$.

Example

Solve the equation by the square root method, $4x^2 = 64$.

A. 4   B. 8   C. ±4   D. ±8

The correct answer is **C**. The correct solution is ±4.

$x^2 = 16$	Divide both sides of the equation by 4.
$x = \pm 4$	Apply the square root to both sides of the equation.

Solving Quadratic Equations by Completing the Square

A quadratic equation in the form $x^2 + bx$ can be solved by a process known as completing the square. The best time to solve by completing the square is when the b term is even.

STEP BY STEP

Step 1. Divide all terms by the coefficient of x^2.

Step 2. Move the number term to the right side of the equation.

Step 3. Complete the square $\left(\frac{b}{2}\right)^2$ and add this value to both sides of the equation.

Step 4. Factor the left side of the equation.

Step 5. Apply the square root to both sides of the equation.

Step 6. Use addition and subtraction properties to move all number terms to the right side of the equation.

Examples

1. **Solve the equation by completing the square, $x^2 - 8x + 12 = 0$.**

   A. -2 and -6 B. 2 and -6 C. -2 and 6 D. 2 and 6

   The correct answer is **D**. The correct solutions are 2 and 6.

$x^2 - 8x = -12$	Subtract 12 from both sides of the equation.
$x^2 - 8x + 16 = -12 + 16$	Complete the square, $\left(-\frac{8}{2}\right)^2 = (-4)^2 = 16.$
	Add 16 to both sides of the equation.
$x^2 - 8x + 16 = 4$	Simplify the right side of the equation.
$(x-4)^2 = 4$	Factor the left side of the equation.
$x - 4 = \pm 2$	Apply the square root to both sides of the equation.
$x = 4 \pm 2$	Add 4 to both sides of the equation.
$x = 4 - 2 = 2,\ x = 4 + 2 = 6$	Simplify the right side of the equation.

2. **Solve the equation by completing the square, $x^2 + 6x - 8 = 0$.**

   A. $-3 \pm \sqrt{17}$ B. $3 \pm \sqrt{17}$ C. $-3 \pm \sqrt{8}$ D. $3 \pm \sqrt{8}$

   The correct answer is **A**. The correct solutions are $-3 \pm \sqrt{17}$.

$x^2 + 6x = 8$	Add 8 to both sides of the equation.
$x^2 + 6x + 9 = 8 + 9$	Complete the square, $\left(\frac{6}{2}\right)^2 = 3^2 = 9.$ Add 9 to both sides of the equation.
$x^2 + 6x + 9 = 17$	Simplify the right side of the equation.
$(x + 3)^2 = 17$	Factor the left side of the equation.
$x + 3 = \pm\sqrt{17}$	Apply the square root to both sides of the equation.
$x = -3 \pm \sqrt{17}$	Subtract 3 from both sides of the equation.

Solving Quadratic Equations by Factoring

Factoring can only be used when a quadratic equation is factorable; other methods are needed to solve quadratic equations that are not factorable.

> **STEP BY STEP**
> **Step 1.** Simplify if needed by clearing any fractions and parentheses.
> **Step 2.** Write the equation in standard form, $ax^2 + bx + c = 0$.
> **Step 3.** Factor the quadratic equation.
> **Step 4.** Set each factor equal to zero.
> **Step 5.** Solve the linear equations using inverse operations.

The quadratic equation will have two solutions if the factors are different or one solution if the factors are the same.

Examples

1. **Solve the equation by factoring, $x^2 - 13x + 42 = 0$.**

   A. $-6, -7$ B. $-6, 7$ C. $6, -7$ D. $6, 7$

   The correct answer is **D**. The correct solutions are 6 and 7.

$(x-6)(x-7) = 0$	Factor the equation.
$(x-6) = 0$ or $(x-7) = 0$	Set each factor equal to 0.
$x-6 = 0$	Add 6 to both sides of the equation to solve for the first factor.
$x = 6$	
$x-7 = 0$	Add 7 to both sides of the equation to solve for the second factor.
$x = 7$	

2. **Solve the equation by factoring, $9x^2 + 30x + 25 = 0$.**

   A. $-\frac{5}{3}$ B. $-\frac{3}{5}$ C. $\frac{3}{5}$ D. $\frac{5}{3}$

   The correct answer is **A**. The correct solution is $-\frac{5}{3}$.

$(3x + 5)(3x + 5) = 0$	Factor the equation.
$(3x + 5) = 0$ or $(3x + 5) = 0$	Set each factor equal to 0.
$(3x + 5) = 0$	Set one factor equal to zero since both factors are the same.
$3x + 5 = 0$	Subtract 5 from both sides of the equation and divide both sides of the equation by 3 to solve.
$3x = -5$	
$x = -\frac{5}{3}$	

Solving Quadratic Equations by the Quadratic Formula

Many quadratic equations are not factorable. Another method of solving a quadratic equation is by using the quadratic formula. This method can be used to solve any quadratic equation in the form . Using the coefficients a, b, and c, the quadratic formula is $x = \frac{-b \pm \sqrt{b^2 - 4ac}}{2a}$. The values are substituted into the formula, and applying the order of operations finds the solution(s) to the equation.

The solution of the quadratic formula in these examples will be exact or estimated to three decimal places. There may be cases where the exact solutions to the quadratic formula are used.

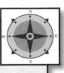

> **KEEP IN MIND**
> Watch the negative sign in the formula. Remember that a number squared is always positive.

Examples

1. Solve the equation by the quadratic formula, $x^2 - 5x - 6 = 0$.

    A. –6 and –1   B. 6 and –1   C. –6 and 1   D. 6 and 1

    The correct answer is **B**. The correct solutions are 6 and –1.

    $x = \frac{-(-5) \pm \sqrt{(-5)^2 - 4(1)(-6)}}{2(1)}$ Substitute 1 for a, –5 for b, and –6 for c.

    $x = \frac{5 \pm \sqrt{25 - (-24)}}{2}$ Apply the exponent and perform the multiplication.

    $x = \frac{5 \pm \sqrt{49}}{2}$ Perform the subtraction.

    $x = \frac{5 \pm 7}{2}$ Apply the square root.

    $x = \frac{5+7}{2}$, $x = \frac{5-7}{2}$ Separate the problem into two expressions.

    $x = \frac{12}{2} = 6$, $x = \frac{-2}{2} = -1$ Simplify the numerator and divide.

2. Solve the equation by the quadratic formula, $2x^2 + 4x - 5 = 0$.

    A. – 0.87 and –2.87   B. 0.87 and –2.87   C. – 0.87 and 2.87   D. 0.87 and 2.87

    The correct answer is **B**. The correct solutions are 0.87 and -2.87.

    $x = \frac{-4 \pm \sqrt{4^2 - 4(2)(-5)}}{2(2)}$ Substitute 2 for a, 4 for b, and –5 for c.

    $x = \frac{-4 \pm \sqrt{16 - (-40)}}{4}$ Apply the exponent and perform the multiplication.

    $x = \frac{-4 \pm \sqrt{56}}{4}$ Perform the subtraction.

    $x = \frac{-4 \pm 7.48}{4}$ Apply the square root.

    $x = \frac{-4+7.48}{4}$, $x = \frac{-4-7.48}{4}$ Separate the problem into two expressions.

    $x = \frac{3.48}{4} = 0.87$, $x = \frac{-11.48}{4} = -2.87$ Simplify the numerator and divide.

Let's Review!

There are four methods to solve a quadratic equation algebraically:

- The square root method is used when there is a squared variable term and a constant term.
- Completing the square is used when there is a squared variable term and an even variable term.
- Factoring is used when the equation can be factored.
- The quadratic formula can be used for any quadratic equation.

POLYNOMIALS

This lesson introduces adding, subtracting, and multiplying polynomials. It also explains polynomial identities that describe numerical expressions.

Adding and Subtracting Polynomials

A **polynomial** is an expression that contains exponents, variables, constants, and operations. The exponents of the variables are only whole numbers, and there is no division by a variable. The operations are addition, subtraction, multiplication, and division. Constants are terms without a variable. A polynomial of one term is a **monomial**; a polynomial of two terms is a **binomial**; and a polynomial of three terms is a **trinomial**.

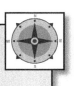

KEEP IN MIND

The solution is an expression, and a value is not calculated for the variable.

To add polynomials, combine like terms and write the solution from the term with the highest exponent to the term with the lowest exponent. To simplify, first rearrange and group like terms. Next, combine like terms.

$$(3x^2 + 5x{-}6) + (4x^3{-}3x + 4) = 4x^3 + 3x^2 + (5x{-}3x) + (-6 + 4) = 4x^3 + 3x^2 + 2x{-}2$$

To subtract polynomials, rewrite the second polynomial using an additive inverse. Change the minus sign to a plus sign, and change the sign of every term inside the parentheses. Then, add the polynomials.

$$(3x^2 + 5x{-}6){-}(4x^3{-}3x + 4) = (3x^2 + 5x{-}6) + (-4x^3 + 3x{-}4) = -4x^3 + 3x^2 + (5x + 3x) + (-6{-}4)$$
$$= -4x^3 + 3x^2 + 8x{-}10$$

Examples

1. **Perform the operation, $(2y^2{-}5y + 1) + (-3y^2 + 6y + 2)$.**

    A. $y^2 + y + 3$ B. $-y^2{-}y + 3$ C. $y^2{-}y + 3$ D. $-y^2 + y + 3$

    The correct answer is **D.** The correct solution is $-y^2 + y + 3$.

    $$(2y^2{-}5y + 1) + (-3y^2 + 6y + 2) = (2y^2{-}3y^2) + (-5y + 6y) + (1 + 2) = -y^2 + y + 3$$

2. **Perform the operation, $(3x^2y + 4xy{-}5xy^2){-}(x^2y{-}3xy{-}2xy^2)$.**

    A. $2x^2y{-}7xy + 3xy^2$

    B. $2x^2y + 7xy + 3xy^2$

    C. $2x^2y + 7xy{-}3xy^2$

    D. $2x^2y{-}7xy{-}3xy^2$

    The correct answer is **C.** The correct solution is $2x^2y + 7xy{-}3xy^2$.

    $$(3x^2y + 4xy{-}5xy^2){-}(x^2y{-}3xy{-}2xy^2) = (3x^2y + 4xy{-}5xy^2) + (-x^2y + 3xy + 2xy^2)$$
    $$= (3x^2y{-}x^2y) + (4xy + 3xy) + (-5xy^2 + 2xy^2) = 2x^2y + 7xy{-}3xy^2$$

Multiplying Polynomials

Multiplying polynomials comes in many forms. When multiplying a monomial by a monomial, multiply the coefficients and apply the multiplication rule for the power of an exponent.

BE CAREFUL!

Make sure that you apply the distributive property to all terms in the polynomials.

$$4xy(3x^2y) = 12x^3y^2.$$

When multiplying a monomial by a polynomial, multiply each term of the polynomial by the monomial.

$$4xy(3x^2y{-}2xy^2) = 4xy(3x^2y) + 4xy(-2xy^2) = 12x^3y^2{-}8x^2y^3.$$

When multiplying a binomial by a binomial, apply the distributive property and combine like terms.

$$(3x{-}4)(2x + 5) = 3x(2x + 5){-}4(2x + 5) = 6x^2 + 15x{-}8x{-}20 = 6x^2 + 7x{-}20$$

When multiplying a binomial by a trinomial, apply the distributive property and combine like terms.

$$(x + 2)(3x^2{-}2x + 3) = (x + 2)(3x^2) + (x + 2)(-2x) + (x + 2)(3) = 3x^3 + 6x^2{-}2x^2{-}4x + 3x + 6 = 3x^3 +$$

$$4x^2{-}x + 6$$

Examples

1. **Multiply, $3xy^2(2x^2y)$.**

   A. $6x^2y^2$ B. $6x^3y^2$ C. $6x^3y^3$ D. $6x^2y^3$

   The correct answer is **C**. The correct solution is $6x^3y^3$. $3xy^2(2x^2y) = 6x^3y^3$.

2. **Multiply, $-2xy(3xy{-}4x^2y^2)$.**

   A. $-6x^2y^2 + 8x^3y^3$ B. $-6x^2y^2{-}8x^3y^3$ C. $-6xy + 8x^3y^3$ D. $-6xy{-}8x^3y^3$

   The correct answer is **A**. The correct solution is $-6x^2y^2 + 8x^3y^3$.

   $$-2xy(3xy{-}4x^2y^2) = -2xy(3xy){-}2xy(-4x^2y^2) = -6x^2y^2 + 8x^3y^3$$

Polynomial Identities

BE CAREFUL!

Pay attention to the details of each polynomial identity and apply them appropriately.

There are many polynomial identities that show relationships between expressions.

- Difference of two squares: $a^2{-}b^2 = (a{-}b)(a + b)$
- Square of a binomial: $(a + b)^2 = a^2 + 2ab + b^2$
- Square of a binomial: $(a{-}b)^2 = a^2 {-}2ab + b^2$
- Sum of cubes: $a^3 + b^3 = (a + b)(a^2{-}ab + b^2)$
- Difference of two cubes: $a^3{-}b^3 = (a{-}b)(a^2 + ab + b^2)$

Examples

1. **Apply the polynomial identity to rewrite $x^2 + 6x + 9$.**

   A. $x^2 + 9$ B. $(x^2 + 3)^2$ C. $(x + 3)^2$ D. $(3x)^2$

   The correct answer is **C**. The correct solution is $(x + 3)^2$. The expression $x^2 + 6x + 9$ is rewritten as $(x + 3)^2$ because the value of a is x and the value of b is 3.

2. **Apply the polynomial identity to rewrite $8x^3 - 1$.**

   A. $(2x + 1)(4x^2 + 2x - 1)$ C. $(2x + 1)(4x^2 - 2x + 1)$

   B. $(2x - 1)(4x^2 - 2x - 1)$ D. $(2x - 1)(4x^2 + 2x + 1)$

   The correct answer is **D**. The correct solution is $(2x - 1)(4x^2 + 2x + 1)$. The expression $8x^3 - 1$ is rewritten as $(2x - 1)(4x^2 + 2x + 1)$ because the value of a is $2x$ and the value of b is 1.

Let's Review!

- Adding, subtracting, and multiplying are commonly applied to polynomials. The key step in applying these operations is combining like terms.
- Polynomial identities require rewriting polynomials into different forms.

Ratios, Proportions, and Percentages

This lesson reviews percentages and ratios and their application to real-world problems. It also examines proportions and rates of change.

Percentages

A **percent** or **percentage** represents a fraction of some quantity. It is an integer or decimal number followed by the symbol %. The word *percent* means "per hundred." For example, 50% means 50 per 100. This is equivalent to half, or 1 out of 2.

Converting between numbers and percents is easy. Given a number, multiply by 100 and add the % symbol to get the equivalent percent. For instance, 0.67 is equal to $0.67 \times 100 = 67\%$, meaning 67 out of 100. Given a percent, eliminate the % symbol and divide by 100. For instance, 23.5% is equal to $23.5 \div 100 = 0.235$.

Although percentages between 0% and 100% are the most obvious, a percent can be any real number, including a negative number. For example, $1.35 = 135\%$ and $-0.872 = -87.2\%$. An example is a gasoline tank that is one-quarter full: one-quarter is $\frac{1}{4}$ or 0.25, so the tank is 25% full. Another example is a medical diagnostic test that has a certain maximum normal result. If a patient's test exceeds that value, its representation can be a percent greater than 100%. For instance, a reading that is 1.22 times the maximum normal value is 122% of the maximum normal value. Likewise, when measuring increases in a company's profits as a percent from one year to the next, a negative percent can represent a decline. That is, if the company's profits fell by one-tenth, the change was −10%.

Example

If 15 out of every 250 contest entries are winners, what percentage of entries are winners?

A. 0.06%	B. 6%	C. 15%	D. 17%

The correct answer is **B**. First, convert the fraction $\frac{15}{250}$ to a decimal: 0.06. To get the percent, multiply by 100% (that is, multiply by 100 and add the % symbol). Of all entries, 6% are winners.

Ratios

A **ratio** expresses the relationship between two numbers and is expressed using a colon or fraction notation. For instance, if 135 runners finish a marathon but 22 drop out, the ratio of finishers to non-finishers is 135:22 or $\frac{135}{22}$. These expressions are equal.

> **BE CAREFUL!**
> Avoid confusing standard ratios with odds (such as "3:1 odds"). Both may use a colon, but their meanings differ. In general, a ratio is the same as a fraction containing the same numbers.

Ratios also follow the rules of fractions. Performing arithmetic operations on ratios follows the same procedures as on fractions. Ratios should also generally appear in lowest terms. Therefore, the constituent numbers in a ratio represent the relative quantities of each side, not absolute quantities. For example, because the ratio 1:2 is equal to 2:4, 5:10, and 600:1,200, ratios are insufficient to determine the absolute number of entities in a problem.

Example

If the ratio of women to men in a certain industry is 5:4, how many people are in that industry?

A. 9   B. 20   C. 900   D. Not enough information

The correct answer is **D.** The ratio 5:4 is the industry's relative number of women to men. But the industry could have 10 women and 8 men, 100 women and 80 men, or any other breakdown whose ratio is 5:4. Therefore, the question provides too little information to answer. Had it provided the total number of people in the industry, it would have been possible to determine how many women and how many men are in the industry.

> **KEY POINT**
> Mathematically, ratios act just like fractions. For example, the ratio 8:13 is mathematically the same as the fraction $\frac{8}{13}$.

Proportions

A **proportion** is an equation of two ratios. An illustrative case is two equivalent fractions:

$$\frac{21}{28} = \frac{3}{4}$$

This example of a proportion should be familiar: going left to right, it is the conversion of one fraction to an equivalent fraction in lowest terms by dividing the numerator and denominator by the same number (7, in this case).

Equating fractions in this way is correct, but it provides little information. Proportions are more informative when one of the numbers is unknown. Using a question mark (?) to represent an unknown number, setting up a proportion can aid in solving problems involving different scales. For instance, if the ratio of maple saplings to oak saplings in an acre of young forest is 7:5 and that acre contains 65 oaks, the number of maples in that acre can be determined using a proportion: $\frac{7}{5} = \frac{?}{65}$

Note that to equate two ratios in this manner, the numerators must contain numbers that represent the same entity or type, and so must the denominators. In this example, the numerators represent maples and the denominators represent oaks.

$$\frac{7 \text{ maples}}{5 \text{ oaks}} = \frac{? \text{ maples}}{65 \text{ oaks}}$$

Recall from the properties of fractions that if you multiply the numerator and denominator by the same number, the result is an equivalent fraction. Therefore, to find the unknown in this proportion, first divide the denominator on the right by the denominator on the left. Then, multiply the quotient by the numerator on the left.

$65 \div 5 = 13$

$$\frac{7 \times 13}{5 \times 13} = \frac{?}{65}$$

The unknown (?) is $7 \times 13 = 91$. In the example, the acre of forest has 91 maple saplings.

> **DID YOU KNOW?**
> When taking the reciprocal of both sides of a proportion, the proportion still holds. When setting up a proportion, ensure that the numerators represent the same type and the denominators represent the same type.

Example

If a recipe calls for 3 parts flour to 2 parts sugar, how much sugar does a baker need if she uses 12 cups of flour?

A. 2 cups   B. 3 cups   C. 6 cups   D. 8 cups

The correct answer is **D**. The baker needs 8 cups of sugar. First, note that "3 parts flour to 2 parts sugar" is the ratio 3:2. Set up the proportion using the given amount of flour (12 cups), putting the flour numbers in either the denominators or the numerators (either will yield the same answer): $\frac{3}{2} = \frac{12}{?}$

Since $12 \div 3 = 4$, multiply 2×4 to get 8 cups of sugar.

Rates of Change

Numbers that describe current quantities can be informative, but how they change over time can provide even greater insight into a problem. The rate of change for some quantity is the ratio of the quantity's difference over a specific time period to the length of that period. For example, if an automobile increases its speed from 50 mph to 100 mph in 10 seconds, the rate of change of its speed (its acceleration) is

$$\frac{100 \text{ mph} - 50 \text{ mph}}{10 \text{ s}} = \frac{50 \text{ mph}}{10 \text{ s}} = 5 \text{ mph per second} = 5 \text{ mph/s}$$

The basic formula for the rate of change of some quantity is $\frac{x_f - x_i}{t_f - t_i}$, where t_f is the "final" (or ending) time and t_i is the "initial" (or starting) time. Also, x_f is the (final) quantity at (final) time t_f, and x_i is the (initial) quantity at (initial) time t_i. In the example above, the final time is 10 seconds and the initial time is 0 seconds—hence the omission of the initial time from the calculation.

According to the rules of fractions, multiplying the numerator and denominator by the same number yields an equivalent fraction, so you can reverse the order of the terms in the formula:

$$\frac{x_f - x_i}{t_f - t_i} = \frac{-1}{-1} \times \frac{x_f - x_i}{t_f - t_i} = \frac{x_i - x_f}{t_i - t_f}$$

The key to getting the correct rate of change is to ensure that the first number in the numerator and the first number in the denominator correspond to each other (that is, the quantity from the numerator corresponds to the time from the denominator). This must also be true for the second number.

TEST TIP

To convert a quantity's rate of change to a percent, divide it by the quantity at the *initial* time and multiply by 100%. To convert to a ratio, just skip the multiplication step.

Example

If the population of an endangered frog species fell from 2,250 individuals to 2,115 individuals in a year, what is that population's annual rate of increase?

 A. −135%   B. −6%   C. 6%   D. 135%

The correct answer is **B**. The population's rate of increase was −6%. The solution in this case involves two steps. First, calculate the population's annual rate of change using the formula. It will yield the change in the number of individuals.

$$\frac{2{,}115 - 2{,}250}{1 \text{ year} - 0 \text{ year}} = -135 \text{ per year}$$

Second, divide the result by the initial population. Finally, convert to a percent.

$$\frac{-135 \text{ per year}}{2{,}250} = -0.06 \text{ per year}$$

$$(-0.06 \text{ per year}) \times 100\% = -6\% \text{ per year}$$

Since the question asks for the *annual* rate of increase, the "per year" can be dropped. Also, note that the answer must be negative to represent the decreasing population.

Let's Review!

- A percent—meaning "per hundred"—represents a relative quantity as a fraction or decimal. It is the absolute number multiplied by 100 and followed by the % symbol.
- A ratio is a relationship between two numbers expressed using fraction or colon notation (for example, $\frac{3}{2}$ or 3:2). Ratios behave mathematically just like fractions.
- An equation of two ratios is called a proportion. Proportions are used to solve problems involving scale.
- Rates of change are the speeds at which quantities increase or decrease. The formula $\frac{x_f - x_i}{t_f - t_i}$ provides the rate of change of quantity x over the period between some initial (i) time and final (f) time.

POWERS, EXPONENTS, ROOTS, AND RADICALS

This lesson introduces how to apply the properties of exponents and examines square roots and cube roots. It also discusses how to estimate quantities using integer powers of 10.

Properties of Exponents

An expression that is a repeated multiplication of the same factor is a **power**. The **exponent** is the number of times the **base** is multiplied. For example, 6^2 is the same as 6 times 6, or 36. There are many rules associated with exponents.

Property	Definition	Examples
Product Rule (Same Base)	$a^m \times a^n = a^{m+n}$	$4^1 \times 4^4 = 4^{1+4} = 4^5 = 1024$
		$x^1 \times x^4 = x^{1+4} = x^5$
Product Rule (Different Base)	$a^m \times b^m = (a \times b)^m$	$2^2 \times 3^2 = (2 \times 3)^2 = 6^2 = 36$
		$3^3 \times x^3 = (3 \times x)^3 = (3x)^3 = 27x^3$
Quotient Rule (Same Base)	$\frac{a^m}{a^n} = a^{m-n}$	$\frac{4^4}{4^2} = 4^{4-2} = 4^2 = 16$
		$\frac{x^6}{x^3} = x^{6-3} = x^3$
Quotient Rule (Different Base)	$\frac{a^m}{b^m} = \left(\frac{a}{b}\right)^m$	$\frac{4^4}{3^4} = \left(\frac{4}{3}\right)^4$
		$\frac{x^6}{y^6} = \left(\frac{x}{y}\right)^6$
Power of a Power Rule	$(a^m)^n = a^{mn}$	$(2^2)^3 = 2^{2\times3} = 2^6 = 64$
		$(x^5)^8 = x^{5\times8} = x^{40}$
Zero Exponent Rule	$a^0 = 1$	$64^0 = 1$
		$y^0 = 1$
Negative Exponent Rule	$a^{-m} = \frac{1}{a^m}$	$3^{-3} = \frac{1}{3^3} = \frac{1}{27}$
		$\frac{1}{x^{-3}} = x^3$

For many exponent expressions, it is necessary to use multiplication rules to simplify the expression completely.

Examples

1. **Simplify $(3^2)^3$.**

   A. 18

   B. 216

   C. 243

   D. 729

   The correct answer is **D**. The correct solution is 729 because $(3^2)^3 = 3^{2\times3} = 3^6 = 729$.

> **KEEP IN MIND**
>
> The expressions
> $(-2)^2 = (-2) \times (-2) = 4$ and
> $-2^2 = -(2 \times 2) = -4$ have different results because of the location of the negative signs and parentheses. For each problem, focus on each detail to simplify completely and correctly.

2. **Simplify $(2x^2)^4$.**

   A. $2x^8$ B. $4x^4$ C. $8x^6$ D. $16x^8$

   The correct answer is **D.** The correct solution is $16x^8$ because $(2x^2)^4 = 2^4(x^2)^4 = 2^4 x^{2\times4} = 16x^8$.

3. **Simplify $\left(\frac{x^{-2}}{y^2}\right)^3$.**

   A. $\frac{1}{x^6y^6}$ B. $\frac{x^6}{y^6}$ C. $\frac{y^6}{x^6}$ D. x^6y^6

   The correct answer is **A.** The correct solution is $\frac{1}{x^6y^6}$ because $\left(\frac{x^{-2}}{y^2}\right)^3 = \left(\frac{1}{x^2y^2}\right)^3 = \frac{1}{x^{2\times3}y^{2\times3}} = \frac{1}{x^6y^6}$.

Square Root and Cube Roots

The **square** of a number is the number raised to the power of 2. The **square root** of a number, when the number is squared, gives that number. $10^2 = 100$, so the square of 100 is 10, or $\sqrt{100} = 10$. **Perfect squares** are numbers with whole number square roots, such as 1, 4, 9, 16, and 25.

Squaring a number and taking a square root are opposite operations, meaning that the operations undo each other. This means that $\sqrt{x^2} = x$ and $(\sqrt{x})^2 = x$. When solving the equation $x^2 = p$, the solutions are $x = \pm\sqrt{p}$ because a negative value squared is a positive solution.

The **cube** of a number is the number raised to the power of 3. The **cube root** of a number, when the number is cubed, gives that number. $10^3 = 1000$, so the cube of 1,000 is 10, or $\sqrt[3]{1000} = 10$. **Perfect cubes** are numbers with whole number cube roots, such as 1, 8, 27, 64, and 125.

KEEP IN MIND

Most square roots and cube roots are not perfect roots.

Cubing a number and taking a cube root are opposite operations, meaning that the operations undo each other. This means that $\sqrt[3]{x^3} = x$ and $\left(\sqrt[3]{x}\right)^3 = x$. When solving the equation $x^3 = p$, the solution is $x = \sqrt[3]{p}$.

If a number is not a perfect square root or cube root, the solution is an approximation. When this occurs, the solution is an irrational number. For example, $\sqrt{2}$ is the irrational solution to $x^2 = 2$.

Examples

1. **Solve $x^2 = 121$.**

   A. –10, 10   B. –11, 11   C. –12, 12   D. –13, 13

   The correct answer is **B.** The correct solution is –11, 11 because the square root of 121 is 11. The values of –11 and 11 make the equation true.

2. **Solve $x^3 = 125$.**

   A. 1   B. 5   C. 10   D. 25

   The correct answer is **B.** The correct solution is 5 because the cube root of 125 is 5.

Express Large or Small Quantities as Multiples of 10

Scientific notation is a large or small number written in two parts. The first part is a number between 1 and 10. In these problems, the first digit will be a single digit. The number is followed by a multiple to a power of 10. A positive integer exponent means the number is greater than 1, while a negative integer exponent means the number is smaller than 1.

KEEP IN MIND

A positive exponent in scientific notation represents a large number, while a negative exponent represents a small number.

The number 3×10^4 is the same as $3 \times 10,000 = 30,000$.

The number 3×10^{-4} is the same as $3 \times 0.0001 = 0.0003$.

For example, the population of the United States is about 3×10^8, and the population of the world is about 7×10^9. The population of the United States is 300,000,000, and the population of the world is 7,000,000,000. The world population is about 20 times larger than the population of the United States.

Examples

1. **The population of China is about 1×10^9, and the population of the United States is about 3×10^8. How many times larger is the population of China than the population of the United States?**

   A. 2   B. 3   C. 4   D. 5

   The correct answer is **B**. The correct solution is 3 because the population of China is about 1,000,000,000 and the population of the United States is about 300,000,000. So the population is about 3 times larger.

2. **A red blood cell has a length of 8×10^{-6} meter, and a skin cell has a length of 3×10^{-5} meter. How many times larger is the skin cell?**

   A. 1   B. 2   C. 3   D. 4

   The correct answer is **D**. The correct solution is 4 because 3×10^{-5} is 0.00003 and 8×10^{-6} is 0.000008. So, the skin cell is about 4 times larger.

Let's Review!

- The properties and rules of exponents are applicable to generate equivalent expressions.
- Only a few whole numbers out of the set of whole numbers are perfect squares. Perfect cubes can be positive or negative.
- Numbers expressed in scientific notation are useful to compare large or small numbers.

CHAPTER 7 FUNCTIONS PRACTICE QUIZ

1. Multiply, $(x-1)(x^2 + 2x + 3)$.

   A. $x^3 + x^2 + x - 3$

   B. $x^3 - x^2 - x - 3$

   C. $x^3 + x^2 - x - 3$

   D. $x^3 - x^2 + x - 3$

2. Apply the polynomial identity to rewrite $9x^2 - 30x + 25$.

   A. $(3x + 5)(3x - 5)$

   B. $(3x - 5)^2$

   C. $(3x - 5)(3x - 1)$

   D. $(3x - 5)(3x + 1)$

3. Perform the operation, $(3y^2 + 4y) - (5y^3 - 2y^2 + 3)$.

   A. $-5y^3 + y^2 + 4y - 3$

   B. $-5y^3 + 5y^2 + 4y + 3$

   C. $-5y^3 + y^2 + 4y + 3$

   D. $-5y^3 + 5y^2 + 4y - 3$

4. Solve $x^3 = 343$.

   A. 6

   B. 7

   C. 8

   D. 9

5. One online seller has about 6×10^8 online orders, and another online seller has about 5×10^7 online orders. How many times more orders does the first company have?

   A. 12

   B. 15

   C. 20

   D. 32

6. Simplify $\frac{x^2 y^{-2}}{x^{-3} y^3}$.

   A. $\frac{x^5}{y^5}$

   B. $\frac{y^5}{x^5}$

   C. $\frac{1}{x^5 y^5}$

   D. $x^5 y^5$

7. What is 15% of 64?

   A. 5:48

   B. 15:64

   C. 48:5

   D. 64:15

8. Which number satisfies the proportion $\frac{378}{?} = \frac{18}{7}$?

   A. 18

   B. 147

   C. 972

   D. 2,646

9. If a tree grows an average of 4.2 inches in a day, what is the rate of change in its height per month? Assume a month is 30 days.

   A. 0.14 inches per month

   B. 4.2 inches per month

   C. 34.2 inches per month

   D. 126 inches per month

10. Solve the equation by the quadratic formula, $11x^2 - 14x + 4 = 0$.

    A. -0.84 and -0.43

    B. 0.84 and -0.43

    C. -0.84 and 0.43

    D. 0.84 and 0.43

11. Solve the equation by any method, $3x^2 - 5 = 22$.

    A. 0

    B. ± 1

    C. ± 2

    D. ± 3

12. Solve the equation by the square root method, $5x^2 + 10 = 10$.

    A. 0

    B. 1

    C. 2

    D. 3

CHAPTER 7 FUNCTIONS
PRACTICE QUIZ — ANSWER KEY

1. A. The correct solution is $x^3 + x^2 + x - 3$.

$(x-1)(x^2 + 2x + 3) = (x-1)(x^2) + (x-1)(2x) + (x-1)(3) = x^3 - x^2 + 2x^2 - 2x + 3x - 3 = x^3 + x^2 + x - 3$

See Lesson: Polynomials.

2. B. The correct solution is $(3x-5)^2$. The expression $9x^2 - 30x + 25$ is rewritten as $(3x-5)^2$ because the value of a is $3x$ and the value of b is 5. **See Lesson: Polynomials.**

3. D. The correct solution is $-5y^3 + 5y^2 + 4y - 3$.

$(3y^2 + 4y) - (5y^3 - 2y^2 + 3) = (3y^2 + 4y) + (-5y^3 + 2y^2 - 3) = -5y^3 + (3y^2 + 2y^2) + 4y - 3 = -5y^3 + 5y^2 + 4y - 3$

See Lesson: Polynomials.

4. B. The correct solution is 7 because the cube root of 343 is 7. **See Lesson: Powers, Exponents, Roots, and Radicals.**

5. A. The correct solution is 12 because the first company has about 600,000,000 orders and the second company has about 50,000,000 orders. So, the first company is about 12 times larger. **See Lesson: Powers, Exponents, Roots, and Radicals.**

6. A. The correct solution is $\frac{x^5}{y^5}$ because $\frac{x^2 y^2}{x^{-3} y^3} = x^{2-(-3)} y^{-2-3} = x^5 y^{-5} = \frac{x^5}{y^5}$. **See Lesson: Powers, Exponents, Roots, and Radicals.**

7. C. Either set up a proportion or just note that this question is asking for a fraction of a specific number: 15% (or $\frac{3}{20}$) of 64. Multiply $\frac{3}{20}$ by 64 to get $\frac{48}{5}$, or 48:5. **See Lesson: Ratios, Proportions, and Percentages.**

8. B. The number 147 satisfies the proportion. First, divide 378 by 18 to get 21. Then, multiply 21 by 7 to get 147. Check your answer by dividing 147 by 7: the quotient is also 21, so 147 satisfies the proportion. **See Lesson: Ratios, Proportions, and Percentages.**

9. D. The rate of change is 126 inches per month. One approach is to set up a proportion.

$$\frac{1 \text{ day}}{4.2 \text{ inches}} = \frac{30 \text{ days}}{?}$$

Since 1 month is equivalent to 30 days, multiply the rate of change per day by 30 to get the rate of change per month. 4.2 inches multiplied by 30 is 126 inches. Thus, the growth rate is 126 inches per month. **See Lesson: Ratios, Proportions, and Percentages.**

10. D. The correct solutions are 0.84 and 0.43.

$$x = \frac{-(-14) \pm \sqrt{(-14)^2 - 4(11)(4)}}{2(11)}$$ Substitute 11 for a, –14 for b, and 4 for c.

$$x = \frac{14 \pm \sqrt{196 - 176}}{22}$$ Apply the exponent and perform the multiplication.

$$x = \frac{14 \pm \sqrt{20}}{22}$$ Perform the subtraction.

$$x = \frac{14 \pm 4.47}{22}$$ Apply the square root.

$$x = \frac{14 + 4.47}{22}, \; x = \frac{14 - 4.47}{22}$$ Separate the problem into two expressions.

$$x = \frac{18.47}{22} = 0.84, \; x = \frac{9.53}{22} = 0.43$$ Simplify the numerator and divide.

See Lesson: Solving Quadratic Equations.

11. D. The correct solutions are ±3. Solve this equation by the square root method.

$3x^2 = 27$	Add 5 to both sides of the equation.
$x^2 = \pm 9$	Divide both sides of the equation by 3.
$x = \pm 3$	Apply the square root to both sides of the equation.

See Lesson: Solving Quadratic Equations.

12. A. The correct solution is 0.

$5x^2 = 0$	Subtract 10 from both sides of the equation.
$x^2 = 0$	Divide both sides of the equation by 5.
$x = 0$	Apply the square root to both sides of the equation.

See Lesson: Solving Quadratic Equations.

SECTION III. READING

Chapter 8 Key Ideas and Details

Main Ideas, Topic Sentences, and Supporting Details

To read effectively, you need to know how to identify the most important information in a text. You must also understand how ideas within a text relate to one other.

Main Ideas

The central or most important idea in a text is the **main idea**. As a reader, you need to avoid confusing the main idea with less important details that may be interesting but not central to the author's point.

The **topic** of a text is slightly different than the main idea. The topic is a word or phrase that describes roughly what a text is about. A main idea, in contrast, is a complete sentence that states the topic and explains what an author wants to say about it.

All types of texts can contain main ideas. Read the following informational paragraph and try to identify the main idea:

> The immune system is the body's defense mechanism. It fights off harmful bacteria, viruses, and substances that attack the body. To do this, it uses cells, tissues, and organs that work together to resist invasion.

The topic of this paragraph is the immune system. The main idea can be expressed in a sentence like this: "This paragraph defines and describes the immune system." Ideas about organisms and substances that invade the body are not the central focus. The topic and main idea must always be directly related to every sentence in the text, as the immune system is here.

Read the persuasive paragraph below and consider the topic and main idea:

> Football is not a healthy activity for kids. It causes head injuries that harm the ability to learn and achieve. It causes painful bodily injuries that can linger into adulthood. It teaches aggressive behavioral habits that make life harder for players after they have left the field.

The topic of this paragraph is youth football, and the main idea is that kids should not play the game. Note that if you are asked to state the main idea of a persuasive text, it is your job to be objective. This means you should describe the author's opinion, not make an argument of your own in response.

Both of the example paragraphs above state their main idea explicitly. Some texts have an implicit, or suggested, main idea. In this case, you need to figure out the main idea using the details as clues.

FOR EXAMPLE

The following fictional paragraph has an implicit main idea:

Daisy parked her car and sat gripping the wheel, not getting out. A few steps to the door. A couple of knocks. She could give him the news in two words. She'd already decided what she was going to do, so it didn't matter what he said, not really. Still, she couldn't make her feet carry her to the door.

The main idea here is that Daisy feels reluctant to speak to someone. This point is not stated outright, but it is clear from the details of Daisy's thoughts and actions.

Topic Sentences

Many paragraphs identify the topic and main idea in a single sentence. This is called a **topic sentence,** and it often appears at the beginning of a paragraph. However, a writer may choose to place a topic sentence anywhere in the text.

Some paragraphs contain an introductory sentence to grab the reader's attention before clearly stating the topic. A paragraph may begin by asking a rhetorical question, presenting a striking idea, or showing why the topic is important. When authors use this strategy, the topic sentence usually comes second:

> Have you ever wondered how your body fights off a nasty cold? **It uses a complex defense mechanism called the immune system.** The immune system fights off harmful bacteria, viruses, and substances that attack the body. To do this, it uses cells, tissues, and organs that work together to resist invasion.

Here, the first sentence grabs the attention, and the second, **boldfaced** topic sentence states the main idea. The remaining sentences provide further information, explaining what the immune system does and identifying its basic components.

COMPARE!

The informational paragraph above contains a question that grabs the attention at the beginning. The writer could convey the same information with a little less flair by omitting this device. The version you read in Section 1 does exactly this. (The topic sentence below is **boldfaced.**)

The immune system is the body's defense mechanism. It fights off harmful bacteria, viruses, and substances that attack the body. To do this, it uses cells, tissues, and organs that work together to resist invasion.

Look back at the football paragraph from Section 1. Which sentence is the topic sentence?

Sometimes writers wait until the end of a paragraph to reveal the main idea in a topic sentence. When you're reading a paragraph that is organized this way, you may feel like you're reading a bit of a puzzle. It's not fully clear what the piece is about until you get to the end:

> It causes head injuries that harm the ability to learn and achieve. It causes painful bodily injuries that can linger through the passage of years. It teaches aggressive behavioral habits that make life harder for players after they have left the field. **Football is not a healthy activity for kids.**

Note that the topic—football—is not actually named until the final, **boldfaced** topic sentence. This is a strong hint that this final sentence is the topic sentence. Other paragraphs with this structure may contain several examples or related ideas and then tie them together with a summary statement near the end.

Supporting Details

The **supporting details** of a text develop the main idea, contribute further information, or provide examples.

All of the supporting details in a text must relate back to the main idea. In a text that sets out to define and describe the immune system, the supporting details could explain how the immune system works, define parts of the immune system, and so on.

> **Main Idea:** The immune system is the body's defense mechanism.
>
> **Supporting Detail:** It fights off harmful bacteria, viruses, and substances that attack the body.
>
> **Supporting Detail:** To do this, it uses cells, tissues, and organs that work together to resist invasion.

The above text could go on to describe white blood cells, which are a vital part of the body's defense system against disease. However, the supporting details in such a text should *not* drift off into descriptions of parts of the body that make no contribution to immune response.

Supporting details may be facts or opinions. A single text can combine both facts and opinions to develop a single main idea.

> **Main Idea:** Football is not a healthy activity for kids.
>
> **Supporting Detail:** It teaches aggressive behavioral habits that make life harder for players after they have left the field.
>
> **Supporting Detail:** In a study of teenage football players by Dr. Sophia Ortega at Harvard University, 28% reported involvement in fights or other violent incidents, compared with 19% of teenage boys who were not involved in sports.

The first supporting detail above states an opinion. The second is still related to the main idea, but it provides factual information to back up the opinion. Further development of this paragraph could contain other types of facts, including information about football injuries and anecdotes about real players who got hurt playing the game.

Let's Review!

- The main idea is the most important piece of information in a text.
- The main idea is often expressed in a topic sentence.
- Supporting details develop the main idea, contribute further information, or provide examples.

SUMMARIZING TEXT AND USING TEXT FEATURES

Effective readers need to know how to identify and restate the main idea of a text through summary. They must also follow complex instructions, figure out the sequence of events in a text that is not presented in order, and understand information presented in graphics.

Summary Basics

A **summary** is a text that restates the ideas from a different text in a new way. Every summary needs to include the main idea of the original. Some summaries may include information about the supporting details as well.

The content and level of detail in a summary vary depending on the purpose. For example, a journalist may summarize a recent scientific study in a newspaper profile of its authors. A graduate student might briefly summarize the same study in a paper questioning its conclusions. The journalist's version would likely use fairly simple language and restate only the main points. The student's version would likely use specialized scientific vocabulary and include certain supporting details, especially the ones most applicable to the argument the student intends to make later.

The language of a summary must be substantially different from the original. It should not retain the structure and word choice of the source text. Rather, it should provide a completely new way of stating the ideas.

Read the passage below and the short summary that follows:

> **Original:** There is no need for government regulations to maintain a minimum wage because free market forces naturally adjust wages on their own. Workers are in short supply in our thriving economy, and businesses must offer fair wages and working conditions to attract labor. Business owners pay employees well because common sense dictates that they cannot succeed any other way.

> **Effective Summary:** The author argues against minimum wage laws. He claims free market forces naturally keep wages high in a healthy economy with a limited labor supply.

KEY POINT!

Many ineffective summaries attempt to imitate the structure of the original text and change only individual words. This makes the writing process difficult, and it can lead to unintentional plagiarism.

Ineffective Summary (Plagiarism): It is unnecessary for government regulations to create a minimum wage because capitalism adjusts wages without help. Good labor is rare in our excellent economy, and businesses need to offer fair wages and working conditions in order to attract workers.

The above text is an example of structural plagiarism. Summary writing does not just involve rewriting the original words one by one. An effective summary restates the main ideas of the text in a wholly original way.

The effective summary above restates the main ideas in a new but objective way. Objectivity is a key quality of an effective summary. A summary does not exaggerate, judge, or distort the author's original ideas.

> **Not a Summary:** The author makes a wild and unsupportable claim that minimum wage laws are unnecessary because market forces keep wages high without government intervention.

Although the above text might be appropriate in persuasive writing, it makes its own claims and judgments rather than simply restating the original author's ideas. It would not be an effective sentence in a summary.

In some cases, particularly dealing with creative works like fiction and poetry, summaries may mention ideas that are clearly implied but not stated outright in the original text. For example, a mobster in a thriller novel might turn to another character and say menacingly, "I wouldn't want anything to happen to your sweet little kids." A summary of this passage could objectively say the mobster had threatened the other character. But everything in the summary needs to be clearly supportable in the text. The summary could not go on to say how the other character feels about the threat unless the author describes it.

Attending to Sequence and Instructions

Events happen in a sequence. However, many written texts present events out of order to create an effect on the reader. Nonfiction writers such as journalists and history writers may use this strategy to create surprise or bring particular ideas to the forefront. Fiction writers may interrupt the flow of a plot to interweave bits of a character's history or to provide flashes of insight into future events. Readers need to know how to untangle this presentation of events and figure out what actually happened first, second, and third. Consider the following passage:

> The man in dark glasses was looking for something. He checked his pockets. He checked his backpack. He walked back to his car, unlocked the doors, and inspected the area around the seats. Shaking his head, he re-locked the doors and rubbed his forehead in frustration. When his hand bumped his sunglasses, he finally realized where he had put them.

This passage does not mention putting the sunglasses on until the end, but it is clear from context that the man put them on first, before beginning his search. You can keep track of sequence by paying attention to time words like *when* and *before,* noticing grammatical constructions *he had* that indicate when events happened, and making common sense observations like the fact that the man is wearing his dark glasses in the first sentence.

Sequence is also an important aspect of reading technical and functional documents such as recipes and other instructions. If such documents present many steps in a large text block without illustrations or visual breaks, you may need to break them down and categorize them yourself. Always read all the steps first and think about how to follow them before jumping in.

To see why, read the pancake recipe below:

> Combine flour, baking powder, sugar, and salt. Break the eggs into a separate bowl. Add milk and oil to the beaten eggs. Combine dry and liquid ingredients and stir. While you are doing the above, put a small amount of oil into a pan and heat it on medium heat. When it is hot, spoon batter onto the pan.

To follow directions like these effectively, a reader must break them down into categories, perhaps even rewriting them in a numbered list and noting when to start steps like heating the pan, which may be worth doing in a different order than it appears above.

Interpreting Graphics

Information is often presented in pictures, graphs, or diagrams. These **graphic elements** may provide information to back up an argument, illustrate factual information or instructions, or present key facts and statistics.

When you read charts and graphs, it is important to look carefully at all the information presented, including titles and labels, to be sure that you are interpreting the visuals correctly.

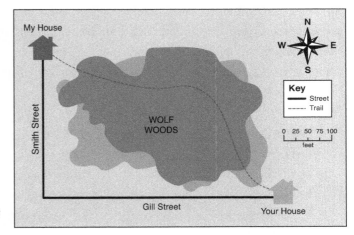

Diagram

A diagram presents a picture with labels that shows the parts of an object or functions of a

mechanism. The diagram of a knee joint below shows the parts of the knee. Like many diagrams, it is placed in relation to a larger object—in this case, a leg—to clarify how the labeled parts fit into a larger context.

Flowchart

A flowchart shows a sequence of actions or decisions involved in a complex process. A flowchart usually begins with an oval-shaped box that asks a yes-no question or gives an instruction. Readers follow arrows indicating possible responses. This helps readers figure out how to solve a problem, or it illustrates how a complex system works.

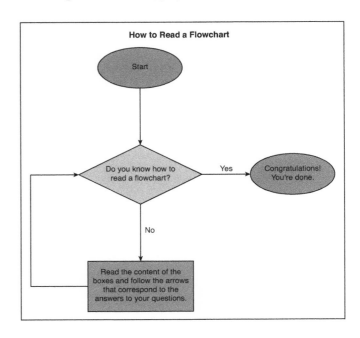

Bar Graph

A bar graph uses bars of different sizes to represent numbers. Larger bars show larger numbers to convey the magnitude of differences between two numeric values at a glance. In this case, each rectangle shows the number of candy bars of different types that a particular group of people ate.

Pie Chart

A pie chart is useful for representing all of something—in this case, the whole group of people surveyed about their favorite kind of pie. Larger wedges mean larger percentages of people liked a particular kind of pie. Percentage values may be written directly on the chart or in a key to the side.

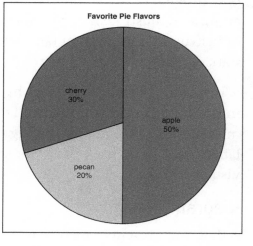

Let's Review!

- A summary restates the main ideas of a text in different words.
- A summary should objectively restate ideas in the present tense and give credit to the original author.
- Effective readers need to mentally reconstruct the basic sequence of events authors present out of order.
- Effective readers need to approach complex instructions by grouping steps into categories or considering how best to approach the steps.
- Information may be presented graphically in the form of diagrams, flowcharts, graphs, or charts.

UNDERSTANDING PRIMARY SOURCES, MAKING INFERENCES, AND DRAWING CONCLUSIONS

Effective readers must understand the difference between types of sources and choose credible sources of information to support research. Readers must also consider the content of their reading materials and draw their own conclusions.

Primary Sources

When we read and research information, we must differentiate between different types of sources. Sources are often classified depending on how close they are to the original creation or discovery of the information they present.

Primary sources include firsthand witness accounts of events, research described by the people who conducted it, and any other original information. Contemporary researchers can often access mixed media versions of primary sources such as video and audio recordings, photographs of original work, and so on. Note that original content is still considered primary even if it is reproduced online or in a book.

> **Examples:** Diaries, scientific journal articles, witness testimony, academic conference presentations, business memos, speeches, letters, interviews, and original literature and artwork.

Secondary sources respond to, analyze, summarize, or comment on primary sources. They add value to a discussion of the topic by giving readers new ways to think about the content. However, they may also introduce errors or layers of bias. Secondary sources may be very good sources of information, but readers must evaluate them carefully.

> **Examples:** Biographies, books and articles that summarize research for wider audiences, analyses of original literature and artwork, histories, political commentary.

Tertiary sources compile information in a general, highly summarized, and sometimes simplified way. Their purpose is not to add anything to the information, but rather to present the information in an accessible manner, often for audiences who are only beginning to familiarize themselves with a topic.

> **Examples:** Encyclopedias, guidebooks, literature study guides.

Source Materials in Action

Primary sources are often considered most trustworthy because they are closest to the original material and least likely to contain errors. However, readers must take a common sense approach to evaluating trustworthiness. For example, a single letter written by one biased witness of a historical event may not provide as much insight into what really happened as a secondary account by a historian who has considered the points of view of a dozen firsthand witnesses.

Tertiary sources are useful for readers attempting to gain a quick overview of understanding about a subject. They are also a good starting point for readers looking for keywords and subtopics to use for further research of a subject. However, they are not sufficiently detailed or credible to support an article, academic paper, or other document intended to add valuable analysis and commentary on a subject.

Evaluating Credibility

Not everything you read is equally trustworthy. Many sources contain mistakes, faulty reasoning, or deliberate misinformation designed to manipulate you. Effective readers seek out information from **credible**, or trustworthy, sources.

There is no single formula for determining credibility. Readers must make judgment calls based on individual texts and their purpose.

FOR EXAMPLE

Most sources should attempt to be objective. But if you're reading an article that makes an argument, you do not need to demand perfect objectivity from the source. The purpose of a persuasive article is to defend a point of view. As long as the author does this openly and defends the point of view with facts, logic, and other good argumentative techniques, you may trust the source.

Other sources may seem highly objective but not be credible. For example, some scientific studies meet all the criteria for credibility below except the one about trustworthy publishers. If a study is funded or conducted by a company that stands to profit from it, you should treat the results with skepticism no matter how good the information looks otherwise.

Sources and References

Credible texts are primary sources or secondary sources that refer to other trustworthy sources. If the author consults experts, they should be named, and their credentials should be explained. Authors should not attempt to hide where they got their information. Vague statements like "studies show" are not as trustworthy as statements that identify who completed a study.

Objectivity

Credible texts usually make an effort to be objective. They use clear, logical reasoning. They back arguments up with facts, expert opinions, or clear explanations. The assumptions behind the arguments do not contain obvious stereotypes.

Emotional arguments are acceptable in some argumentative writing, but they should not be manipulative. For example, photos of starving children may be acceptable for raising awareness of a famine, but they need to be respectful of both the victims and the audience—not just there for shock value.

Date of Publication

Information changes quickly in some fields, especially the sciences and technology. When researching a fast-changing topic, look for sources published in the last ten years.

Author Information

If an author and/or a respected organization take public credit for information, it is more likely to be reliable. Information published anonymously on the Internet may be suspicious because nobody is clearly responsible for mistakes. Authors with strong credentials such as university professors in a given field are more trustworthy than authors with no clear resume.

Publisher Information

Information published by the government, a university, a major national news organization, or another respected organization is often more credible. On the Internet, addresses ending in .edu or .gov may be more trustworthy than .com addresses. Publishers who stand to profit or otherwise benefit from the content of a text are always questionable.

> **BE CAREFUL!**
> Strong credentials only make a source more trustworthy if the credentials are related to the topic. A Columbia University Professor of Archeology is a credible source on ancient history. But if she writes a parenting article, it's not necessarily more credible than a parenting article by someone without a flashy university title.

Professionalism

Credible sources usually look professional and present information free of grammatical errors or major factual errors.

Making Inferences and Drawing Conclusions

In reading—and in life—people regularly make educated guesses based on limited information. When we use the information we have to figure out something nobody has told us directly, we are making an **inference**. People make inferences every day.

> **Example:** You hear a loud thump. Then a pained voice says, "Honey, can you bring the first aid kit?"

From the information above, it is reasonable to infer that the speaker is hurt. The thumping noise, the pain in the speaker's voice, and the request for a first aid kit all suggest this conclusion.

When you make inferences from reading, you use clues presented in the text to help you draw logical conclusions about what the author means. Before you can make an inference, you must read the text carefully and understand the explicit, or overt, meaning. Next, you must look for clues to any implied, or suggested, meanings behind the text. Finally, consider the clues in light of your prior knowledge and the author's purpose, and draw a conclusion about the meaning.

> As soon as Raizel entered the party, someone handed her a plate. She stared down at the hot dog unhappily.
>
> "What?" asked an unfamiliar woman nearby with an edge to her voice. "You don't eat dead animal?"

From the passage above, it would be reasonable to infer that the unfamiliar woman has a poor opinion of vegetarians. Several pieces of information suggest this: her combative tone, the edge in her voice, and the mocking question at the end.

When you draw inferences from a text, make sure your conclusion is truly indicated by the clues provided.

> Author Glenda Davis had high hopes for her children's book *Basketball Days*. But when the novel was released with a picture of a girl on the cover, boys refused to pick it up. The author reported this to her publisher, and the paperback edition was released with a new cover—this time featuring a dog and a basketball hoop. After that, many boys read the book. And Davis never heard anyone complain that the main character was a girl.

The text above implies that boys are reluctant to read books with a girl on the cover. A hasty reader might stop reading early and conclude that boys are reluctant to read about girls—but this inference is not suggested by the full text.

BE CAREFUL!

Before you make a conclusion about a text, consider it in light of your prior knowledge and the clues presented.

After reading the paragraph above, you might suspect that Raizel is a vegetarian. But the text does not fully support that conclusion. There are many reasons why Raizel might not want to eat a hot dog.

Perhaps she is keeping kosher, or she has social anxiety that makes it difficult to eat at parties, or she simply isn't hungry. The above inference about the unfamiliar woman's dislike for vegetarians is strongly supported. But you'd need further evidence before you could safely conclude that Raizel is actually a vegetarian.

Let's Review!

- Effective readers must consider the credibility of their sources.
- Primary sources are usually considered the most trustworthy.
- Readers must often make inferences about ideas that are implied but not explicitly stated in a text.

CHAPTER 8 KEY IDEAS AND DETAILS PRACTICE QUIZ

1. Which type of graphic element would be most helpful for teaching the names of the parts of a bicycle?

   A. Diagram
   B. Pie chart
   C. Bar graph
   D. Flowchart

Read the following sentence and answer questions 2-4.

Numerous robotic missions to Mars have revealed tantalizing evidence of a planet that may once have been capable of supporting life.

2. Imagine this sentence is a *supporting detail* in a well-developed paragraph. Which of the following sentences would best function as a *topic sentence*?

   A. Venus is an intensely hot planet surrounded by clouds full of drops of sulfuric acid.
   B. Of all the destinations within human reach, Mars is the planet most similar to Earth.
   C. Liquid water—a necessary ingredient of life—may once have flowed on the planet's surface.
   D. Space research is a costly, frivolous exercise that brings no clear benefit to people on Earth.

3. Imagine this sentence is the *topic sentence* of a well-developed paragraph. Which of the following sentences would best function as a *supporting detail*?

   A. Of all the destinations within human reach, Mars is the planet most similar to Earth.
   B. Venus is an intensely hot planet surrounded by clouds full of drops of sulfuric acid.
   C. Space research is a costly, frivolous exercise that brings no clear benefit to people on Earth.
   D. Liquid water—a necessary ingredient of life—may once have flowed on the planet's surface.

4. How could this sentence function as a *supporting detail* in a persuasive text arguing that space research is worth the expense and effort because it teaches us more about Earth and ourselves?

   A. By using statistics to back up an argument that needs support to be believed
   B. By showing how a space discovery could earn money for investors here on Earth
   C. By providing an example of a space discovery that enhances our understanding of life
   D. By developing the main idea that no space discovery can reveal information about Earth

The bar graph below provides information about book sales for a book called *The Comings,* which is the first book in a trilogy. Study the image and answer questions 5-6.

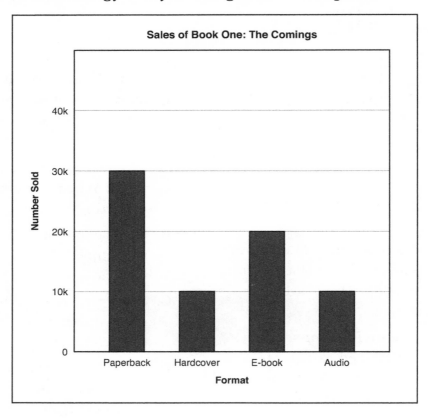

5. Which type of book has sold the most copies?

   A. E-book
   B. Hardcover
   C. Paperback
   D. Audio book

6. The marketing director for *The Comings* wants to use a different strategy for publishing book two in the series. Which argument does the bar graph *best* support?

   A. The first book in the trilogy has only sold 10,000 copies.

   B. The second book in the trilogy should not be released in hardcover.

   C. The second book in the trilogy should only be released as an e-book.

   D. The second and third books in the trilogy should be combined into one.

Study the infographic below and answer questions 7-9.

https://www.cdc.gov/nccdphp/dch/images/infographics/getmoving_15-18.png

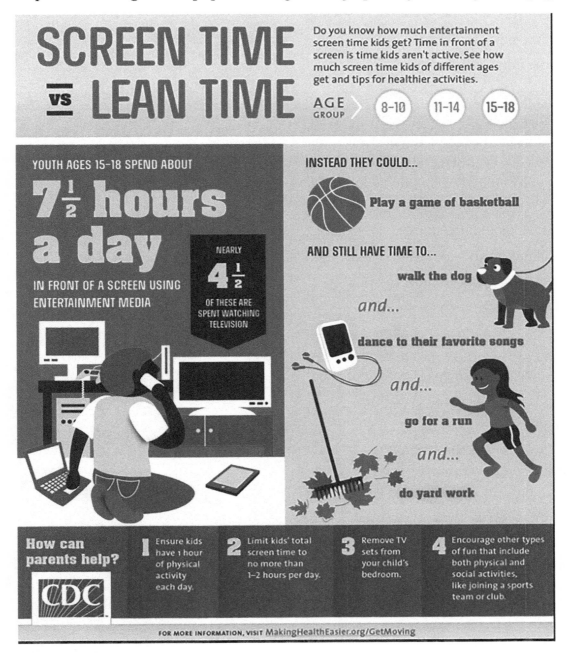

Resources:

American Academy of Pediatrics (AAP):

Childhood obesity calls to action

Screen Time Policy Statement

CDC: Strategies to Prevent Obesity

Screen-Free Week

7. Which of the following is not a sign that the infographic is credible?

   A. The use of verifiable facts

   B. The list of source materials

   C. The professional appearance

   D. The inclusion of an author's name

8. Zetta is unsure of the credibility of this source and has never heard of the Centers for Disease Control (CDC). Which fact could help her decide to trust it?

   A. The CDC is located in Atlanta.

   B. The CDC has a .gov web address.

   C. The CDC creates many infographics.

   D. The CDC is also listed as a source consulted.

9. What could a skeptical reader do to verify the facts on the infographic?

   A. Interview one teenager to ask about his or her screen time

   B. Follow the links for the sources and determine their credibility

   C. Check a tertiary source like Wikipedia to verify the information

   D. Find different values for screen time on someone's personal blog

Chapter 8 Key Ideas and Details Practice Quiz – Answer Key

1. A. A diagram illustrates complex visual ideas, so it could show which part of a bicycle is which and how they fit together. **See Lesson: Summarizing Text and Using Text Features.**

2. B. The sentence above conveys factual information about Mars in an excited tone that suggests a positive interest in the subject. This makes it most likely to fit into an informational paragraph sharing facts about Mars. **See Lesson: Main Ideas, Topic Sentences, and Supporting Details.**

3. D. If the above sentence were a topic sentence, its supporting details would likely share information to develop the idea that Mars may have supported life in the past. **See Lesson: Main Ideas, Topic Sentences, and Supporting Details.**

4. C. The sentence above could act as an example to show how space discoveries teach us about Earth and ourselves. **See Lesson: Main Ideas, Topic Sentences, and Supporting Details.**

5. C. Larger bars in a bar graph indicate higher numbers. This book has sold more paperback copies than any other. **See Lesson: Summarizing Text and Using Text Features.**

6. B. The bar graph shows fewer hardcover sales than any other kind. This could help support an argument that later books should only be released in electronic and paperback forms. **See Lesson: Summarizing Text and Using Text Features.**

7. D. It is usually a good sign if an author is clearly named in a source. Although this source is authored by an organization, the CDC, instead of a single author, there are many other signs it is credible. **See Lesson: Understanding Primary Sources, Making Inferences, and Drawing Conclusions.**

8. B. When presenting this type of information, a government organization with a .gov web address is typically considered a reputable source. **See Lesson: Understanding Primary Sources, Making Inferences, and Drawing Conclusions.**

9. B. One way to verify facts is to check the sources an author used. Verifying facts elsewhere may also be a good idea, but it is important to use reputable primary or secondary sources. **See Lesson: Understanding Primary Sources, Making Inferences, and Drawing Conclusions.**

Chapter 9 Craft and Structure

Formal and Informal Language

In English, there is formal language that is used most often in writing, and informal language that is most often used in speaking, but there are situations where one is more appropriate than the other. This lesson will cover differentiating contexts for (1) formal language and (2) informal language.

Formal Language

Formal language is often associated with writing for professional and academic purposes, but it is also used when giving a speech or a lecture. An essay written for a class will always use **formal language**. **Formal language** is used in situations where people are not extremely close and when one needs to show respect to another person. Certain qualities and contexts differentiate **formal language** from informal language.

Formal language does not use contractions.

- It doesn't have that - It does not have that.
- He's been offered a new job - He has been offered a new job.

Formal language also uses complete sentences.

- So much to tell you - I have so much to tell you.
- Left for the weekend - We left for the weekend.

Formal language includes more formal and polite vocabulary.

- The class starts at two - The class commences at two.
- I try to be the best person I can be - I endeavor to be the best person I can be.

Formal language is not personal and normally does not use the pronouns "I" and "We" as the subject of a sentence.

- I argue that the sky is blue - This essay argues that the sky is blue.
- We often associate green with grass - Green is often associated with grass.

Formal language also does not use slang.

- It's raining cats and dogs - It is raining heavily.
- Patients count on doctors to help them - Patients expect doctors to help them.

Informal Language

Informal language is associated with speaking, but is also used in text messages, emails, letters, and postcards. It is the language a person would use with their friends and family.

Informal language uses contractions.

- I can't go to the movie tomorrow.
- He doesn't have any manners.

Informal language can include sentence fragments.

- See you
- Talk to you later

Informal language uses less formal vocabulary such as slang.

- The dog drove me up the wall.
- I was so hungry I could eat a horse.
- I can always count on you.

Informal language is personal and uses pronouns such as "I" and "We" as the subject of a sentence.

- I am in high school.
- We enjoy going to the beach in the summer.

Let's Review!

- **Formal language** is used in professional and academic writing and talks. It does not have contractions, uses complete sentences, uses polite and formal vocabulary, not slang, and is not personal and generally does not use the pronouns "I" and "We" as the subject of a sentence.
- **Informal language** is used in daily life when communicating with friends and family through conversations, text messages, emails, letters, and postcards. It uses contractions, can be sentence fragments, uses less formal vocabulary and slang, and is personal and uses pronouns such as "I" and "We" as the subject of a sentence.

TONE, MOOD, AND TRANSITION WORDS

Authors use language to show their emotions and to make readers feel something too. They also use transition words to help guide the reader from one idea to the next.

Tone and Mood

The **tone** of a text is the author's or speaker's attitude toward the subject. The tone may reflect any feeling or attitude a person can express: happiness, excitement, anger, boredom, or arrogance.

Readers can identify tone primarily by analyzing word choice. The reader should be able to point to specific words and details that help to establish the tone.

> **Example:** The train rolled past miles and miles of cornfields. The fields all looked the same. They swayed the same. They produced the same dull nausea in the pit of my stomach. I'd been sent out to see the world, and so I looked, obediently. What I saw was sameness.

Here, the author is expressing boredom and dissatisfaction. This is clear from the repetition of words like "same" and "sameness." There's also a sense of unpleasantness from phrases like "dull nausea" and passivity from words like "obediently."

Sometimes an author uses an ironic tone. Ironic texts often mean the opposite of what they actually say. To identify irony, you need to rely on your prior experience and common sense to help you identify texts with words and ideas that do not quite match.

> **Example:** With that, the senator dismissed the petty little problem of mass shootings and returned to the really important issue: his approval ratings.

> **BE CAREFUL!**
>
> When you're asked to identify the tone of a text, be sure to keep track of *whose* tone you're supposed to identify, and which part of the text the question is referencing. The author's tone can be different from that of the characters in fiction or the people quoted in nonfiction.
>
> **Example:** The reporter walked quickly, panting to catch up to the senator's entourage. "Senator Biltong," she said. "Are you going to take action on mass shootings?"
>
> "Sure, sure. Soon," the senator said vaguely. Then he turned to greet a newcomer. "Ah ha! Here's the man who can fix my approval ratings!" And with that, he returned to the really important issue: his popularity.
>
> *
>
> In the example above, the author's tone is ironic and angry. But the tone of the senator's dialogue is different. The line beginning with the words "Sure, sure" has a distracted tone. The line beginning with "Ah ha!" has a pleased tone.

Here the author flips around the words most people would usually use to discuss mass murder and popularity. By calling a horrific issue "petty" and a trivial issue "important," the author highlights what she sees as a politician's backwards priorities. Except for the phrase "mass shootings," the words here are light and airy—but the tone is ironic and angry.

A concept related to tone is **mood**, or the feelings an author produces in the reader. To determine the mood of a text, a reader can consider setting and theme as well as word choice and tone. For example, a story set in a haunted house may produce an unsettled or frightened feeling in a reader.

Tone and mood are often confused. This is because they are sometimes the same. For instance, in an op-ed article that describes children starving while food aid lies rotting, the author may use an outraged tone and simultaneously arouse an outraged mood in the reader.

However, tone and mood can be different. When they are, it's useful to have different words to distinguish between the author's attitude and the reader's emotional reaction.

> **Example:** I had to fly out of town at 4 a.m. for my trip to the Bahamas, and my wife didn't even get out of bed to make me a cup of coffee. I told her to, but she refused just because she'd been up five times with our newborn. I'm only going on vacation for one week, and she's been off work for a month! She should show me a little consideration.

Here, the tone is indignant. The mood will vary depending on the reader, but it is likely to be unsympathetic.

Transitions

Authors use connecting words and phrases, or **transitions**, to link ideas and help readers follow the flow of their thoughts. The number of possible ways to transition between ideas is almost limitless.

Below are a few common transition words, categorized by the way they link ideas.

Transitions	Examples
Time and sequence transitions orient the reader within a text. They can also help show when events happened in time.	*First, second, next, now, then, at this point, after, afterward, before this, previously, formerly, thereafter, finally, in conclusion*
Addition or emphasis transitions let readers know the author is building on an established line of thought. Many place extra stress on an important idea.	*Moreover, also, likewise, furthermore, above all, indeed, in fact*
Example transitions introduce ideas that illustrate a point.	*For example, for instance, to illustrate, to demonstrate*
Causation transitions indicate a cause-and-effect relationship.	*As a result, consequently, thus*
Contrast transitions indicate a difference between ideas.	*Nevertheless, despite, in contrast, however*

Transitions may look different depending on their function within the text. Within a paragraph, writers often choose short words or expressions to provide transitions and smooth the flow. Between paragraphs or larger sections of text, transitions are usually longer. They may use some of the key words or ideas above, but the author often goes into detail restating larger concepts and explaining their relationships more thoroughly.

Between Sentences: Students who cheat do not learn what they need to know. *As a result,* they get farther behind and face greater temptation to cheat in the future.

Between Paragraphs: *As a result of the cheating behaviors described above,* students find themselves in a vicious cycle.

Longer transitions like the latter example may be useful for keeping the reader clued in to the author's focus in an extended text. But long transitions should have clear content and function. Some long transitions, such as the very wordy "due to the fact that" take up space without adding more meaning and are considered poor style.

Let's Review!
- Tone is the author's or speaker's attitude toward the subject.
- Mood is the feeling a text creates in the reader.
- Transitions are connecting words and phrases that help readers follow the flow of a writer's thoughts.

THE AUTHOR'S PURPOSE AND POINT OF VIEW

In order to understand, analyze, and evaluate a text, readers must know how to identify the author's purpose and point of view. Readers also need to attend to an author's language and rhetorical strategies.

Author's Purpose

When writers put words on paper, they do it for a reason. This reason is the author's **purpose**. Most writing exists for one of three purposes: to inform, to persuade, or to entertain.

TEST TIP

You may have learned about a fourth purpose for writing: conveying an emotional experience. Many poems as well as some works of fiction, personal essays, and memoirs are written to give the reader a sense of how an event or moment might feel. This type of text is rarely included on placement tests, and if it is, it tends to be lumped in with literature meant to entertain.

If a text is designed to share knowledge, its purpose is to **inform**. Informational texts include technical documents, cookbooks, expository essays, journalistic newspaper articles, and many nonfiction books. Informational texts are based on facts and logic, and they usually attempt an objective tone. The style may otherwise vary; some informational texts are quite dry, whereas others have an engaging style.

If a text argues a point, its purpose is to **persuade**. A persuasive text attempts to convince a reader to believe a certain point of view or take a certain action. Persuasive texts include op-ed newspaper articles, book and movie reviews, project proposals, and argumentative essays. Key signs of persuasive texts include judgments, words like *should*, and other signs that the author is sharing opinions.

If a text is primarily for fun, its purpose is to **entertain**. Entertaining texts usually tell stories or present descriptions. Entertaining texts include novels, short stories, memoirs, and some poems. Virtually all stories are lumped into this category, even if they describe unpleasant experiences.

CONNECTIONS

You may have read elsewhere that readers can break writing down into the following basic categories. These categories are often linked to the author's purpose.

Narrative writing tells a story and is usually meant to entertain.
Expository writing explains an idea and is usually meant to inform.
Technical writing explains a mechanism or process and is usually meant to inform.
Persuasive writing argues a point and, as the label suggests, is meant to persuade.

A text can have more than one purpose. For example, many traditional children's stories come with morals or lessons. These are meant both to entertain children and persuade them to behave in ways society considers appropriate. Also, commercial nonfiction texts like popular science books are often written in an engaging or humorous style. The purpose of such a text is to inform while also entertaining the reader.

Point of View

Every author has a general outlook or set of opinions about the subject. These make up the author's **point of view.**

To determine point of view, a reader must recognize implicit clues in the text and use them to develop educated guesses about the author's worldview. In persuasive texts, the biggest clue is the author's explicit argument. From considering this argument, a reader can usually make some inferences about point of view. For instance, if an author argues that parents should offer kids opportunities to exercise throughout the day, it would be reasonable to infer that the author has an overall interest in children's health, and that he or she is troubled by the idea of kids pursuing sedentary behaviors like TV watching.

It is more challenging to determine point of view in a text meant to inform. Because the writer does not present an explicit argument, readers must examine assumptions and word choice to determine the writer's point of view.

> **Example:** Models suggest that at the current rate of global warming, hurricanes in 2100 will move 9 percent slower and drop 24 percent more rain. Longer storm durations and rainfall rates will likely translate to increased economic damage and human suffering.

It is reasonable to infer that the writer of this passage has a general trust for science and scientists. This writer assumes that global warming is happening, so it is clear he or she is not a global warming denier. Although the writer does not suggest a plan to prevent future storm damage, the emphasis on negative effects and the use of negative words like "damage" and "suffering" suggest that the author is worried about global warming.

Texts meant to entertain also contain clues about the author's point of view. That point of view is usually evident from the themes and deeper meanings. For instance, a memoirist who writes an upbeat story about a troubled but loving family is likely to believe strongly in the power of love. Note, however, that in this type of work, it is not possible to determine point of view merely from one character's words or actions. For instance, if a character says, "Your mother's love doesn't matter much if she can't take care of you," the reader should *not* automatically assume the writer agrees with that statement. Narrative writers often present a wide range of characters with varying outlooks on life. A reader can only determine the author's point of view by considering the work as a whole. The attitudes that are most emphasized and the ones that win out in the end are likely to reflect the author's point of view.

Rhetorical Strategies

Rhetorical strategies are the techniques an author uses to support an argument or develop a main idea. Effective readers need to study the language of a text and determine how the author is supporting his or her points.

One strategy is to appeal to the reader's reason. This is the foundation of effective writing, and it simply means that the writer relies on factual information and the logical conclusions that follow from it. Even persuasive writing uses this strategy by presenting facts and reasons to back up the author's opinions.

Ineffective: Everyone knows *Sandra and the Lumps* is the best band of the new millennium.

Effective: The three most recent albums by *Sandra and the Lumps* are the first, second, and third most popular records released since the turn of the millennium.

Another strategy is to establish trust. A writer can do this by choosing credible sources and by presenting ideas in a clear and professional way. In persuasive writing, writers may show they are trustworthy by openly acknowledging that some people hold contradicting opinions and by responding fairly to those positions. Writers should never attack or misrepresent their opponents' position.

Ineffective: People who refuse to recycle are too lazy to protect their children's future.

Effective: According to the annual Throw It Out Questionnaire, many people dislike the onerous task of sorting garbage, and some doubt that their effort brings any real gain.

A final strategy is to appeal to the reader's emotions. For instance, a journalist reporting on the opioid epidemic could include a personal story about an addict's attempts to overcome substance abuse. Emotional content can add a human dimension to a story that would be missing if the writer only included statistics and expert opinions. But emotions are easily manipulated, so writers who use this strategy need to be careful. Emotions should never be used to distort the truth or scare readers into agreeing with the writer.

Ineffective: If you don't take action on gun control, you're basically killing children.

Effective: Julie was puzzling over the Pythagorean Theorem when she heard the first gunshot.

Let's Review!

- Every text has a purpose.
- Most texts are meant to inform, persuade, or entertain.
- Texts contain clues that imply an author's outlook or set of opinions about the subject.
- Authors use rhetorical strategies to appeal to reason, establish trust, or invoke emotions.

CHAPTER 9 CRAFT AND STRUCTURE PRACTICE QUIZ

1. **Which of the following sentences uses the MOST informal language?**

   A. The house creaked at night.

   B. I ate dinner with my friend.

   C. It's sort of a bad time.

   D. The water trickled slowly.

2. **In which of the following situations would it be best to use informal language?**

   A. In a seminar

   B. Writing a postcard

   C. Talking to your boss

   D. Participating in a professional conference

3. **Which of the following sentences uses the MOST formal language?**

   A. Thanks for letting me know.

   B. I want to thank you for telling me.

   C. I appreciate you telling me about this issue.

   D. Thank you for bringing this issue to my attention.

Read the passage below and answer questions 4-6.

The train was the most amazing thing ever even though it didn't go "choo choo." The toddler pounded on the railing of the bridge and supplied the sound herself. "Choo choo! Choo choooooo!" she shouted as the train cars whizzed along below.

In the excitement, she dropped her favorite binky.

Later, when she noticed the binky missing, all the joy went out of the world. The wailing could be heard three houses down. The toddler's usual favorite activities were garbage—even waving to Hank the garbage man, which she refused to do, so that Hank went away looking mildly hurt. It was clear the little girl would never, ever, ever recover from her loss.

Afterward, she played at the park.

4. **Which adjectives best describe the tone of the passage?**

   A. Ironic, angry

   B. Earnest, angry

   C. Ironic, humorous

   D. Earnest, humorous

5. **Which sentence from the passage is clearly ironic?**

   A. "Choo choo! Choo choooooo!" she shouted as the train cars whizzed along below.

   B. Later, when she noticed the binky missing, all the joy went out of the world.

   C. The wailing could be heard three houses down.

   D. Afterward, she played at the park.

6. The author of the passage first establishes the ironic tone by:

   A. describing the child's trip to play at the park.

   B. calling the train "the most amazing thing ever."

   C. pretending that the child can make the sounds "choo chooooo!"

   D. claiming inaccurately that the lost binky was the child's "favorite."

7. What is the most likely purpose of a popular science book describing recent advances in genetics?

   A. To decide   C. To persuade

   B. To inform   D. To entertain

8. Which phrase describes the set of techniques an author uses to support an argument or develop a main idea?

   A. Points of view

   B. Logical fallacies

   C. Statistical analyses

   D. Rhetorical strategies

9. What is the most likely purpose of an article that claims some genetic research is immoral?

   A. To decide   C. To persuade

   B. To inform   D. To entertain

CHAPTER 9 CRAFT AND STRUCTURE PRACTICE QUIZ – ANSWER KEY

1. C. *It's sort of a bad time.* The sentence has contractions and uses informal and slang words. **See Lesson: Formal and Informal Language.**

2. B. *Writing a postcard.* It is an informal mode of communication between close friends and relatives. **See Lesson: Formal and Informal Language.**

3. D. *Thank you for bringing this issue to my attention.* The sentence uses the most formal and polite vocabulary. **See Lesson: Formal and Informal Language.**

4. C. This passage ironically is an ironic, humorous description of a toddler's emotions, written by an adult who has enough experience to know that a toddler's huge emotions will pass. **See Lesson: Tone, Mood, and Transition Words.**

5. B. Authors use irony when their words do not literally mean what they say. The joy does not really go out of the world when a toddler loses her binky—but it may seem that way to the child. **See Lesson: Tone, Mood, and Transition Words.**

6. B. This passage establishes irony in the opening sentence by applying the superlative phrase "the most amazing thing ever" to an ordinary occurrence. **See Lesson: Tone, Mood, and Transition Words.**

7. B. If a book is describing information, its purpose is to inform. **See Lesson: The Author's Purpose and Point of View.**

8. D. The techniques an author uses to support an argument or develop a main idea are called rhetorical strategies. **See Lesson: The Author's Purpose and Point of View.**

9. C. An article that takes a moral position is meant to persuade. **See Lesson: The Author's Purpose and Point of View.**

CHAPTER 10 INTEGRATION OF KNOWLEDGE AND IDEAS

FACTS, OPINIONS, AND EVALUATING AN ARGUMENT

Nonfiction writing is based on facts and real events, but most nonfiction nevertheless expresses a point of view. Effective readers must evaluate the author's point of view and form their own conclusions about the points in the text.

Fact and Opinion

Many texts make an **argument**. In this context, the word *argument* has nothing to do with anger or fighting. It simply means the author is trying to convince readers of something.

Arguments are present in a wide variety of texts. Some relate to controversial issues, for instance by advocating support for a political candidate or change in laws. Others may defend a certain interpretation of facts or ideas. For example, a literature paper may argue that an author's story suggests a certain theme, or a science paper may argue for a certain interpretation of data. An argument may also present a plan of action such as a business strategy.

To evaluate an argument, readers must distinguish between **fact** and **opinion**. A fact is verifiably true. An opinion is someone's belief.

> **Fact:** Seattle gets an average of 37 inches of rain per year.

> **Opinion:** The dark, rainy, cloudy weather makes Seattle an unpleasant place to live in winter.

Meteorologists measure rainfall directly, so the above fact is verifiably true. The statement "it is unpleasant" clearly reflects a feeling, so the second sentence is an opinion.

The difference between fact and opinion is not always straightforward. For instance, a text may present a fact that contains an opinion within it:

> **Fact:** Nutritionist Fatima Antar questions the wisdom of extreme carbohydrate avoidance.

Assuming the writer can prove that this sentence genuinely reflects Fatima Antar's beliefs, it is a factual statement of her point of view. The reader may trust that Fatima Antar really holds this opinion, whether or not the reader is convinced by it.

If a text makes a judgment, it is not a fact:

> **Opinion:** The patient's seizure drug regimen caused horrendous side effects.

The above sentence uses language that different people would interpret in different ways. Because people have varying ideas about what they consider "horrendous," this sentence is an opinion as it is written, even though the actual side effects and the patient's opinion of them could both be verified.

> **COMPARE!**
>
> Small changes to the statement about seizure drugs could turn it into a factual statement:
>
> **Fact:** The patient's seizure drug regiment caused side effects such as migraines, confusion, and dangerously high blood pressure.
>
> The above statement can be verified because the patient and other witnesses could confirm the exact nature of her symptoms. This makes it a fact.
>
> **Fact:** The patient reported that her seizure drug regimen caused horrendous side effects.
>
> This statement can also be verified because the patient can verify that she considers the side effects horrendous. By framing the statement in this way, the writer leaves nothing up to interpretation and is clearly in the realm of fact.

The majority of all arguments contain both facts and opinions, and strong arguments may contain both fact and opinion elements. It is rare for an argument to be composed entirely of facts, but it can happen if the writer is attempting to convince readers to accept factual information that is little-known or widely questioned. Most arguments present an author's opinion and use facts, reasoning, and expert testimony to convince readers.

Evaluating an Argument

Effective readers must evaluate an argument and decide whether or not it is valid. To do this, readers must consider every claim the author presents, including both the main argument and any supporting statements. If an argument is based on poor reasoning or insufficient evidence, it is not valid—even if you agree with the main idea.

> **KEY POINT!**
>
> Most of us want to agree with arguments that reflect our own beliefs. But it is inadvisable to accept an argument that is not properly rooted in good reasoning. Consider the following statements about global climate change:
>
> **Poor Argument:** It just snowed fifteen inches! How can anyone say the world is getting warmer?
>
> **Poor Argument:** It's seventy degrees in the middle of February! How can anyone deny global warming?
>
> Both of these arguments are based on insufficient evidence. Each relies on *one* weather event in *one* location to support an argument that the entire world's climate is or is not changing. There is not nearly enough information here to support an argument on either side.

Beware of any argument that presents opinion information as fact.

False Claim of Fact: I know vaccines cause autism because my niece began displaying autism symptoms after receiving her measles vaccine.

The statement above states a controversial idea as fact without adequate evidence to back it up. Specifically, it makes a false claim of cause and effect about an incident that has no clear causal relationship.

Any claim that is not supported by sufficient evidence is an example of **faulty reasoning**.

Type of Faulty Reasoning	Definition	Example	Explanation
Circular Reasoning	Restating the argument in different words instead of providing evidence	Baseball is the best game in the world because it is more fun than any other game.	Here, everything after the word *because* says approximately the same thing as everything before it. It looks like the author is providing a reason, but no evidence has actually been offered.
Either/Or Fallacy	Presenting an issue as if it involves only two choices when in fact it is not so simple	Women should focus on motherhood, not careers.	This statement assumes that women cannot do both. It also assumes that no woman needs a career in order to provide for her children.
Overgeneralizations	Making a broad claim based on too little evidence	All elderly people have negative stereotypes of teenagers.	This statement lumps a whole category of people into a group and claims the whole group shares the same belief—always an unlikely prospect.

Most texts about evaluating arguments focus on faulty reasoning and false statements of fact. But arguments that attempt to misrepresent facts as opinions are equally suspicious. A careful reader should be skeptical of any text that denies clear physical evidence or questions the truth of events that have been widely verified.

Assumptions and Biases

A well-reasoned argument should be supported by facts, logic, and clearly explained opinions. But most arguments are also based on **assumptions,** or unstated and unproven ideas about what is true. Consider the following argument:

Argument: To improve equality of opportunity for all children, schools in underprivileged areas should receive as much taxpayer funding as schools in wealthy districts.

This argument is based on several assumptions. First is the assumption that all children should have equal opportunities. Another is that taxpayer-funded public schools are the best way to provide these opportunities. Whether or not you disagree with either of these points, it is worth noting that the second idea in particular is not the only way to proceed. Readers who examine the assumptions behind an argument can sometimes find points of disagreement even if an author's claims and logic are otherwise sound.

Examining an author's assumptions can also reveal a writer's biases. A **bias** is a preconceived idea that makes a person more likely to show unfair favor for certain thoughts, people, or groups. Because every person has a different experience of the world, every person has a different set of biases. For example, a person who has traveled widely may feel differently about world political events than someone who has always lived in one place.

Virtually all writing is biased to some degree. However, effective writing attempts to avoid bias as much as possible. Writing that is highly biased may be based on poor assumptions that render the entire argument invalid.

Highly biased writing often includes overgeneralizations. Words like *all, always, never,* and so on may indicate that the writer is overstating a point. While these words can exist in true statements, unbiased writing is more likely to qualify ideas using words like *usually, often,* and *rarely.*

Another quality of biased writing is excessively emotional word choice. When writers insult people who disagree with them or engage the emotions in a way that feels manipulative, they are being biased.

Biased: Power-hungry politicians don't care that their standardized testing requirements are producing a generation of overanxious, incurious, impractical kids.

Less biased: Politicians need to recognize that current standardized testing requirements are causing severe anxiety and other negative effects in children.

Biased writing may also reflect stereotypical thinking. A **stereotype** is a particularly harmful type of bias that applies specifically to groups of people. Stereotypical thinking is behind racism, sexism, homophobia, and so on. Even people who do not consider themselves prejudiced can use language that reflects common stereotypes. For example, the negative use of the word *crazy* reflects a stereotype against people with mental illnesses.

Historically, writers in English have used male nouns and pronouns to indicate all people. Revising such language for more inclusivity is considered more effective in contemporary writing.

Biased: The history of the human race proves that man is a violent creature.

Less biased: The history of the human race proves that people are violent.

Let's Review!

- A text meant to convince someone of something is making an argument.
- Arguments may employ both facts and opinions.
- Effective arguments must use valid reasoning.
- Arguments are based on assumptions that may be reasonable or highly biased.
- Almost all writing is biased to some degree, but strong writing makes an effort to eliminate bias.

EVALUATING AND INTEGRATING DATA

Effective readers do more than absorb and analyze the content of sentences, paragraphs, and chapters. They recognize the importance of features that stand out in and around the text, and they understand and integrate knowledge from visual features like maps and charts.

Text Features

Elements that stand out from a text are called **text features**. Text features perform many vital functions.

- **Introducing the Topic and Organizing Information**

> **COMPARE!**
> The title on a fictional work does not always state the topic explicitly. While some titles do this, others are more concerned with hinting at a theme or setting up the tone.

  - *Titles* – The title of a nonfiction text typically introduces the topic. Titles are guiding features of organization because they give clues about what is and is not covered. The title of this section, "Text Features," covers exactly that—not, for example, implicit ideas.
  - *Headings and Subheadings* – Headings and subheadings provide subtopic information about supporting points and let readers scan to see how information is organized. The subheadings of this page organize text features according to the functions they perform.

- **Helping the Reader Find Information**

  - *Table of Contents* – The table of contents of a long work lists chapter titles and other large-scale information so readers can predict the content. This helps readers to determine whether or not a text will be useful to them and to find sections relevant to their research.
  - *Index* – In a book, the index is an alphabetical list of topics covered, complete with page numbers where the topics are discussed. Readers looking for information on one small subtopic can check the index to find out which pages to view.
  - *Footnotes and Endnotes* – When footnotes and endnotes list sources, they allow the reader to find and evaluate the information an author is citing.

- **Emphasizing Concepts**

  - *Formatting Features* – Authors may use formatting features such as *italics*, **boldfacing** or underlining to emphasize a word, phrase, or other important information in a text.
  - *Bulleting and numbering* – Bullet points and numbered lists set off information and allow readers to scan for bits of information they do not know. It also helps to break down a list of steps.

- **Presenting Information and Illustrating Ideas**

  - *Graphic Elements* – Charts, graphs, diagrams, and other graphic elements present data succinctly, illustrate complex ideas, or otherwise convey information that would be difficult to glean from text alone.

- **Providing Peripheral Information**

  - *Sidebars* – Sidebars are text boxes that contain information related to the topic but not essential to the overall point.

  - *Footnotes and Endnotes* – Some footnotes and endnotes contain information that is not essential to the development of the main point but may nevertheless interest readers and researchers.[1]

> **FUN FACT!**
>
> Online, a sidebar is sometimes called a *doobly doo*.
>
> P.S. This is an example of a sidebar.

Maps and Charts

To read maps and charts, you need to understand what the labels, symbols, and pictures mean. You also need to know how to make decisions using the information they contain.

Maps

Maps are stylized pictures of places as seen from above. A map may have a box labeled "Key" or "Legend" that provides information about the meanings of colors, lines, or symbols. On the map below, the key shows that a solid line is a road and a dotted line is a trail.

There may also be a line labeled "scale" that helps you figure out how far you need to travel to get from one point on the map to another. In the example below, an inch is only 100 feet, so a trip from one end to the other is not far.

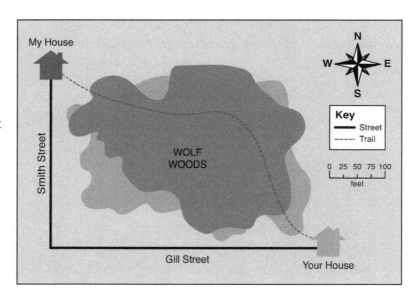

Some maps, including the example above, have compasses that show directions. If no compass is pictured, assume the top of the map is north.

---

[1] Anthony Grafton's book *The Footnote: A Curious History* is an in-depth history of the origins and development of the footnote. (Also, this is an example of a footnote.)

Charts

Nutrition Facts Labels

Nutrition facts labels are charts many people see daily, but not everyone knows how to read them. The top third of the label lists calorie counts, serving sizes, and amount of servings in a package. If a package contains more than one serving, a person who eats the entire contents of the package may be consuming many times the number of calories listed per serving.

The label below lists the content of nutrients such as fats and carbohydrates, and so on. According to the label, a person who eats one serving of the product in the package will ingest 30 mg of cholesterol, or 10% of the total cholesterol he or she should consume in a day.

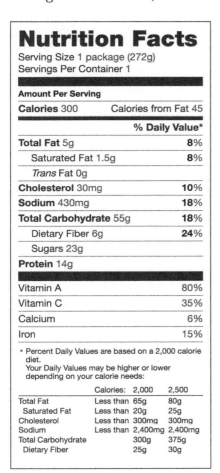

KEEP IN MIND . . .

The percentages on a Nutrition Facts label do not (and are not meant to) add up to 100. Instead, they show how much of a particular nutrient is contained in a serving of the product, as a proportion of a single person's Daily Value for that nutrient. The Daily Value is the total amount of a nutrient a person is supposed to eat in a day, based on a 2000-calorie diet.

In general, a percentage of 5% or less is considered low, whereas a percentage of 20% or more is considered high. A higher percentage can be good or bad, depending on whether or not a person should be trying to get more of a particular ingredient. People need to get plenty of vitamins, minerals, and fiber. In contrast, most people need to limit their intake of fat, cholesterol, and sodium.

Tables

Tables organize information into vertical columns and horizontal rows. Below is a table that shows how much water falls on areas of various sizes when it rains one inch. It shows, for instance, that a 40'x70' roof receives 1,743 gallons of rain during a one-inch rainfall event.

Area	Area (square miles)	Area (square kilometers)	Amount of water (gallons)	Amount of water (liters)
My roof 40x70 feet	.0001	.000257	1,743 gallons	6,601 liters
1 acre (1 square mile = 640 acres)	.00156	.004	27,154 gallons	102,789 liters
1 square mile	1	2.6	17.38 million gallons	65.78 million liters
Atlanta, Georgia	132.4	342.9	2.293 billion gallons	8.68 billion liters
United States	3,537,438	9,161,922	61,474 billion gallons	232,700 billion liters

Let's Review!

- Readers must understand how and why text features make certain information stand out from the text.
- Readers must understand and interpret the content of maps and charts.

Types of Passages, Text Structures, Genre and Theme

To read effectively, you must understand what kind of text you are reading and how it is structured. You must also be able to look behind the text to find its deeper meanings.

Types of Passages

There are many ways of breaking texts down into categories. To do this, you need to consider the author's **purpose**, or what the text exists to do. Most texts exist to inform, persuade, or entertain. You also need to consider what the text does—whether it tells a story, describes facts, or develops a point of view.

Type of Passage	Examples
Narrative writing tells a story. The story can be fictional, or it can describe real events. The primary purpose of narrative writing is to entertain.	• An autobiography • A memoir • A short story • A novel
Expository writing provides an explanation or a description. Many academic essays and informational nonfiction books are expository writing. Stylistically, expository writing is highly varied. Although the explanations can be dry and methodical, many writers use an artful or entertaining style. Expository writing is nonfiction. Its primary purpose is to inform.	• A book about a historical event • An essay describing the social impacts of a new technology • A description of changing gender roles in marriages • A philosophical document exploring the nature of truth.
Technical writing explains a complex process or mechanism. Whereas expository writing is often academic, technical writing is used in practical settings such as businesses. The style of a technical document is almost always straightforward and impersonal. Technical writing is nonfiction, and its purpose is to inform.	• Recipes • Instructions • User manuals • Process descriptions
Persuasive writing makes an argument. It asks readers to believe something or do something. Texts that make judgments, such as movie reviews, are persuasive because they are attempting to convince readers to accept a point of view. Texts that suggest a plan are also persuasive because they are trying to convince readers to take an action. As the name "persuasive writing" indicates, the author's primary purpose is to persuade.	• Op-ed newspaper articles • Book reviews • Project proposals • Advertisements • Persuasive essays

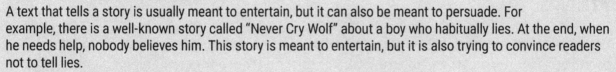

BE CAREFUL!

Many texts have more than one purpose.

A text that tells a story is usually meant to entertain, but it can also be meant to persuade. For example, there is a well-known story called "Never Cry Wolf" about a boy who habitually lies. At the end, when he needs help, nobody believes him. This story is meant to entertain, but it is also trying to convince readers not to tell lies.

Similarly, many explanatory texts are meant to inform readers in an entertaining way. For example, a nonfiction author may describe a scientific topic using humor and wacky examples to make it fun for popular audiences to read.

Also, expository writing can look similar to persuasive writing, especially when it touches on topics that are controversial or emotional. For example, if an essay says social media is changing society, many readers assume it means social media is changing society *in a negative way.* If the writing makes this kind of value judgment or uses words like *should,* it is persuasive writing. But if the author is merely describing changes, the text is expository.

Text Structures

Authors rarely present ideas within a text in a random order. Instead, they organize their thoughts carefully. To read effectively, you must be able to recognize the **structure** of a text. That is, you need to identify the strategies authors use to organize their ideas. The five most common text structures are listed below.

Text Structure	Examples
In a **sequence** text, an author explains what happened first, second, third, and so on. In other words, a sequence text is arranged in **chronological order**, or time order. This type of text may describe events that have already happened or events that may happen in the future.	• A story about a birthday party. • A historical paper about World War II. • A list of instructions for baking a cake. • A series of proposed steps in a plan for business expansion.
A **compare/contrast** text explains the similarities and differences between two or more subjects. Authors may compare and contrast people, places, ideas, events, cultures, and so on.	• An essay describing the similarities and differences between women's experiences in medieval Europe and Asia. • A section in an op-ed newspaper article explaining the similarities and differences between two types of gun control.
A **cause/effect** text describes an event or action and its results. The causes and effects discussed can be actual or theoretical. That is, the author can describe the results of a historical event or predict the results of a possible future event.	• An explanation of ocean acidification and the coral bleaching that results. • A paper describing a proposed new law and its likely effects on the economy.
A **problem-solution** text presents a problem and outlines a solution. Sometimes it also predicts or analyzes the results of the solution. The solution can be something that already happened or a plan the author is proposing. Note that a problem can sometimes be expressed in terms of a wish or desire that the solution fulfills.	• An explanation of the problems smallpox caused and the strategies scientists used to eradicate it. • A business plan outlining a group of potential customers and the strategy a company should use to get their business.

Text Structure	Examples
A **description** text creates a mental picture for the reader by presenting concrete details in a coherent order. Description texts are usually arranged spatially. For instance, authors may describe the subject from top to bottom, or they may describe the inside first and then the outside, etc.	• An explanation of the appearance of a character in a story. • A paragraph in a field guide detailing the features of a bird. • A section on an instruction sheet describing how the final product should look.

KEEP IN MIND . . .

The text structures above do not always work in isolation. Authors often combine two or more structures within one text. For example, a business plan could be arranged in a problem-solution structure as the author describes what the business wants to achieve and how she proposes to achieve it. The "how" portion could also use a sequence structure as the author lists the steps to follow first, second, third, and so on.

CONNECTIONS

Different types of texts can use the same structures.

1. A story about a birthday party is a narrative, and its purpose is to entertain.
2. A historical paper about a war is an expository text meant to inform.
3. A list of instructions for baking a cake is a technical text meant to inform.
4. A series of proposed steps in a plan for business expansion is a persuasive text meant to persuade.

If all of these texts list ideas in chronological order, explaining what happened (or what may happen in the future) first, second, third, and so on, they are all using a sequence structure.

Genre and Theme

Literature can be organized into categories called **genres**. The two major genres of literature are fiction and nonfiction.

Fiction is made up. It can be broken down into many sub-genres, or sub-categories. The following are some of the common ones:

- Short story – Short work of fiction.
- Novel – Book-length work of fiction.
- Science fiction – A story set in the future
- Romance – A love story
- Mystery – A story that answers a concrete question, often about who committed a crime
- Mythology – A traditional story that reflects cultural traditions and beliefs but does not usually teach an explicit lesson
- Legends – Traditional stories that are presented as histories, even though they often contain fantastical or magical elements
- Fables – Traditional stories meant to teach an explicit lesson

COMPARE!

The differences between myths and fables are sometimes hard to discern.

Myths are often somewhat religious in nature. For instance, stories about Ancient Greek gods and goddesses are myths. These stories reflect cultural beliefs, for example by showing characters being punished for failing to please their gods. But the lesson is implicit. These stories do not usually end with a moral lesson that says to readers, "Do not displease the gods!"

Fables are often for children, and they usually end with a sentence stating an explicit moral. For example, there's a story called "The Tortoise and the Hare," in which a tortoise and a hare agree to have a race. The hare, being a fast animal, gets cocky and takes a lot of breaks while the tortoise plods slowly toward the finish line without stopping. Because the tortoise keeps going, it eventually wins. The story usually ends with the moral, "Slow and steady win the race."

Nonfiction is true. Like fiction, it can be broken down into many sub-genres. The following are some of the common ones:

- Autobiography and memoir – The author's own life story
- Biography – Someone else's life story (not the author's)
- Histories – True stories about real events from the past
- Criticism and reviews – A response or judgment on another piece of writing or art
- Essay – A short piece describing the author's outlook or point of view.

CONNECTIONS

Everything under "Fiction" and several items under "Nonfiction" above are examples of narrative writing. We use labels like "narrative" and "persuasive" largely when we discuss writing tasks or the author's purpose. We could use these labels here too, but at the moment we're more concerned with the words that are most commonly used in discussions about literature's deeper meanings.

Literature reflects the human experience. Texts from different genres often share similar **themes**, or deeper meanings. Texts from different cultures do too. For example, a biography of a famous civil rights activist may highlight the same qualities of heroism and interconnectedness that appear in a work of mythology from Ancient India. Other common themes in literature may relate to war, love, survival, justice, suffering, growing up, and other experiences that are accessible to virtually all human beings.

Many students confuse the term *theme* with the term *moral*. A **moral** is an explicit message contained in the text, like "Don't lie" or "Crime doesn't pay." Morals are a common feature of fables and other traditional stories meant to teach lessons to children. Themes, in contrast, are implicit. Readers must consider the clues in the story and figure out themes for themselves. Because of this, themes are debatable. For testing purposes, questions focus on themes that are clearly and consistently indicated by clues within the text.

Let's Review!

- Written texts can be organized into the following categories: narrative, expository, technical, and persuasive.
- Texts of all categories may use the following organizational schemes or structures: sequence, compare/contrast, cause/effect, problem-solution, description.
- Literature can be organized into genres including fiction, nonfiction, and many sub-genres.
- Literature across genres and cultures often reflects the same deeper meanings, or themes.

CHAPTER 10 INTEGRATION OF KNOWLEDGE AND IDEAS
PRACTICE QUIZ

1. **Which of the following is *not* a function of text features?**

   A. Introducing the topic

   B. Emphasizing a concept

   C. Making the theme explicit

   D. Providing peripheral information

2. **If a map does not have a compass, north is:**

   A. up.   C. right.

   B. down.   D. left.

3. **The purpose of an index is to tell readers:**

   A. how to find sources that back up key ideas in the text.

   B. who wrote the text and what his or her credentials are.

   C. where to find information on a given subject within a book.

   D. why the author believes the main idea of a text is important.

Read the following passage and answer questions 4-5.

Overworked public school teachers are required by law to spend extra time implementing Individual Educational Plans for students with learning and attention challenges. This shortchanges children who are actually engaged in their education by depriving them of an equal amount of individualized attention.

4. **What assumption behind this passage reflects negative stereotypical thinking?**

   A. Public school teachers are generally overworked and underpaid.

   B. Students with learning disabilities are not engaged in their education.

   C. Laws require teachers to provide accommodations to certain students.

   D. Teachers have a finite amount of attention to divide between students.

5. **The above argument is invalid because the author:**

   A. suggests that some students do not need as much attention because they learn the material more quickly.

   B. uses derogatory and disrespectful word choice to describe people who think, learn, and process information differently.

   C. describes public school teachers in a negative way that makes it seem as though they have no interest in helping students.

   D. professes an interest in equality for all students while simultaneously suggesting some students are more worthy than others.

6. Which statement, if true, is a fact?

    A. The 1918 flu pandemic killed more people than World War I.

    B. The 1918 flu pandemic was more devastating than World War I.

    C. The 1918 flu pandemic was a terrifying display of nature's power.

    D. The 1918 flu pandemic caused greater social instability than the plague.

Read the following passage and answer questions 7-9.

There is inherent risk associated with the use of Rip Gym facilities. Although all Rip Gym customers sign a Risk Acknowledgment and Consent Form before gaining access to our grounds and equipment, litigation remains a possibility if customers suffer injuries due to negligence. Negligence complaints may include either staff mistakes or avoidable problems with equipment and facilities. It is therefore imperative that all Rip Gym employees follow the Safety Protocol in the event of a customer complaint.

Reports of Unsafe Equipment and Environs

Rip Gym employees must always respond promptly and seriously to any customer report of a hazard in our equipment or facilities, even if the employee judges the complaint frivolous. **Customers may not use rooms or equipment that have been reported unsafe until the following steps have been taken, in order, to confirm and/or resolve the problem.**

1. Place "Warning," "Out of Order," or "Off Limits" signs in the affected area or on the affected equipment, as appropriate. **Always follow this step first, before handling paperwork or attempting to resolve the reported problem.**

2. Fill out a Hazard Complaint Form. Include the name of the customer making the complaint and the exact wording of the problems being reported.

3. Visually check the area or equipment in question to verify the problem.

    a) If the report appears to be **accurate** and a resolution is necessary, proceed to step 4.

    b) If the report appears to be **inaccurate**, consult the manager on duty.

4. Determine whether you are qualified to correct the problem. Problems **all** employees are qualified to correct are listed on page 12 of the Employee Handbook.

    a) Employees who have **not** undergone training for equipment repair and maintenance must....

7. This passage is best described as a(n):

    A. narrative text.

    B. technical text.

    C. expository text.

    D. persuasive text.

8. **Which term best describes the structure of the opening paragraph?**

   A. Sequence

   B. Description

   C. Problem-solution

   D. Compare/contrast

9. **Which term best describes the structure of the section under the subheading "Reports of Unsafe Equipment and Environs"?**

   A. Sequence

   B. Description

   C. Cause/effect

   D. Compare/contrast

Chapter 10 Integration of Knowledge and Ideas
Practice Quiz – Answer Key

1. C. Although the title of a fictional work may hint at a theme, a theme is a message that is, by definition, not stated explicitly. **See Lesson: Evaluating and Integrating Data.**

2. A. By convention, north on a map is up. Mapmakers include a compass if they break this convention for some reason. **See Lesson: Evaluating and Integrating Data.**

3. C. An index lists subtopics of a book along with page numbers where those topics will be covered. **See Lesson: Evaluating and Integrating Data.**

4. B. The writer of this passage suggests implicitly that only students without learning and attention challenges are engaged in their education. This assumption reflects a negative stereotype that renders the entire argument faulty. **See Lesson: Facts, Opinions, and Evaluating an Argument.**

5. B. The author of the passage uses the phrase "students with learning and attention challenges" to refer to students who think and learn differently. This is not derogatory, but even so, the passage implies that people who experience these differences are less engaged in their education. **See Lesson: Facts, Opinions, and Evaluating an Argument.**

6. A. All of these statements contain beliefs or feelings that are subject to interpretation except the statement about the number of people killed in the 1918 flu pandemic compared to World War I. This is a verifiable piece of information, or a fact. **See Lesson: Facts, Opinions, and Evaluating an Argument.**

7. B. This is a technical text written to inform the reader about a complex process. **See Lesson: Types of Passages, Text Structures, Genre and Theme.**

8. C. The opening paragraph has a problem-solution structure. The problem it describes involves risks of injury and litigation, and the solution is that employees follow a process designed to minimize those risks. **See Lesson: Types of Passages, Text Structures, Genre and Theme.**

9. A. The step-by-step instructions under the subheading follow a sequential structure. Note key words and phrases such as "first" and "in order." **See Lesson: Types of Passages, Text Structures, Genre and Theme.**

SECTION IV. SCIENCE

CHAPTER 11 HUMAN ANATOMY AND PHYSIOLOGY: ORGANIZATION OF SYSTEMS

ORGANIZATION OF THE HUMAN BODY

Human anatomy and physiology is the study of the structures and functions of the human body.

Levels of Organization and Body Cavities

The body can be studied at seven structural levels: **chemical, organelle, cell, tissue, organ, organ system,** and **organism**.

- **Chemical:** The chemical level involves interactions among atoms and their combination into molecules.
- **Organelle:** An organelle is a small structure contained within a cell that performs one or more specific functions.
- **Cell:** Cells are the basic functional units of life. All cells share many characteristics, but they differ in structure and function.
- **Tissue:** A tissue is a group of cells with similar structures and functions.
- **Organ:** An organ is composed of two or more tissue types that together perform one or more common function.
- **Organ system:** An organ system is a group of organs classified as a unit because of a common function or set of functions.
- **Organism:** An organism is any living thing considered as a whole. Organisms can have anywhere from a single cell to trillions of cells.

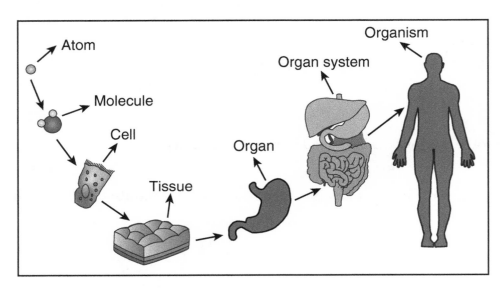

Body Cavities

The human body has many cavities, some of which open to the exterior. A **cavity** is a fluid-filled space in the body that holds and protects internal organs. The **ventral cavity** (front of the body) contains three major cavities:

- The **thoracic cavity** is surrounded by the rib cage and separated from the abdominal cavity by the diaphragm. It is divided into right and left halves by a structure called the mediastinum. It contains the esophagus, trachea, thymus gland, heart, and both lungs, along with other structures.
- The **abdominal cavity** is bounded by the abdominal muscles below the thoracic cavity and contains the stomach, intestines, liver, spleen, pancreas, and kidneys.
- The **pelvic cavity** is enclosed by the bones of the pelvis and contains the urinary bladder, part of the intestines, and the internal reproductive organs. The abdominal and pelvic cavities are sometimes referred to as the abdominopelvic cavity.

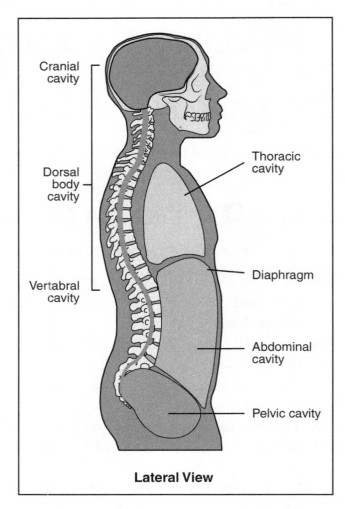

Lateral View

The **dorsal cavity** is the back of the human body, and it is subdivided into two cavities: cranial and spinal.

- The **cranial cavity** contains the brain.
- The **spinal cavity** contains the spinal cord.

Example

Which of the following organs is located in the pelvic cavity?

A. Heart   B. Intestines   C. Liver   D. Pancreas

The correct answer is **B**. The intestines are located in both the abdominal and pelvic cavities.

Terminology and the Body Planes and Regions

Directional terms refer to the body in the **anatomical position**, regardless of its actual position. The term *anatomical position* refers to a person standing erect with the feet forward, arms hanging to the sides, and the palms of the hands facing forward.

Terminology

Term	Definition
Inferior	A structure below another
Superior	A structure above another
Anterior	Toward the front of the body
Posterior	Toward the back of the body
Dorsal	Toward the back
Ventral	Toward the front
Proximal	Closer to the point of attachment to the body than another structure
Distal	Farther from the point of attachment to the body
Lateral	Away from the midline of the body
Medial	Toward the middle or midline of the body
Superficial	Toward or on the surface
Deep	Away from the surface
Anterosuperior	In front or above
Midline	A median line
Supine position	Lying flat with face and torso facing upward
Prone position	Lying face down

Body Planes

Sectioning the body is a way to look inside and observe the body's structures. The following are the major planes of the body:

- The **sagittal plane** runs vertically through the body and separates the body into right and left parts.
- The **midsagittal plane** divides the body into two equal halves.
- The **transverse plane** runs parallel to the surface of the ground and divides the body into superior and inferior planes.
- The **coronal plane**, sometimes called the frontal plane, runs vertically from left to right and divides the body into anterior and posterior parts.

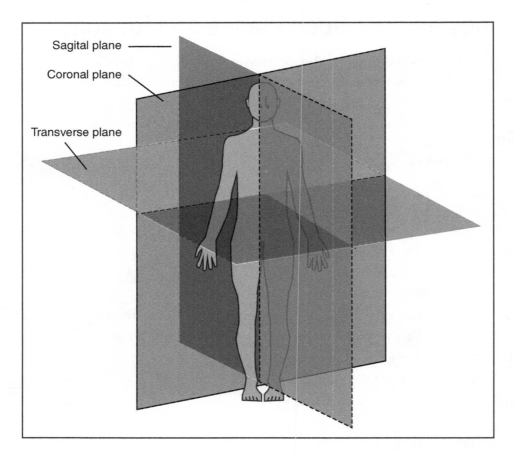

Body Regions

The body is divided into the following four regions:

- **Upper limb:** The upper limb includes the arm, forearm, wrist, and hand.
- **Lower limb:** The lower limb is divided into the thigh, leg, ankle, and foot.
- **Central region:** The central region includes the neck and trunk.
- **Head region:** The head region includes the entire head.

Example

The wrist is _____ to the shoulder.

   A. distal   B. lateral   C. median   D. superior

The correct answer is **A.** The wrist is farther from the point of attachment than the shoulder is, so it is distal to the shoulder.

Human Tissues

A **tissue** is a group of cells with similar structure and function and similar extracellular substances located between the cells. The table below describes the four primary tissues found in the human body.

Tissue	Structure	Function	Example
Connective	characterized by extracellular material that separate cells from one another	enclosing and separating connecting tissues to one another supportive and moving storing cushioning and insulating transporting protecting	cells of the immune system and blood
Epithelial	classified according to the number of cell layers and shapes	protecting underlying structures acting as barriers permitting the passage of substances secreting substances	skin, linings of internal organs
Muscle	cells of muscles resemble long threads and are called *fibers*	providing movement	heart, organs of digestive system
Neural	cells are composed of dendrites, cell bodies, and axons	coordinating and controlling many body activities	brain, spinal cord

Four Types of Tissue

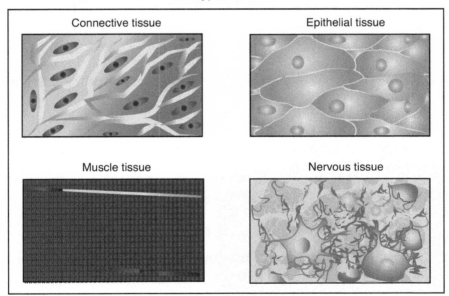

Example

Which type of tissue controls when the heart beats?

A. Connective   B. Epithelial   C. Muscle   D. Nervous

The correct answer is **D.** Although the muscle tissue is responsible for the actual movement of the heart, the neural tissue "tells" the heart when to beat.

Homeostasis and Feedback Mechanisms

Homeostasis is the existence and maintenance of a relatively constant environment within the body. Each cell of the body is surrounded by a small amount of fluid, and the normal functions of each cell depend on the maintenance of its fluid environment within a narrow range of conditions, including temperature, volume, and chemical content. These conditions are known as **variables**. For example, body temperature is a variable that can increase in a hot environment or decrease in a cold environment.

There are two types of feedback mechanisms in the human body: negative and positive.

Negative Feedback

Most systems of the body are regulated by **negative feedback mechanisms**, which maintain homeostasis. *Negative* means that any deviation from the set point is made smaller or is resisted. The maintenance of normal blood pressure is a negative-feedback mechanism. Normal blood pressure is important because it is responsible for moving blood from the heart to tissues.

Positive Feedback

Positive-feedback mechanisms are not homeostatic and are rare in healthy individuals. *Positive* means that when a deviation from a normal value occurs, the response of the system is to make the deviation even greater. Positive feedback therefore usually creates a cycle leading away from homeostasis and, in some cases, results in death. Inadequate delivery of blood to cardiac muscle is an example of positive feedback.

Example

Childbirth is a response to hormones in a woman's body. What type of feedback mechanism is at work during childbirth?

    A. Neutral feedback

    B. Positive feedback

    C. Negative feedback

    D. Need more information

The correct answer is **B**. During childbirth, the frequency and strength of the contractions increases until the contractions are powerful enough to deliver the baby.

Let's Review!

- The body can be studied at seven structural levels.
- The human body has multiple body cavities.
- Directional terms refer to the body in the anatomical position.
- Sectioning the body is a way to look inside and observe the body's structures.
- The four primary tissues found in the human body are connective, epithelial, muscular and nervous.
- Homeostasis is the existence and maintenance of a relatively constant environment within the body.
- The two types of feedback mechanisms in the human body are negative and positive feedback mechanisms.

THE CARDIOVASCULAR SYSTEM

This lesson introduces the anatomy of blood and its connection to the cardiovascular system. Explore the parts that make up the cardiovascular system and how this system functions.

Anatomy of Blood

Blood is a type of fluid connective tissue that circulates throughout the body, carrying substances to and away from bodily tissues. It has a pH of about 7.4 and is more viscous than water. Blood consists of three types of formed elements, an extracellular matrix called **plasma,** molecules, cell fragments, and debris. The formed elements consist of red blood cells, white blood cells, and platelets. They are also referred to as **erythrocytes**, **leukocytes**, and **thrombocytes**, respectively. The following table details key characteristics of these elements.

Characteristic	Red Blood Cells	White Blood Cells	Platelets
Scientific Name	Erythrocytes	Leukocytes	Thrombocytes
Size (Diameter)	0.008 mm	0.02 mm	0.003 mm
Function	Participate in gas exchange, primarily with oxygen and carbon dioxide	Protect the body from foreign substances by eliciting an immune response	Aid in blood clotting and wound healing

Plasma is different from other types of connective tissue because it is a fluid. Consisting of about 92% water, formed elements remain suspended in the matrix where they are circulated throughout the body.

> **DID YOU KNOW?**
> The average volume of blood in the human body, for a 70-kilogram person, is 5 liters. Blood accounts for roughly 8% of a person's body weight.

Consider the following image, which illustrates the composition of blood in a person's blood sample. When a blood sample is spun in a centrifuge, less-dense plasma floats on top of a reddish mass that consists of red blood cells. There is also a thin white layer called the **buffy coat** that consists of white blood cells and platelets. This layer is found between the reddish mass and plasma layers.

> **KEEP IN MIND**
> Blood viscosity is indirectly proportional to blood flow throughout the body. If the viscosity of blood is high, blood flow decreases. When blood viscosity is low, or blood is thin, blood flow increases.

Example

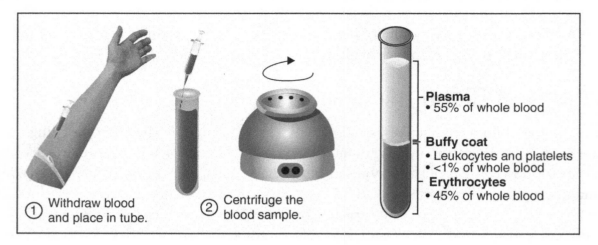

Plasma
• 55% of whole blood

Buffy coat
• Leukocytes and platelets
• <1% of whole blood

Erythrocytes
• 45% of whole blood

① Withdraw blood and place in tube.

② Centrifuge the blood sample.

A laboratory technician needs to determine the leukocyte count in a patient. From which part of a blood sample are these cells extracted?

A. Water   B. Buffy coat   C. Liquid plasma   D. Reddish mass

The correct answer is **B.** Buffy coat contains white blood cells (or leukocytes) and platelets in blood.

Functions of Blood

Transportation, regulation, and protection are three primary functions of blood. Blood transports the following substances throughout the body:

- Gases: Blood delivers oxygen from the lungs to all cells in the body. It also transports carbon dioxide to the lungs for elimination from the body.
- Nutrients: Blood transports nutrients from the digestive tract and storage sites in the body to various places in the body.
- Wastes: Blood transports waste products to the liver, where they are excreted as bile. Waste products also travel by blood to the kidneys when they need to be excreted as urine.
- Hormones: Blood transports hormones from the glands where they are produced to their target organs.

> **KEEP IN MIND**
> Albumin is the main protein in blood, accounting for roughly 60% of the plasma proteins in blood. It plays a role in water balance and functions as a carrier protein, shuttling certain molecules throughout the body.

Although blood's primary function is to distribute substances throughout the body, it also has regulatory functions. These functions include the regulation of body temperature, chemical balance, and water balance. Blood ensures the right body temperature is maintained with help from plasma and the speed of blood flow. Plasma is able to absorb or give off heat. As shown in the following image, when blood vessels expand, or **vasodilate**, blood flows slowly, causing heat loss. This occurs when the temperature of the external environment is high. If external environmental temperatures are low, blood vessels contract, or **vasoconstrict**, causing less heat to be released.

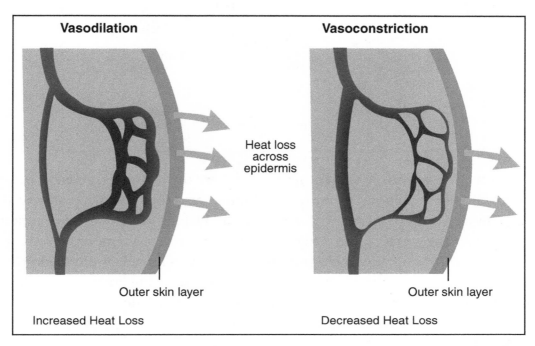

Blood also functions as a form of protection, defending the body against foreign invaders or **pathogens** that harm the body. As blood circulates through the body, it carries white blood cells and **antibodies** that destroy any pathogens they encounter. With the help of platelets and plasma proteins, blood also protects the body from extensive blood loss if a blood vessel is damaged.

Example

Platelets are important because they

    A. give blood its natural color.

    B. repair broken blood vessels.

    C. transport nutrients to the cells.

    D. protect the body against infection.

The correct answer is **B**. At the site of injury or damage to a blood vessel, platelets help repair the damaged area.

Hemostasis

Recall that a function of platelets and plasma proteins is to repair damaged blood vessels. When blood vessels are damaged, a physiological process called hemostasis is activated. **Hemostasis** helps maintain blood in its fluid state and stops blood from leaking out of a damaged blood vessel through clot formation. As shown in the image below, there are three steps of hemostasis.

Steps of Hemostasis

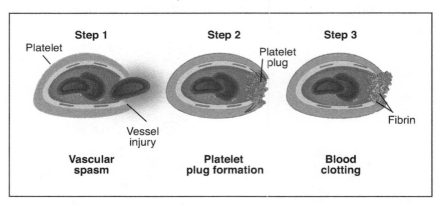

The first step is **vascular spasm**, or vasoconstriction, where the blood vessels constrict to reduce blood loss. Reducing blood loss for several hours, this process works best with small blood vessels. The second step is platelet plug formation. Platelets adhere to the epithelial wall of the blood vessel and aggregate by sticking together. This creates a temporary seal over the damaged site. In the third step, **blood coagulation** occurs. Also known as **blood clotting**, this process is a series of events that strengthen the platelet plug by using fibrin threads to form a mesh around the plug. The protein mesh functions as a molecular glue, securing the plug to the damaged site. Red blood cells and platelets remain trapped at the damaged site, forming a clot that facilitates wound healing.

Example

What happens after platelets aggregate at a damaged blood vessel site?

  A. The site of the wound is healed.

  B. The damaged blood vessel constricts.

  C. The platelets stick together and form a plug.

  D. Red blood cells are recruited to the injured site.

The correct answer is **C**. After the platelets aggregate at the damaged site, they stick together to form a plug. Next, blood coagulation occurs when a fibrin mesh forms around the platelet aggregate.

Blood Grouping and Agglutination

There are several different types or groups of blood, and the major groups are A, B, AB, and O. Blood group is a way to classify blood according to inherited differences of red blood cell **antigens** found on the surface of a red blood cell. The type of antibody in blood also identifies a particular blood group. **Antibodies** are proteins found in the plasma. They function as part of the body's natural defense to recognize foreign substances and alert the immune system.

Depending on which antigen is inherited, parental offspring will have one of the four major blood groups. Collectively, the following major blood groups comprise the ABO system:

- Blood group A: Displays type A antigens on the surface of a red blood cell and contains B antibodies in the plasma.
- Blood group B: Displays type B antigens on the red blood cell's surface and contains A antibodies in the plasma.
- Blood group O: Does not display A or B antigens on the surface of a red blood cell. Both A and B antibodies are in the plasma.
- Blood group AB: Displays type A and B antigens on the red blood cell's surface, but neither A nor B antibodies are in the plasma.

> **KEEP IN MIND**
> A person can be a universal blood donor or acceptor. A universal blood donor has type O blood, while a universal blood acceptor has type AB blood.

In addition to antigens, the **Rh factor** protein may exist on a red blood cell's surface. Because this protein can be either present (+) or absent (-), it increases the number of major blood groups from four to eight: A+, A-, B+, B-, O+, O-, AB+, and AB-. The following table summarizes what blood types a person can receive or donate.

Blood Group	Can accept blood from	Can donate blood to
A	A, O	A, AB
B	B, O	B, AB
AB	AB, A, B, O	AB
O	O	AB, A, B, O

When determining an individual's blood type, a sample of blood is mixed with an antiserum. If **agglutination**, or clumping, occurs during this process, the antibody has found an antigen with which to interact. This means there are antigens on the surface of the red blood cell to which the antibodies can bind. Evidence of agglutination is used to interpret the final blood type result from a sample.

Example

People with type O blood can accept blood from people with _____ blood.

A. type O   B. type B   C. type AB   D. type A

The correct answer is **A**. People with type O blood are universal donors but can accept blood only from people with type O blood.

Cardiovascular Anatomy

The **cardiovascular system** circulates substances throughout the body using blood as a transporting mechanism. The organs of the cardiovascular system work together to supply cells and tissues with oxygen and nutrients and remove cellular wastes such as carbon dioxide. Blood, heart, and blood vessels form this system.

Because blood circulation is a closed loop system, blood is contained within the heart or blood vessels at all times. There are three types of blood vessels: arteries, veins, and capillaries. **Arteries** carry blood away from the heart, toward organs and tissues. **Veins** carry blood toward the heart, away from organs and tissues. Arteries branch into smaller blood vessels called **arterioles**, which further divide into capillaries. As shown in the following image, **capillaries** are tiny vessels that form a network around tissues. Veins branch into venules before further dividing into capillaries.

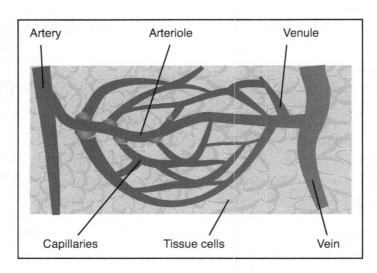

The heart is found between the lungs in the middle of the chest. It rests behind and slightly to the left of the sternum, or breastbone. The human heart is a muscular organ composed primarily of cardiac muscle. It consists of four chambers: two upper chambers called the **atria** and two lower chambers called the **ventricles**. The atria are separated from the ventricles by a muscular structure called the **septum**. Three layers make up the heart wall. These are the **pericardium** or outer layer, the **myocardium** or middle layer, and the **endocardium** or innermost layer. Most cardiac muscle tissue is found in the myocardium.

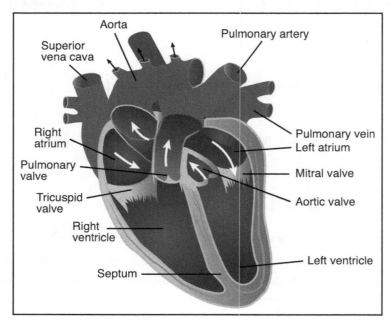

DID YOU KNOW?

Capillaries have thin walls and a very large surface area. Because of the capillaries' thin walls, blood flow slows to facilitate exchanges between blood and the body's tissues.

In addition to the four chambers, the heart has four valves that regulate blood flow into and out of the heart:

- **Tricuspid valve** regulates blood flow between the right atrium and right ventricle.
- **Pulmonary valve** regulates blood flow from the right ventricle into the pulmonary artery.
- **Mitral valve** regulates blood flow from the left atrium into the left ventricle.
- **Aortic valve** regulates blood flow from the left ventricle to the **aorta**. The aorta is the largest artery in the body.

Example

Which heart layer is composed primarily of cardiac muscle?

A. Myocardium   B. Pericardium   C. Septum   D. Sternum

The correct answer is **A**. The heart is composed of three layers, the middle of which is the myocardium. The myocardium contains cardiac muscle tissue.

Circulation and the Cardiac Cycle

Blood continually flows in one direction, beginning in the heart and proceeding to the arteries, arterioles, and capillaries. When blood reaches the capillaries, exchanges occur between blood and tissues. After this exchange happens, blood is collected into venules, which feed into veins and eventually flow back to the heart's atrium. The heart must relax between two heartbeats for blood circulation to begin. Two types of circulatory processes occur in the body:

Systemic circulation
1. The pulmonary vein pushes oxygenated blood into the left atrium.
2. As the atrium relaxes, oxygenated blood drains into the left ventricle through the mitral valve.
3. The left ventricle pumps oxygenated blood to the aorta.
4. Blood travels through the arteries and arterioles before reaching the capillaries that surround the tissues.

Pulmonary circulation
1. Deoxygenated blood is sent back to the heart via the veins and pooled into the right atrium.
2. Blood travels through the superior vena cava and drains into the right ventricle.
3. The right ventricle contracts, causing the blood to be pushed through the pulmonary valve into the pulmonary artery.

4. Deoxygenated blood becomes oxygenated in the lungs.

5. Oxygenated blood returns from the lungs to the left atrium through the pulmonary veins.

The following image shows the heart's role in systemic and pulmonary circulation.

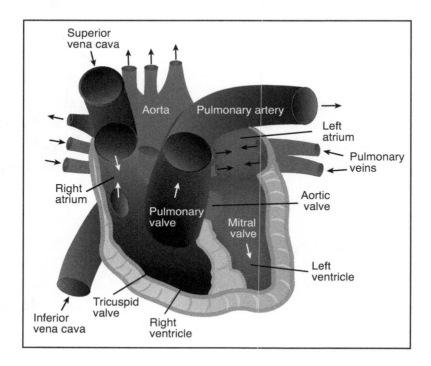

The complete cycle beginning with atrial contraction and ending with ventricular contraction is called the **cardiac cycle**. When the heart contracts and pumps blood into systemic circulation, this is called **systole**. **Diastole** refers to the period of relaxation when the heart chambers fill with blood.

KEEP IN MIND

Blood flow is regulated by many mechanisms in the body. This regulated variable is also directly proportional to blood pressure. If blood volume increases, blood pressure increases. The opposite occurs if blood pressure decreases.

Because the heart is a muscle, it transmits electrical impulses that cause the heart to contract. This electrical activity can be recorded using an **electrocardiogram**, or EKG. An EKG is a graph that shows the heart's rate and rhythm over a period of time. As shown in the following image of an EKG, waves in the graph have different meanings.

The first wave on an EKG is the P wave. This indicates atrial contraction or systole. The QRS complex represents the combination of Q, R, and S waves. This indicates ventricular systole or contraction. The T wave indicates ventricular diastole. The flat line between the S and T wave is the ST segment.

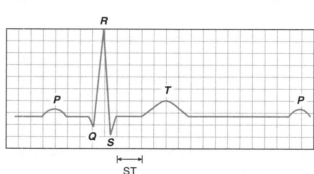

Example

What segment of the electrocardiogram is associated with atrial systole?

A. P wave   B. S wave   C. ST segment   D. QRS complex

The correct answer is **A.** Atrial systole occurs when the atrium contracts. On an EKG, atrial systole is indicated by a P wave.

Let's Review!

- Blood is a type of connective tissue composed of formed elements, plasma, and other substances.
- Erythrocytes, leukocytes, and thrombocytes are the formed elements that make up blood.
- Blood transports substances throughout the body, regulates physiological processes, and protects the body.
- There are four common blood groups that are determined by inherited differences in antigens on red blood cells.
- Agglutination, or clumping, can be used to help interpret the blood type of a blood sample.
- The cardiovascular system circulates blood throughout the body in a closed loop structure.
- The heart is a muscular organ with four chambers: two atria and two ventricles.
- Deoxygenated blood flows through pulmonary circulation, and oxygenated blood flows through systemic circulation.
- The cardiac cycle refers to the contraction and relaxation states of the atria and ventricles.
- An electrocardiogram, or EKG, is used to record heart beat and rhythm.

THE RESPIRATORY SYSTEM

This lesson introduces the anatomy of the respiratory system and how each organ within this system functions. It also discusses the mechanics of breathing and respiration.

Anatomy of the Respiratory System

Every living thing requires oxygen for survival. Humans can live for days without water and for weeks without food. But they can only survive a few minutes without air. The respiratory system's primary function is to bring oxygen into the body, in exchange for carbon dioxide. As shown in the following image, organs of the respiratory system include the nose, nasal cavity, mouth, larynx, pharynx, lungs, and diaphragm.

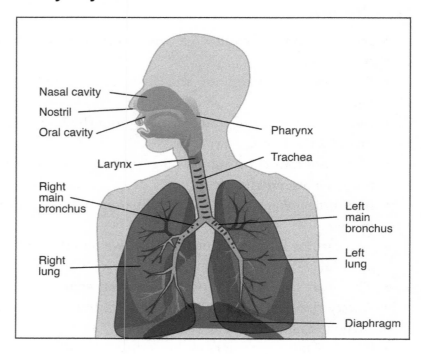

The respiratory organs can be divided into the upper and lower respiratory tract. The **upper respiratory tract** includes the nasal cavity, pharynx, and larynx. The trachea, bronchus, and lungs belong to the **lower respiratory tract**. The **nasal cavity** opens to the nose. The nose and nasal cavity warm and moisten air as a person breathes. As a defensive mechanism, tiny nose hairs and mucus produced by the epithelial mucosa cells in the nose help prevent particles in the air from entering the lungs.

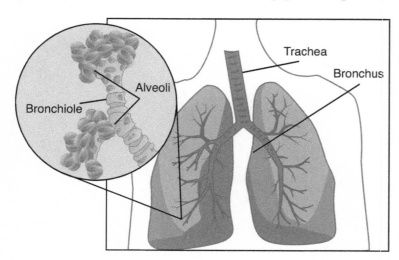

Behind the nasal cavity is the **pharynx**. Both food and air pass through this long tube. Just below the pharynx is the **larynx**, or voice box. It channels air to the trachea and pushes food past the **epiglottis**, which covers the trachea during swallowing to prevent food from entering the lungs. Once food passes the epiglottis, it moves toward the esophagus. When air reaches the **trachea**, or windpipe, it travels down a long tube that branches into **bronchi**. The bronchi enter the lungs. As shown in the image, the bronchi branch into **bronchioles** before reaching tiny air sacs in the lung called **alveoli**. Gas exchange occurs in the alveolar region.

The **diaphragm** is a muscle that plays a large role in breathing. It is found at the base of the lungs and spreads across the bottom of the rib cage, forming the chest cavity. The human body has two lungs that vary in size and weight. The right lung, which is larger and heavier, has three lobes. The left lung has two lobes.

DID YOU KNOW?
The total surface area of the alveoli in the lungs is roughly the size of a tennis court. Such a large surface area is needed to facilitate gas exchange and ensure the body is oxygenated at all times.

Example

Which organ uses hairs to filter out particles that try to enter the lungs?

A. Alveoli   B. Bronchus   C. Larynx   D. Nose

The correct answer is **D.** The nose is part of the upper respiratory tract. Because it is the site where air enters the body, nose hairs help prevent airborne particles from entering the lungs.

Respiratory Functions and Breathing Mechanics

Recall that the primary function of the respiratory system is to provide oxygen to and remove carbon dioxide from the body. In addition to gas exchange, the respiratory system enables a person to breathe. Breathing, or inhalation, is essential to life. It is the mechanism that provides oxygen to the body. Without oxygen, cells are unable to perform their functions necessary to keep the body alive.

The primary muscle of **inspiration** is the diaphragm. Known as the chest cavity, this dome-shaped structure flattens when it contracts. The rib cage moves outward, allowing outside air to be drawn into the lungs. During relaxation, the diaphragm returns to its dome shape and the rib cage moves back to its natural position. This causes the chest cavity to push air out of the lungs.

The respiratory system can be functionally divided into two parts:

- **Air-conducting portion:** Air is delivered to the lungs. This region consists of the upper and lower respiratory tract—specifically, the larynx, trachea, bronchi, and bronchioles.
- **Gas exchange portion:** Gas exchange takes place between the air and the blood. This portion includes the lungs, alveoli, and capillaries.

Alveolus Gas Exchange

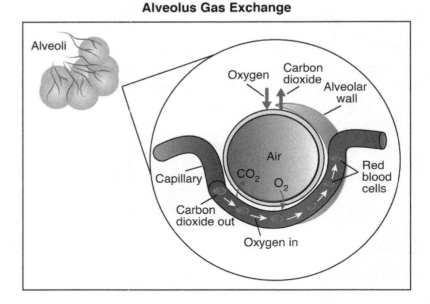

Oxygen from the air enters the body through the respiratory system. But the cardiovascular system circulates oxygen throughout the body via the blood. As shown in the image, alveoli are surrounded by a capillary bed in the lung.

This anatomical structure allows blood to absorb oxygen and transport it through a network of blood vessels to cells in various tissues throughout the body. During the process of gas exchange, the blood system absorbs carbon dioxide from cells and carries it to the respiratory system, where it is exhaled from the body.

The respiratory system works closely with both the cardiovascular and nervous systems to maintain blood gas and pH **homeostasis**. The body must regulate blood pH levels. When there is too much carbon dioxide in the blood, it is acidic (that is, its

BE CAREFUL!

When regulating blood gas and pH homeostasis levels, carbon dioxide, not oxygen, must be closely monitored.

pH value is too low). If there is not enough carbon dioxide in the blood, it will be too alkaline (its pH value will be too high).

Example

What structure is directly involved in gas exchange?

A. Alveolus   B. Bronchiole   C. Pharynx   D. Trachea

The correct answer is **A.** The alveolus is a tiny air sac found in the lung. Its primary function is to help the respiratory system perform gas exchange.

The Mechanics of Respiration

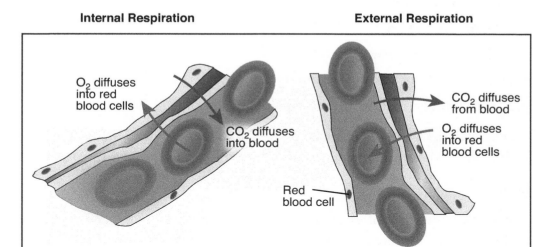

As shown in the image, the process of gas exchange between the outside air and the body is called **respiration**. It occurs on two levels: internal and external.

- **External respiration** occurs between the lungs and blood. When a person inhales, alveoli fill with oxygen through **diffusion**. Oxygen content is much higher than carbon dioxide levels. While in the alveoli region, blood becomes oxygen-rich. Once oxygenated, the blood leaves the lungs and travels through the left side of the heart, where it is pumped into circulation.

STEP-BY-STEP

The following four steps summarize external respiration:

Step 1. Air moves in and out of the lungs, which is called pulmonary ventilation.

Step 2. Gases are exchanged between air and blood in the lungs by diffusion.

Step 3. Gases are transported by circulation of the blood, with help from the heart.

Step 4. Gases are exchanged by diffusion between blood and tissues throughout the body.

- **Internal respiration** occurs between the blood and tissues. Once blood enters circulation, it reaches the capillaries. Oxygen diffuses through the capillaries into the cells. Carbon dioxide diffuses from the cells into the capillaries. Because carbon dioxide content is higher than oxygen content in blood at this point, it is called oxygen-poor blood. This oxygen-poor blood travels to the right side of the heart. It moves through the pulmonary circuit, where external respiration begins.

Example

What happens during internal respiration?

    A. Air is inhaled into the body.

    B. Oxygen-rich blood travels to the heart.

    C. Air moves into and out of the pulmonary circuit.

    D. Oxygen is exchanged for carbon dioxide in circulation.

The correct answer is **D.** During internal respiration, oxygen-poor blood is created as oxygen diffuses into the cells in exchange for carbon dioxide.

Let's Review!

- The respiratory system supplies oxygen to the body and removes carbon dioxide.
- Blood pH levels are regulated by the respiratory, cardiovascular, and nervous systems.
- Respiratory organs are anatomically divided into the upper and lower tract.
- Breathing is a mechanical process that provides oxygen, which is essential to all living things.
- Internal respiration involves gas exchange between blood and body tissues.
- External respiration is a gas exchange that happens between blood and the lungs.

THE GASTROINTESTINAL SYSTEM

This lesson introduces the structures and functions of the digestive system.

Anatomy of the Digestive System

The following are the functions of the digestive system:

1. Take in food.
2. Break down food.
3. Absorb digested molecules.
4. Provide nutrients.
5. Eliminate wastes.

The digestive system consists of the **digestive tract**, which is a tube extending from the mouth to the anus, and the associated organs, which secrete fluids into the digestive tract. The term **gastrointestinal tract** technically refers to only the stomach and intestines.

The Path of Food

Food takes the path outlined below as it moves through the body.

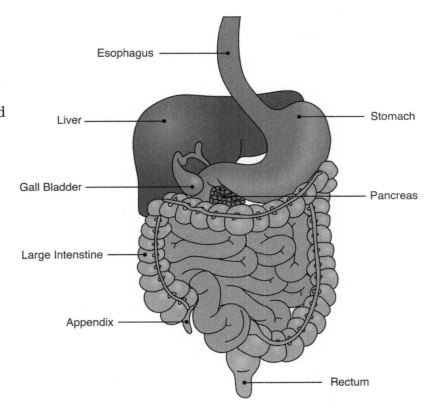

- The **oral cavity**, or the mouth, is the first part of the digestive system. It is bounded by the lips and cheeks and contains the teeth and tongue. Its primary function is to masticate, or chew, and moisten the food.
- The **pharynx**, or throat, connects the mouth to the esophagus.
- The **esophagus** is a muscular tube about 25 centimeters long. Food travels down it to the cardiac sphincter of the stomach.
- The **stomach** is an enlarged segment of the digestive tract.
- The opening of the stomach is the **cardiac sphincter**.
- The muscular layer of the stomach is different from other regions because it has folds called **rugae** that increase the surface area.

- The exit of the stomach is the **pyloric sphincter**.

- The **small intestine** is about 6 meters long and consists of three parts: duodenum, jejunum, and ileum.

  - The duodenum has more **villi** (finger-like projections), has a larger diameter, and is thicker than the other two parts.
  - This increases the surface area in the duodenum, which allows for more absorption of nutrients.
  - The small intestine is the primary site for diffusion of nutrients into the blood.

- The **large intestine** consists of the cecum, colon, rectum, and anal canal. The cecum is located where the small and large intestine meet.

  - The colon is about 1.5 to 1.8 meters long and consists of four parts: the ascending, transverse, descending, and sigmoid colon.
  - The primary function of the large intestine is to compress the waste and collect any excess water that can be recycled.

Example

Digestive organs include structures such as villi and rugae. Which of the following is a purpose they serve?

    A. Increase surface area

    B. Increase blood supply

    C. Increase mucus secretion

    D. Increase bacterial content

The correct answer is **A**. Structures such as the rugae and villi increase surface area. This allows for greater absorption.

Accessory Organs

Accessory organs contribute to the process of digestion. Food does not pass through these organs, but they play critical roles in the digestion of food. The accessory organs are listed below.

The **liver** weighs about 1.36 kilograms and is located in the upper-right quadrant of the abdomen. It is divided into two major lobes: the right lobe and left lobe. The liver has multiple functions:

- **Digestion:** Bile salts emulsify and help break down fats into fatty acids and glycerol.
- **Excretion:** Bile contains excretory products from the hemoglobin breakdown.
- **Nutrient storage:** The liver removes sugar from the blood and stores fats, vitamins, copper, and iron
- **Nutrient conversion:** The liver converts some nutrients into others. For example, it coverts amino acids to lipids or glucose

- **Detoxification of harmful chemicals:** The liver removes ammonia from the blood and converts it to urea.
- **Synthesis of new molecules:** The liver synthesizes new blood proteins such as albumins and fibrinogens.

The **pancreas** is a complex organ composed of both endocrine and exocrine tissues that perform several functions:

- It secretes bicarbonate ions, which neutralize acids.
- It secretes digestive enzymes that are important to all classes of foods.
- It produces insulin and glucagon, which regulate blood sugar levels.

The **gallbladder**, nestled under the liver, stores concentrated bile.

The **tongue** is a large, muscular organ that occupies most of the oral cavity. It moves food in the mouth and, in cooperation with the lips and cheeks, holds the food in place during mastication.

Saliva keeps the oral cavity moist and begins the process of chemical digestion with the enzyme amylase. There are three pairs of **salivary glands**:

- **Parotid** (largest, located in front of the ears)
- **Submandibular** (located below the mandible)
- **Sublingual** (smallest, located in the bottom of oral cavity)

These glands produce saliva, which is a mixture of serous (watery) and mucus fluids that contain digestive enzymes.

Example

Which of the following organs maintains a healthy pH level when a person eats an orange?

A. Gallbladder   B. Liver   C. Pancreas   D. Tongue

The correct answer is **C.** One of the functions of the pancreas is to release bicarbonate ions, which neutralize acids.

Digestion

Digestion is the breakdown of food into molecules that are small enough to be absorbed into the bloodstream. There are two types of digestion: mechanical and chemical. **Mechanical digestion** breaks down large food particles into smaller ones and is evident as a person's teeth grind food into smaller pieces. During **chemical digestion**, digestive enzymes break covalent chemical bonds into organic molecules.

Carbohydrates are broken down into monosaccharides, **proteins** are broken down into amino acids, and **fats or lipids** are broken down into fatty acids and glycerol. Monosaccharides, amino acids, fatty acids, and glycerol molecules are small enough to diffuse across the membranes of the digestive system and enter the bloodstream, to be taken where they are needed.

Absorption begins in the stomach, where small, lipid-soluble molecules, such as alcohol and aspirin, can pass through the stomach epithelium into circulation. Most absorption occurs in the duodenum and jejunum, although some occurs in the ileum. Some molecules can diffuse through the intestinal wall. Others must be transported across the intestinal wall. Transport requires a carrier molecule. If the transport is active, energy is required to move the transported molecule across the intestinal wall.

Enzymes:

Most enzymes are recognizable by the *-ase* ending. Here are some of the most common enzymes:

- **Amylase** is produced in the mouth and breaks down carbohydrates.
- **Pepsin** is produced in the stomach and breaks down proteins.
- **Lipase** is produced in the pancreas and secreted into the small intestine to break down lipids.
- **Peptidase** is produced in the pancreas and secreted into the small intestine to brown down peptides into amino acids.
- **Sucrase** is produced in the small intestine and breaks down sucrose into glucose.
- **Lactase** is produced in the small intestine and breaks down lactose into glucose.

Example
What are the building blocks of carbohydrates?

A. Glycerols

B. Fatty acids

C. Amino acids

D. Monosaccharides

The correct answer is **D**. Monosaccharides are the foundational units of carbohydrates.

Disorders of the Digestive System

The following are disorders of the digestive system.

Stomach:

- **Vomiting** results primarily from irritation of the stomach and small intestine. After the vomiting center has been stimulated, a sequence of events occurs that result in vomiting.
- **Ulcers** occur from a specific bacterium, *Helicobacter pylori*. Ulcers were previously thought to be caused by stress, but they can be treated successfully with antibiotics.
- **Peptic ulcer** is a condition in which the stomach acids digest the mucus lining of the duodenum. These ulcers are sometimes called **duodenal ulcers**. People who experience a great deal of stress tend to secrete as much as 15 percent more HCl than normal, which causes the **chyme**, semifluid food mass, to be highly acidic. There are not enough sodium bicarbonate ions to neutralize the acidic chime, and it eats away at the mucus lining, causing ulcers.

Liver:

- **Cirrhosis** is a disease characterized by damage or death of liver cells, which are replaced by connective tissue. This causes abnormal blood flow in the liver and interferes with normal liver functions.
- **Hepatitis** is an inflammation of the liver. Liver cells can die and be replaced with scar tissue.

Intestine:

- **Irritable bowel disease** is the general term for Crohn's disease or ulcerative colitis.

  - **Crohn's disease** includes a localized inflammatory degeneration that causes the wall of the small intestine to thicken. This disease causes diarrhea, abdominal pain, and weight loss.
  - **Ulcerative colitis** is limited to the mucosa of the large intestine. The involved mucosa exhibits inflammation, including edema, vascular congestion, and hemorrhaging.

- **Irritable bowel syndrome (IBS)** is a disorder of unknown cause in which intestinal mobility is abnormal. Patients exhibit pain in the left lower quadrant, especially after eating, and have alternating bouts of diarrhea and constipation.
- **Malabsorption syndrome** is a spectrum of disorders of the small intestine that result in abnormal nutrient absorption.
- **Appendicitis** is an inflammation of the appendix that usually occurs because of an obstruction.

Example

How is a duodenal ulcer different from an ulcer?

   A. Antibiotics are ineffective with ulcers.

   B. A duodenal ulcer is only found in adults.

   C. An ulcer can occur from a variety of bacteria.

   D. An increase in stomach acids can produce a duodenal ulcer.

The correct answer is **D**. Duodenal ulcers can occur as a result of an increase in the acidic levels in the duodenum. Regular ulcers are caused by bacteria.

Let's Review!

- The digestive system consists of the digestive tract, which is a tube extending from the mouth to the anus, and accessory organs.
- Accessory organs contribute to the process of digestion.
- Food does not pass through the accessory organs.
- Digestion is the breakdown of food into molecules that are small enough to be absorbed into the bloodstream.
- The two types of digestion are mechanical and chemical.

THE REPRODUCTIVE SYSTEM

This lesson covers the human reproductive system. Through sexual intercourse, this system enables internal fertilization and delivery of an infant.

The Male Reproductive System

Like all biological systems, the male reproductive system is comprised of several organs. These organs are located outside or within the pelvis.

The main male reproductive organs are the **penis** and the **testicles**, which are located external to the body. The penis is composed of a long shaft and a bulbous end called the glans penis. The glans penis is usually surrounded by an extension of skin called the foreskin (though this often is removed in a cosmetic procedure called **circumcision**). The penis has three internal compartments (the corpus cavernosum) that contain erectile tissue. When a male is sexually aroused, this tissue becomes suffused with blood, increasing pressure, and the penis becomes larger and erect.

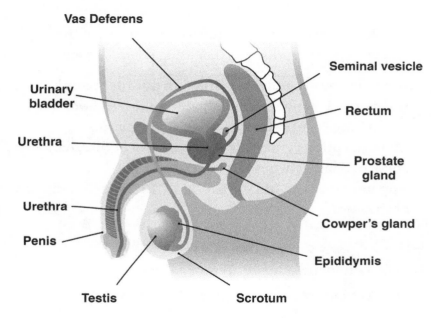

Male Reproductive System

Vas Deferens

Seminal vesicle

Rectum

Urinary bladder

Urethra

Prostate gland

Urethra

Cowper's gland

Penis

Epididymis

Testis

Scrotum

The **testes** (analogous to the female ovaries), or testicles, are retained in a pouch of skin called the **scrotum**, with descends from the base of the penis. The scrotum contains nerves and blood vessels needed to support the testicles' functions. The scrotum also regulates the temperature of the testicles by contracting (drawing the testicles closer to the warmer body) or relaxing (allowing the testicles to move away from the warmer body).

Each testicle (or testis) produces **sperm** (analogous to the female ova), which are passed into a series of coiled tubules called the **epididymis**. The epididymis stores and nurtures sperm until they are passed into the **vas deferens**, a tubule that is about 30 centimeters long, extending from the testicle into the pelvis and ending at the ejaculatory duct. The epididymis and vas deferens are supported by several accessory glands (the seminal vesicles, the prostate gland, and the Cowper glands) that produce fluid components of **semen** and support the sperm cells. During male orgasm, semen passes through the ejaculatory duct into the urethra and is ejaculated from the penis through the urethral opening.

Example

Where is the male reproductive system located?

   A. The male reproductive system is located entirely within the pelvis.

   B. The male reproductive system is located entirely outside the pelvis.

   C. The male reproductive system is located primarily within the pelvis, though some components are outside the pelvis.

   D. The male reproductive system is located primarily outside the pelvis, though some components are located within the pelvis.

The correct answer is **D**. Most of the components of the male reproductive system (penis, scrotum, testes, and epididymis) are external of the body, though some components (vas deferens and accessory glands) are located within the pelvis. The corpus cavernosum extends from within the pelvis into the penis.

The Female Reproductive System

Like all biological systems, the female reproductive system is comprised of several organs. These organs are located within the pelvis or external to the body.

The main female reproductive organs are the **uterus** (the "womb") and the **ovaries**, which are located in the pelvis. The ovaries (analogous to the male testes) produce several important hormones and the **ova** (analogous to the male sperm). After ovulation, the ovum is transported from the ovary to the uterus though the **Fallopian tube**. If sperm are present in the Fallopian tube, **fertilization** may occur. A fertilized **zygote** embeds in the endometrium of the uterus for gestation; an unfertilized ovum passes out of the body during subsequent menstruation.

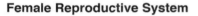

Female Reproductive System

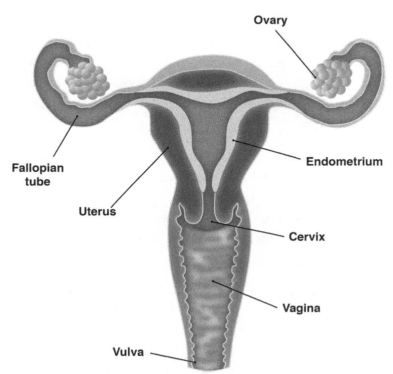

The uterus has a lower opening called the **cervix**, which connects the uterus to the vagina. The female reproductive system has several organs that are external to the body, collectively known as genitals or, specifically, the vulva, including the labia (majora and minora), clitoris, and vaginal opening. When a female is sexually aroused, these external organs become suffused with blood, becoming larger and more erect, and the vagina becomes lubricated.

The uterus performs numerous critical functions during reproduction. It provides mechanical protection, nutritional support, and waste removal for the developing embryo (though a complex interfacing with the embryo's placenta). In addition, it is a powerful, muscular organ that is capable of contractions that push the fetus through the vagina at the time of birth.

Example

An embryo develops into a fetus in the _____.

  A. Fallopian tube   B. ovary   C. uterus   D. vagina

  The correct answer is **C**. The zygote implants into the endometrium (uterine wall) and develops into an embryo; the embryo then develops into a fetus within the uterus.

Reproduction

Human reproduce sexually, with a male partner (the "father") providing sperm and a female partner (the "mother") providing an ovum and all subsequent protection and nourishment until the fetus is delivered.

Post-natal feeding is provided by the female's breasts. Human intercourse consists of the male introducing sperm into the female's reproductive system. Sperm may then pass through the female's reproductive system to the Fallopian tubes where one sperm fertilizes an ovum, creating a zygote. The zygote passes out of the Fallopian tube and implants into the uterine wall to begin gestation. Over nine months, the zygote develops and grows into an **embryo** and then a **fetus**.

At the abdomen, the fetus is connected to the **umbilical cord**, which connects to the **placenta**. The umbilical cord and placenta are formed from fetal tissue. The placenta shares a complex interface with the endometrial lining of the uterus. The endometrium and uterus are maternal tissue. Hormones, food, and fetal waste all pass through the placental/uterine interface and along the umbilical cord. As the fetus grows, the placenta also grows. The fetus is encapsulated in a tough container of fetal tissue, filled with fluid, called the **amniotic sac**.

During the early stages of delivery, the amniotic sac ruptures and the fluid passes through the mother's vagina (this is colloquially known as "water breaking"). Also, the cervix softens and dilates to accommodate the fetus. Powerful muscular contractions of the uterus force the fetus through the cervix and out the vagina, normally with the head emerging first. After the fetus is delivered, hormonal signals in the mother's body cause the endometrial lining to quickly disconnect from the placenta, and the placenta is delivered through the vagina (the "afterbirth").

In some cases, surgical removal of the fetus may be desirable or necessary. This process delivers a live baby and colloquially is known as Caesarean section (or C-section).

Example

An expectant mother's water "breaks" immediately before _____.

    A. childbirth   B. fertilization   C. menstruation   D. puberty

The correct answer is **A.** The amniotic sac ruptures, releasing the amniotic fluid, in the early stages of childbirth. This rupturing releases a large amount of fluid and is colloquially known as "water breaking."

Development

Human newborn infants are unable to care for themselves and survive only with a large amount of parental care extending over at least the first several years of life. At birth, humans have all of the basic structures of the adult reproductive system, though some are undeveloped. At about 10–11 years old in females and about 11–12 years old in males, a child enters **puberty**, during which hormonal changes cause the reproductive system to develop fully. Puberty lasts for about 5–7 years.

Menstruation is a cyclical process occurring in the female body, especially the reproductive system, from about the end of puberty until menopause. During each period of menstruation, fluctuating hormone levels cause the uterus to change in anticipation of receiving a zygote. At the midpoint of the menstrual cycle, an ovum is released from an ovary and travels down the Fallopian tube. If the ovum is not fertilized, it passes out of the body along with the endometrium (lining of the uterus), causing menstrual bleeding. If the ovum is fertilized, the zygote implants in the endometrium and pregnancy follows.

There are significant differences between male and female bodies. The primary differences can be noted in the reproductive organs, but numerous other differences are the result of secondary sex characteristics. Male secondary sex characteristics include facial hair and a generally larger body. Female secondary sex characteristics include enlargement of the breasts and widening of the hips.

Example

Which statement best characterizes the changes that occur during puberty?

A. Puberty is a recurring cycle involving fluctuating levels of hormones.

B. During puberty, the male's penis or the female's vulva develops basic structures.

C. During puberty, males and females reach sexual maturity and develop secondary sex characteristics.

D. Puberty occurs during the first trimester of pregnancy and results in the zygote developing into an embryo.

The correct answer is **C.** Puberty occurs during the early teenage years and results in sexual maturity. It is marked by the development of secondary sex characteristics.

Let's Review!

- The reproductive system enables sexual reproduction in humans.
- Components of the reproductive system are often known by multiple names, some of which are common or "slang" terms; the correct biological or medical terms are always preferred.
- The male reproductive system provides the sperm, the carrier of the genetic contribution from the father.
- The female reproductive system provides the ovum, or egg cell, which contains the genetic contribution from the mother. Additionally, the female reproductive system supports fertilization; provides the mechanical protection and nurturing environment needed for embryogenesis and gestation; and performs the actions necessary for the birth of the infant.
- The male testicles are analogous to the female ovaries. There are other similarities in the male and female reproductive systems.
- Sexual maturity occurs during puberty. Humans are capable of reproduction for several decades.

THE URINARY SYSTEM

This lesson introduces the anatomy of the urinary system and how it functions. This lesson also explores the role of other body systems, particularly the circulatory and endocrine systems, in aiding with urinary excretion, absorption, and filtration.

Anatomy of the Urinary System

Inside the body, the kidney, ureters, bladder, and urethra make up the **urinary system**, which is also called the renal system. The ureters, bladder, and urethra comprise the **urinary tract**. This system has many functions, some of which are outlined below:

- **Waste elimination:** Urea, creatinine, uric acid, and ammonium are the primary types of nitrogenous wastes excreted from the body. The urinary system also detects and excretes excess water from the blood and out of the body.
- **Osmoregulation of blood and water:** There must be a continual balance of water and salt in the blood. The urinary system, specifically the kidneys, help maintain this balance. It also balances levels of metabolites or electrolytes such as sodium, potassium, and calcium.
- **Hormone secretion:** The kidneys secrete several hormones to regulate processes that range from blood pressure and red blood cell production to calcium uptake via vitamin D.

Several of these functions are performed with help from other body systems, specifically the cardiovascular and respiratory systems.

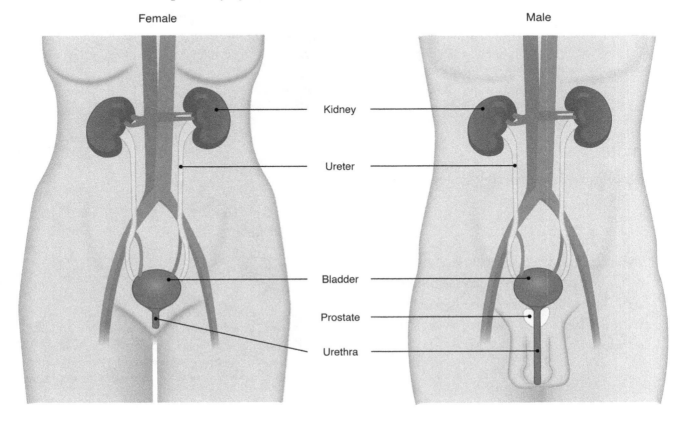

Female   Male

Kidney

Ureter

Bladder

Prostate

Urethra

The following table outlines key characteristics of each organ that is labeled in the image above.

Organ	Shape	Characteristics
Kidney	Resembles beans, reddish-brown in color	The body has two kidneys, which excrete wastes in the urine out of the body.
Ureters	Tubular	Send urine from the kidney to the bladder.
Bladder	Pear (when emptied)	Stores urine until the body expels the fluid from the body. Has three openings: two for the ureters and one for the urethra.
Urethra	Tubular	Site where urine from the urinary bladder travels to an external opening. Removes urine from the body.

The primary organ of the urinary system is the kidney. Blood from the heart flows through the kidneys via the **renal artery**. As blood drains from the kidney, it exits through a series of veins, the most prominent of which is the **renal vein**. When urine is produced, it does not drain through the tubes through which blood flows. Rather, urine flows through two ureters before emptying into the urinary bladder. The following steps outline how the urinary system works:

1. Kidney filters and excretes wastes from blood, producing urine.
2. Urine flows down the ureters.
3. Urine empties into the bladder and is temporarily stored.
4. Bladder, when filled, empties urine out of the body via the urethra.

DID YOU KNOW?

As a person ages, the kidneys and bladder change. This can affect functions such as bladder control and how well the kidneys filter blood. Kidney changes range from a decrease in kidney tissue to decreased filtration capacity. Bladder changes include decreased elasticity (which affects how much urine is stored) and weakened bladder muscles.

Example

Which organ of the urinary system filters blood?

A. Bladder

B. Kidney

C. Ureter

D. Urethra

The correct answer is **B.** There are two kidneys in the body, which are located below the rib cage. The kidneys filter the blood that comes from the heart and remove wastes from the blood.

BE CAREFUL!

The kidneys do not make urine. They help regulate water balance, regulate levels of electrolytes such as sodium and potassium, and eliminate metabolic wastes. Urine is a byproduct of these functions.

Nephrons and Urine Formation

The functional and structural unit of a kidney is a **nephron**. One kidney contains more than one million nephrons. An illustration of these functional units is shown below:

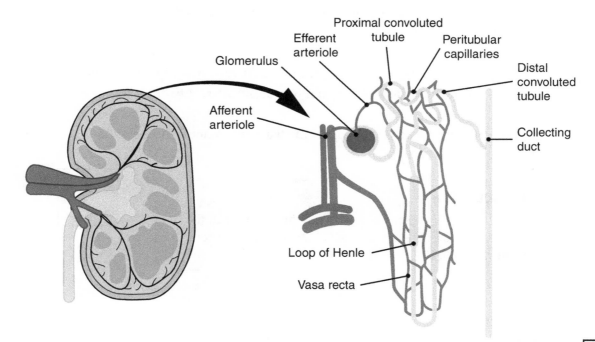

The nephron consists of two parts: the **renal corpuscle** and the **renal tubule**. The renal corpuscle can be divided into the **glomerulus** and **glomerular capsule** (or Bowman's capsule). The glomerulus is a type of capillary bed that functions as a filtration system, filtering solutes as blood enters the kidneys from the renal artery. Surrounding the glomerulus is Bowman's capsule. The renal tubule is a duct that connects to the

> **KEEP IN MIND**
>
> It is helpful to think of each nephron as a tiny filtering structure. Each nephron filters blood and forms urine. With more than one million nephrons in a single kidney, it is no wonder the kidneys are so efficient at filtering and excreting wastes from blood!

glomerulus and terminates at the tip of the medullary pyramid. This tubule is divided into the following four regions: (1) **proximal convoluted tubule**, (2) **loop of Henle**, (3) **distal convoluted tubule**, and (4) **collecting duct**.

The components that make up the nephron filter blood and form urine. The following steps outline the pathway for urine formation. The steps are divided into three processes:

1. Glomerular filtration:
2. Blood enters the kidney though the renal artery.
3. This artery branches off into capillaries, allowing blood to flow into the glomerulus of the nephron.
4. Blood pressure forces water and solutes (smaller than proteins) to diffuse from blood across the capillary walls and through pores of Bowman's capsule into the tubule.

5. Tubular reabsorption:

6. The filtered fluid flows toward the proximal tubule. This is the major site of reabsorption of water and solutes such as glucose, amino acids, and certain ions.

7. The fluid travels to the loop of Henle, which is another site of reabsorption.

8. Next, the fluid reaches the distal convoluted tubule. Reabsorption and secretion take place in this segment.

9. Tubular secretion:

10. In the final segment, the collecting duct, fluid that remains in the duct is called urine. Reabsorption of some water and its return to the bloodstream may happen at this segment.

11. At this site, creatinine and other nitrogenous wastes are actively secreted into the urine so they can be excreted out of the body.

DID YOU KNOW?
About 180 liters of blood pass through the nephrons of the kidney each day. This explains why much of this fluid and its contents must be reabsorbed.

Example

Where does urine form?

A. Loop of Henle

B. Collecting duct

C. Distal convoluted tubule

D. Proximal convoluted tubule

The correct answer is **B**. The nephron is the functional unit of the kidney. This structure consists of four major components: proximal and distal convoluted tubules, loop of Henle, and collecting duct. As blood travels through each of these segments, it is filtered to create urine in the collecting duct.

Urine Excretion and ADH

After blood is filtered through the nephron and the byproduct of urine is produced, urine accumulates in the collecting ducts of the nephron. Eventually, urine enters the ureters, which are muscular tubes. With help from muscle contractions, the ureters contract to move urine into the bladder. Urine is stored until the bladder is about half full.

Upon reaching this level, a neural impulse is transmitted telling a **sphincter** in the bladder to relax and allow urine to exit the bladder. Contraction of this sphincter, which is a muscular tube, is under involuntary control. Urine flows from the bladder into the urethra, which expels

BE CAREFUL!
The urethra in males and females are different sizes due to the reproductive anatomy. The male urethra is about 20 centimeters long. It passes through the length of the penis and terminates at the end of the penis, where urine is removed from the body. The female urethra is about four centimeters long.

urine out of the body. A second sphincter enables urine to leave the body. This process is known as urination.

Recall that the urinary system works closely with the cardiovascular system to filter blood and return important substances back to the bloodstream during tubular reabsorption. To help maintain water and solute concentration either excreted from or reabsorbed by the body, the urinary system works with hormones that are part of the endocrine system to regulate this process. One of these hormones is the **antidiuretic hormone**, also known as ADH. This hormone is secreted from the posterior pituitary gland, which is found at the base of the brain.

One of the most important functions of ADH is to regulate urine concentration and volume by controlling how much water is reabsorbed in the tubules of the nephrons. The following image shows how ADH controls urine formation.

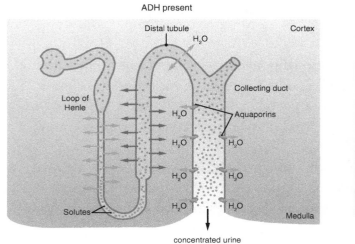

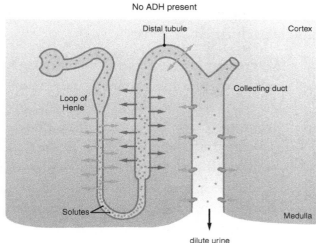

As shown in the image, when ADH is present, there is an increased permeability of water at the distal convoluted tubule and collecting duct. This causes more water to be reabsorbed and retained. It also decreases the volume of urine produced and concentrates the urine. The opposite occurs when ADH is not actively communicating with the kidneys and regulating urine formation.

DID YOU KNOW?
ADH control of urine formation is intimately connected to diabetes insipdus. When people have this disease, ADH does not communicate properly with the kidneys. As a result, symptoms include excessive thirst and frequent urination.

Example

The antidiuretic hormone primarily controls tubular reabsorption of which substance?

    A. Calcium   B. Creatinine   C. Urea   D. Water

The correct answer is **D**. Regulating how much water the body excretes or reabsorbs is a key function of the urinary system. To perform this function, kidneys must communicate with the hormone ADH, which is released from the posterior pituitary gland in the brain.

Urinalysis

Medical professionals can determine diseases that affect the urinary system by conducting a **urinalysis**. This type of test can reveal disease that does not necessarily present observable symptoms. Diseases confirmed through urinalysis include diabetes mellitus, different types of glomerulonephritis, and urinary tract infections. Both macroscopic and microscopic urinalysis can be performed.

- **Macroscopic urinalysis:** The first part of this testing involves visual observation of the urine. Normal fresh urine is pale to dark yellow in color. It is also clear and not cloudy. If the color is turbid or the urine is cloudy, there may be excess protein in the urine or the presence of a bacterial infection. Red or brown urine is considered abnormal. It could indicate that blood is present in the urine.

- An urine dipstick test is another type of macroscopic urinalysis. With this test, a plastic dipstick or paper strip is inserted into the urine sample. There are chemicals on the dipstick that cause it to change color when certain substances are present in the urine (at a specific concentration). Medical professionals can compare the color of the dipstick to a standard chart to analyze a urine sample.

- When the liquid is removed, this sediment is mounted to a microscope slide and analyzed using a microscope. Typically, this test is performed to look at blood cells in the urinary tract, bacteria, parasites, or even tumor cells. This test also helps confirm the diagnosis of various urinary problems like kidney disease, cancer, microbial infections, and liver disease.

- **Microscopic urinalysis:** This type of urinalysis requires the use of a light microscope. Typically, a urine sample is spun down, or centrifuged, in a test tube. This causes a sediment consisting of red blood cells, fat cells, and other large particles to aggregate and separate from the liquid portion of the urine.

Example

What is most likely analyzed during microscopic urinalysis?

   A. Volume of water in urine

   B. Amount of urea excreted

   C. Sodium levels in the urine

   D. Presence of white blood cells

The correct answer is **D**. During microscopic urinalysis, large substances like blood cells and bacteria are separated from the liquid portion of urine. These substances are placed on a microscopic slide and analyzed to make or confirm a diagnosis.

Let's Review!

- The urinary system eliminates wastes from the body, regulates blood and water levels, and secretes hormones that directly influence various physiological processes in the body.
- The circulatory and endocrine systems work with the urinary system to perform various functions.
- Nephrons are functional units and structures of the kidneys that play a large role in filtration, reabsorption, and secretion.
- After blood enters the kidneys through the renal artery, it is filtered in the glomerulus. Then, it travels through the proximal tubule, the loop of Henle, and the distal convoluted tubule before accumulating as urine in the collecting duct.
- The kidneys form urine as a byproduct, which travels through the ureter before being stored in the bladder and eventually excreted from the body via the urethra.
- Urinalysis is a method used to evaluate the quality of urine and help diagnose various urinary health problems.

Chapter 11 Human Anatomy and Physiology: Organization of Systems Practice Quiz 1

1. Platelets are important because they

    A. give blood its natural color.

    B. repair broken blood vessels.

    C. transport nutrients to the cells.

    D. protect the body against infection.

2. What happens after platelets aggregate at a damaged blood vessel site?

    A. The site of the wound is healed.

    B. The damaged blood vessel constricts.

    C. The platelets stick together and form a plug.

    D. Red blood cells are recruited to the injured site.

3. Which of the following enzymes breaks down proteins?

    A. Amylase   C. Pepsin

    B. Lactase   D. Sucrase

4. What is the primary function of the oral cavity?

    A. Diffusion   C. Lubrication

    B. Digestion   D. Mastication

5. Which cavity is surrounded by the rib cage and separated from the abdominal cavity by the diaphragm?

    A. Abdominal   C. Pelvic

    B. Gastric   D. Thoracic

6. _____ are composed of two or more tissue types that together perform one or more common functions.

    A. Cells   C. Organs

    B. Chemicals   D. Tissues

7. Fertilization is the result of _____.

    A. meiosis

    B. childbirth

    C. spermatogenesis

    D. sexual intercourse

8. Humans utilize which type of reproduction?

    A. Binary fission

    B. Parthenogenesis

    C. Sexual reproduction

    D. Asexual reproduction

9. Which organ branches off into the bronchi?

    A. Alveolus   C. Nose

    B. Larynx   D. Trachea

10. **What is the function of the pharynx?**

    A. Allow food and air to pass into the body

    B. Warm and moisten air during inhalation

    C. Create a chest cavity at the base of the lungs

    D. Provide structural support to the alveolar region

11. **Which is a characteristic of the bladder?**

    A. Stores urine

    B. Filters blood

    C. Shaped like a bean

    D. Reddish-brown in color

12. **After being produced by the kidneys, where does urine flow next?**

    A. Ureter   C. Renal vein

    B. Urethra   D. Renal artery

Chapter 11 Human Anatomy and Physiology: Organization of Systems Practice Quiz 1 — Answer Key

1. B. At the site of injury or damage to a blood vessel, platelets help repair the damaged area. **See Lesson: Cardiovascular System.**

2. C. After the platelets aggregate at the damaged site, they stick together to form a plug. Next, blood coagulation occurs when a fibrin mesh forms around the platelet aggregate. **See Lesson: Cardiovascular System.**

3. C. Pepsin is produced in the stomach and breaks down proteins. **See Lesson: Gastrointestinal System.**

4. D. The primary function of the oral cavity is to break up the food through mastication. **See Lesson: Gastrointestinal System.**

5. D. The thoracic cavity is surrounded by the rib cage and is separated from the abdominal cavity by the diaphragm. **See Lesson: Organization of the Human Body.**

6. C. Organs are composed of two or more tissue types that together perform one or more common functions. **See Lesson: Organization of the Human Body.**

7. D. Fertilization results from sexual intercourse. It may result in childbirth. Meiosis and spermatogenesis are precursors to fertilization. **See Lesson: Reproductive System.**

8. C. Humans utilize sexual reproduction. **See Lesson: Reproductive System.**

9. D. The trachea is a hollow tube in the upper respiratory tract that branches off into bronchi, which extend into the lungs. **See Lesson: The Respiratory System.**

10. A. The pharynx is found right behind the nasal cavity. It is a passageway through which food and air flow. **See Lesson: The Respiratory System.**

11. A. The bladder is a sac-like organ that stores urine after it travels through the ureter. Once the bladder reaches half full, the urine is emptied into the urethra and out of the body. **See Lesson: The Urinary System.**

12. A. Urine is a byproduct of the blood that is filtered in the kidneys. This tubular filtrate travels to the ureter, which is a muscular tube that contracts to push urine to the urethra and out of the body. **See Lesson: The Urinary System.**

Chapter 12 Human Anatomy and Physiology: Support and Movement

The Skeletal System

This lesson introduces the anatomy and functions of the skeletal system. This lesson also explores how bone forms, remodels, and constantly changes as a person grows.

Skeletal System Overview

A human is born with roughly 270 bones. As a person grows, this number decreases to approximately 206. This is because many of the bones fuse.

FOR EXAMPLE

Half of the pelvic bone has three separate bones at birth: the ilium, ischium, and pubis. By adulthood, these bones fuse into one bone called the hipbone.

Anatomically, the skeletal system is divided into two major divisions: axial skeleton and appendicular skeleton. The **axial skeleton** consists of the bones of the skull, sternum, vertebral column, and ribcage. The **appendicular skeleton** comprises the bones of the upper and lower extremities and the associated girdles that connect the extremities to the vertebral column. The following table summarizes the number of bones found in each skeletal division.

Axial	80 bones
Inner ear ossicles	6
Skull and hyoid	23
Sternum and ribs	25
Vertebral column	26
Appendicular	126
Pectoral girdle	4
Upper extremities	60
Pelvic girdle	2
Lower extremities	60

Twenty-four of the bones in the vertebral column are called the pre-sacral vertebrae. These consist of 7 cervical, 12 thoracic, and 5 lumbar vertebrae. The last two bones of the vertebral column are the sacrum and coccyx.

The skeletal system consists of **bones**, **cartilage**, and **ligaments** that are tightly bound together to form a strong, yet flexible, framework. Bone is an active form of **connective tissue**. This tissue plays a role in many of the functions of the skeletal system:

- **Support:** Bones and cartilage support body posture because both structures are rigid. They also allow a person to remain upright and provide a framework to which soft tissues like muscles and organs can attach.
- **Movement:** Bones of the skeletal system interact with the muscular system to help he body move. Bones themselves cannot move. But when connected to each other by ligaments, along with the action of muscles, a human body can move.
- **Protection:** The skeletal system protects vital organs from external damage. The skull protects the brain, the vertebral column protects the spinal cord, and the sternum and ribcage protect the lungs.
- **Mineral storage:** Bone functions as a storage site for important minerals like calcium and phosphorus. These minerals are used for a variety of physiological functions in the body.
- **Hematopoiesis:** This is the process bones use to produce red blood cells and stem cells, which differentiate to a variety of different cell types in the body.

The following image illustrates the anatomy of the skeletal system.

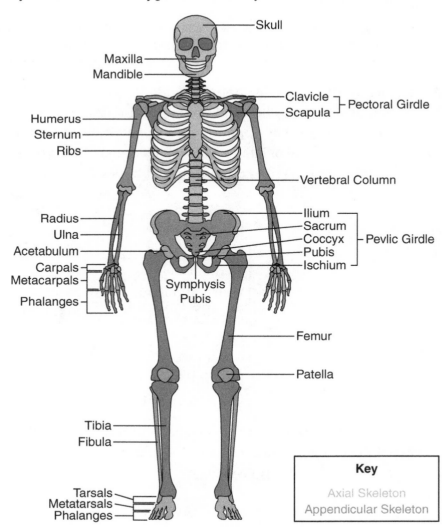

Example

Which of the following is part of the axial skeleton?

A. Carpals   B. Femur   C. Patella   D. Skull

The correct answer is **D**. The axial skeleton consists of bones that do not belong to the upper and lower extremities: the skull, vertebral column, sternum, and ribcage.

Bone Shape and Structure

The overall structure of bone consists of an outer shell called **compact bone**. It encloses another type of bone tissue that is loosely organized called **spongy** or **cancellous bone**. Compact bone is made of units called **osteons**. These structures look like cylinders. They contain a mineral matrix and living bone cells. Each osteon also contains a **Haversian canal** that houses the bone's blood vessels and nerve fibers.

Surrounding the compact bone is a fibrous membrane called the **periosteum**. This consists of blood vessels, nerves, and lymphatic vessels that nourish the compact bone.

There are five types of bones in the human body: long, short, flat, irregular, and sesamoid. The following table details the characteristics of each and where they are found.

> **KEEP IN MIND**
>
> As the name implies, spongy bone is lighter and less dense than compact bone. It is spongy because it consists of open sections called pores. Viewed under a microscope, these sections look like a kitchen sponge.

Bone type	Appearance	Function	Example
Long	Elongated bones; longer than they are wide	Mechanical strength	Femur, tibia, clavicle, humerus, and metacarpals
Flat	Broad bones that are thin	Site of muscle attachment; provide protection	Scapula, hip bone (os coxa), sternum, nasal bone, and occipital/ parietal/ frontal bones of the skull
Irregular	Have a non-uniform shape that cannot be classified as any other bone type	Mechanical support for the body	Vertebrae
Sesamoid	Small bones	Mechanical support; provide protection	Patella (kneecap)
Short	About same width as length	Provide support; little movement	Carpal and tarsal bones of the wrist and feet

To visualize the anatomy of all bone types, it is helpful to view the anatomy of long bone. As shown in the following image, the long bone consists of three major sections: proximal epiphysis, diaphysis, and distal epiphysis.

- **Epiphysis:** This is found at each end of the long bone. It consists primarily of spongy bone with a thin layer of compact bone. Bone growth occurs at the epiphysis.
- **Articular cartilage:** This covers the epiphysis. It decreases frictions at the joints.

- **Diaphysis:** This is the longest part of the long bone. It consists primarily of compact bone.
- **Medullary cavity:** This is found inside the long bone. It is composed of red and yellow bone marrow. Red marrow is where hematopoiesis occurs. Yellow marrow consists primarily of fat cells.

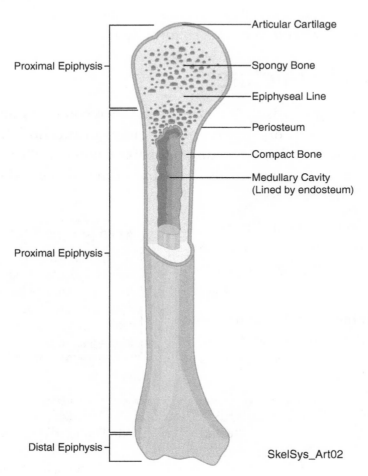

Example

A histologist cracks open a tibia. While viewing the inside, what does he see?

A. Diaphysis B. Soft tissue C. Spongy bone D. Proximal epiphysis

The correct answer is **C.** When looking inside a long bone, such as the tibia, the histologist sees the spongy bone. This is found at the proximal and distal ends of the epiphysis.

Ossification and Bone Remodeling

Although bone is a hard structure, it can grow. This is especially important in childhood. **Ossification** is the process of bone formation that occurs first during embryonic development. This process transforms soft, flexible cartilage to hard bone. It does so by replacing the cartilage with mineral deposits, specifically calcium and phosphorus. Ossification begins in the center of bones and spreads toward the end of the bones.

When a baby is born, a lot of cartilage is still found in the skeleton, particularly in the long bones. But there are **growth plates** at the end of long bones. This region is also made of cartilage. As the child grows, this area of cartilage at the growth plate experiences ossification to elongate the bone, enabling a person to grow taller.

Ossification also plays a role in **bone remodeling**. Mature bone tissue is constantly being broken down through a process called **bone resorption**. Through ossification, new bone tissue replaces this old bone. There are three types of bone cells:

- **Osteocytes:** These are bone cells. They produce collagen and other substances that create the extracellular matrix of bone.
- **Osteoblasts:** These are called bone-forming cells. They are found on the surface of bone and can be stimulated to differentiate into other type of bone cells called osteocytes.
- **Osteoclasts:** These are called bone-resorbing cells. They are found on the surface of bone. They dissolve the bone.

KEEP IN MIND

Bone resorption frees calcium and other minerals from bone for use in the body and clears out older pieces of bone. In doing so, this process promotes the deposition of new bone.

Recall that osteons are found in compact bone. As shown in the following image, the extracellular matrix of bone and osteocytes are found within the osteon. Osteoblasts and osteoclasts are found on the bone surface.

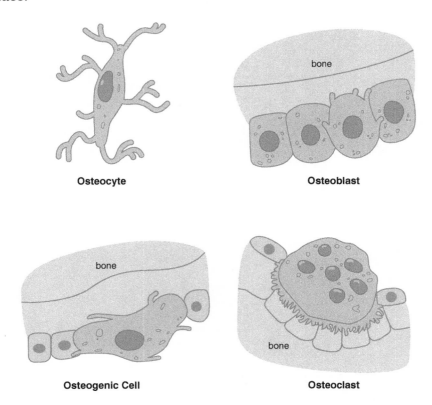

Osteocyte

Osteoblast

Osteogenic Cell

Osteoclast

Example

What bone cell is a bone-forming cell?

A. Osteoblast   B. Osteoclast   C. Osteocyte   D. Osteon

The correct answer is **A**. Osteoblasts are bone-forming cells found on the bone's surface. They help form new bone as older bone is broken down through resorption.

Let's Review!

- The skeletal system provides structural support and protection, aids in movement, serves as a mineral reservoir, and helps produce cells.
- The appendicular skeleton consists of the upper and lower extremities.
- The axial skeleton consists of the skull, sternum, ribcage, and vertebral column.
- The five bone types in the human body are: long, short, flat, irregular, and sesamoid.
- Ossification is a bone-forming process typically performed in childhood.
- Bone remodeling is a process that involves replacing old, mature bone tissue with new bone.
- Osteons are bone cells found in compact bone that contain the Haversian canal, which is the site for blood vessels and nerve fibers.
- Osteoblasts are bone-forming cells, and osteoclasts are bone-dissolving or resorbing cells.
- Osteocytes are bone cells found deep within bone that produce substances like cartilage.

THE MUSCULAR SYSTEM

This lesson introduces the anatomy of the muscular system, including the three different muscle tissues. This lesson also describes the role of the muscular system in movement and the physiology of muscle contraction.

Anatomy of the Muscle

The **muscular system** is responsible for all types of body movement. Additional functions of this system include providing support, stabilizing joints, and generating heat for the body. All muscles consist of specialized cells known as **muscle fibers**, which contract to facilitate body movement. For the body to move, muscles must be attached to bones. Muscles are also attached to internal organs and blood vessels. Thus, most of the body's movements occur because of muscle contraction from muscle fibers.

DID YOU KNOW?
There are over 600 muscles in the body. Muscles are grouped according to characteristics such as size, shape, and location.

The body is comprised of three types of muscles: cardiac, smooth, and skeletal. As shown in the image below, these muscles look different. They also perform different functions.

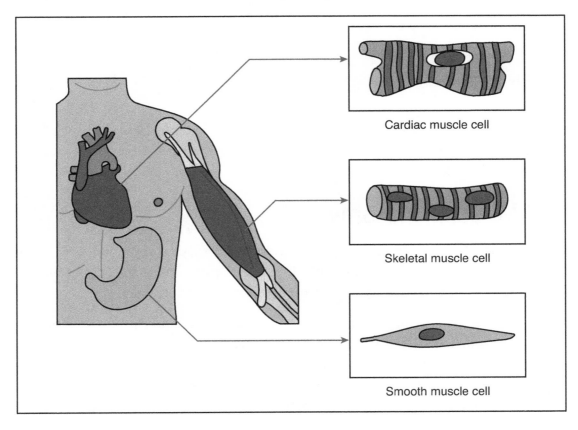

Cardiac muscle cell

Skeletal muscle cell

Smooth muscle cell

- **Cardiac muscle:** This muscle consists of muscle cells that are striated, short, and branched. These cells contain one nucleus, are branched, and are rectangular. Cardiac muscle contraction is an involuntary process, which is why it is under the control of the autonomic nervous system. This muscle is found in the walls of the heart.`

- **Skeletal muscle:** This muscle cell is striated, long, and cylindrical. There are many nuclei in a skeletal muscle cell. Attached to bones in the body, skeletal muscle contracts voluntarily, meaning that it is under conscious control.

> **BE CAREFUL!**
> Skeletal muscles are excited by the nervous system. Cardiac and smooth muscles are stimulated by the nervous system and by circulating hormones.

- **Smooth muscle:** This muscle consists of non-striated muscle cells that are spindle-shaped. Like cardiac muscle cells, smooth muscle cells contain one nucleus. This muscle type is found in the walls of internal organs like the bladder and stomach. Smooth muscle contraction is involuntary and controlled by the autonomic nervous system.

Despite the differences among cardiac, smooth, and skeletal muscles, they share four properties: excitability, contractility (muscle shortening), extensibility (muscle stretching), and elasticity.

Example

What is a purpose of the muscular system?

A. Connects one bone to another

B. Helps the bones of the body move

C. Protects the body from external injury

D. Determines how blood circulates in the body

The correct answer is **B.** One of the primary functions of the muscular system is to aid in movement. Muscles help the bones of the skeletal system move. Muscles contract and relax to facilitate movement.

Skeletal Muscle Anatomy

Bones move with the help of skeletal muscles, through contraction and extension. Skeletal muscles must be attached to the bones to pull on the bones and cause them to move. This movement is performed when the skeletal muscle shortens, or contracts.

As shown in the following image, connective tissue attaches skeletal muscle to bone or other tissues. Skeletal muscle consists of three types of connective tissue. The **endomysium** encases individual skeletal muscle fibers. These muscle fibers are bundled together by a connective tissue called the **perimysium.** Bundles of skeletal muscle fibers are called **fasciculi.** Each fascicle is bundled together by a strong connective tissue called the **epimysium.**

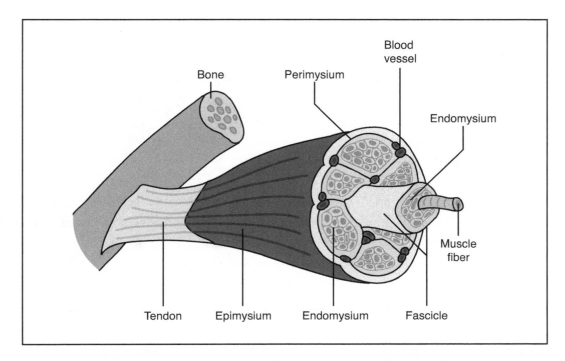

Bone, Perimysium, Blood vessel, Endomysium, Muscle fiber, Tendon, Epimysium, Endomysium, Fascicle

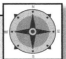

The cell membrane that surrounds a skeletal muscle fiber is called a **sarcolemma**. The cytoplasm of the skeletal muscle fiber is the **sarcoplasm**. One muscle fiber is filled with several long, cylindrical proteins called **myofibrils**, which are the contractile units of the fiber. The smallest contractile unit in a myofibril is a **sarcomere**. Several protein **myofilaments** make up a myofibril. There are two types of myofilaments: thick bands and thin bands. Thick bands, or myofilaments, are made of several protein molecules called **myosin**. Several protein molecules, called **actin**, link together to form the thin bands. These thin actin bands are attached to a **Z-disk** (or Z-line).

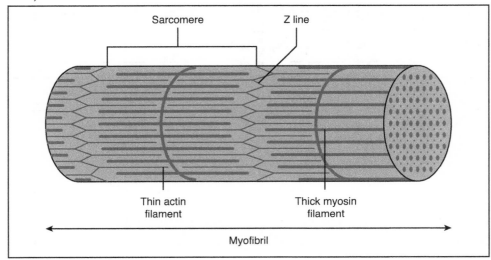

Sarcomere, Z line, Thin actin filament, Thick myosin filament, Myofibril

Example

What is the smallest contractile unit of skeletal muscle?

A. Actin   B. Epimysium   C. Myofibril   D. Sarcomere

The correct answer is **D**. Several contractile units called myofibrils are found within a single muscle fiber. Smaller contractile units called sarcomeres make up a myofibril.

Muscle Contraction

Keep in mind that the dark, striped Z-disc marks where one sarcomere ends and another begins. As shown in the image below, there are light-colored bands called **I-bands** and dark-colored bands called **A-bands**. The Z-line is found in the middle of the I-bands, while the **H zone** is found in the middle of the A-bands. In the middle of the H-zone is the **M line**, which is the center of the sarcomere.

TEST TIP

The following guide can be used to remember the components of the various lines in a skeletal muscle:

A-band	Thick and thin filaments
I-band	Thin filaments only
Z-line	Actin filament attachment site
H-band	Thick filaments only

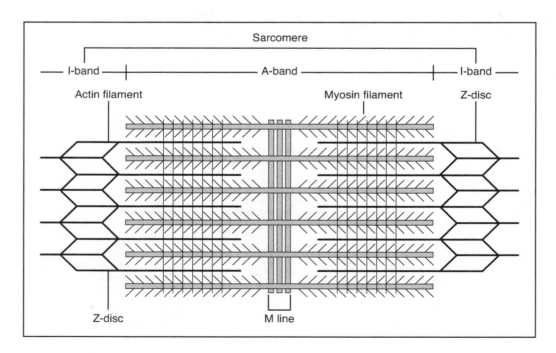

Slide filament theory explains muscle contraction. According to this theory, actin filaments slide past myosin filaments, pulling the actin filaments closer to the center of the sarcomere, or M line. As shown in the image below, this sliding action happens because of interactions between the heads of actin and myosin. The heads of myosin form attachments with the actin myofilaments. These attachments are known as **crossbridges**.

> **KEEP IN MIND**
>
> The head of actin is a round protein shaped like a ball. Several of these round proteins link together to form a long chain, or thin myofilament. Myosin is a thick protein with a head that resembles a golf club. When several myosin proteins join together, they create a myosin filament, where the heads point outward.

With the help of energy in the form of ATP, the myosin heads are energized to attach to binding sites in actin and form a crossbridge. After energy in the myosin head is released, the myosin pulls actin myofilaments closer to the M line. This head can only form another crossbridge when another molecule of ATP attaches to the head, reenergizing it. Calcium also plays an important role in determining when contraction happens. This ion is found in the **sarcoplasmic reticulum**, which surrounds myofibrils.

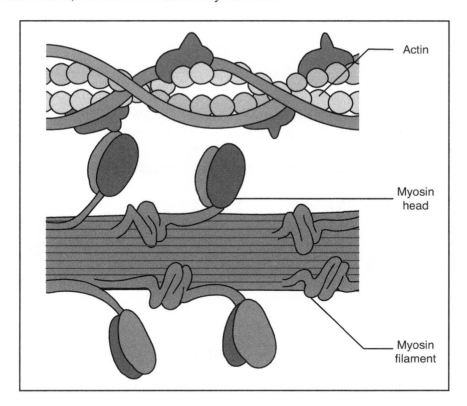

Example

What structure is reenergized with ATP?

A. Actin   B. Myosin   C. Myofibril   D. Sarcomere

The correct answer is **B.** Myosin heads attach to thin actin filaments to form crossbridges. These attachments can only form when the myosin head is energized with ATP.

Coordinating Movement

Ligaments attach bones to bones. Where ligaments connect bones, they form a **joint**. Thus, joints are the site where individual bones meet. There are three types of joints:

- **Immovable:** Also known as fibrous joints, these consist of bones held together by connective tissues. The bones are in very close contact. An example of an immovable joint is the intersection of cranial bones in the skull.
- **Partly movable:** Also known as cartilaginous joints, these consist of bones held together by cartilage. These joints allow some degree of movement. Partly movable joints include the vertebral discs in the spine.
- **Synovial:** These allow the largest freedom of movement because the bones are separated by a joint cavity. Examples of synovial joints are the hip and shoulder.

The muscular system works with the skeletal system to move the body. Thus, the muscles must be attached to bone. **Tendons** attach muscle to bone. Tendons consist of tough connective tissue that is found on either side of the joint where two bones are connected. Tendons work with skeletal muscles to move bones. When muscles contract, they shorten. This pulls on the bones, with the help of the tendon, to allow the body to move.

FOR EXAMPLE

Biceps and triceps muscles in the arm work together to bend and lengthen the elbow. As a biceps muscle contracts, the triceps muscle remains elongated, or relaxed. Thus, the biceps is the flexor and the triceps is the extensor of the elbow joint.

Muscles must work in pairs to move bones at the joint. The muscle that causes a joint to bend is called a **flexor muscle**. The muscle that contracts and causes a joint to straighten is called an **extension muscle**. If one muscle in the pair contracts, the other remains elongated.

Example

How many muscles must work together during contraction and extension?

A. 2　　　　　　　B. 10　　　　　　　C. 206　　　　　　　D. 600

The correct answer is **A.** Muscles work in pairs during contraction and extension. When one muscle contracts, the other extends, or relaxes.

Let's Review!

- A muscle is a fibrous tissue that aids in body movement, provides support, and generates heat energy for the body.
- Cardiac, smooth, and skeletal muscles are the three muscle types found in the body.
- Cardiac and smooth muscle are under involuntary control, while skeletal muscle is under voluntary control.
- Cardiac and skeletal muscles are striated, while smooth muscle is non-striated.

- Three types of muscle tissues comprise a skeletal muscle: epimysium, endomysium, and perimysium.
- A single skeletal muscle fiber consists of several contractile units called myofibrils, which consist of actin and myosin myofilaments.
- According to the slide filament theory, actin and myosin myofilaments form crossbridges to shorten a sarcomere, which shortens a skeletal muscle.
- Tendons attach muscle to bone and help bones move.
- Joints are the regions between bones that influence the degree of flexibility with body movement.
- Skeletal muscles move bones by working in muscle pairs to contract and elongate.

THE INTEGUMENTARY SYSTEM

This lesson introduces the anatomy of the integumentary system, including the system's function. This lesson also describes the effects of aging and cancer on the integumentary system.

The Skin's Many Layers

The **integumentary system** is a body system comprised of the skin and accessory structures, including the hair, sebaceous and sweat glands, and nails. This system protects the body, maintains homeostasis, and provides sensory information about the external environment.

The largest organ in the integumentary system is the skin. Often not thought of as an organ, the skin is made of four different tissues that work together to perform a variety of functions such as preventing toxic substances from entering the body and regulating body temperature.

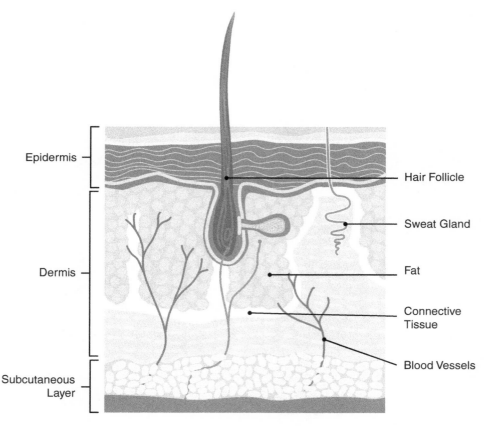

As shown in the image, the skin consists of several layers. These layers are divided into three regions: epidermis, dermis, and subcutaneous tissue. The **epidermis** is the outermost layer composed of **keratin** and stratified squamous epithelium tissue. Keratin is made of keratinocytes, which toughen and waterproof skin. Other cell types that make up the epidermis are melanocytes, which give skin its color, merkel cells, and Langerhans cells. The epidermis can have either four or five layers depending on where it is located on the body. As shown in the following image, these layers consist of the stratum basale (innermost layer), stratum spinosum, stratum granulosum, stratum lucidum, and stratum corneum.

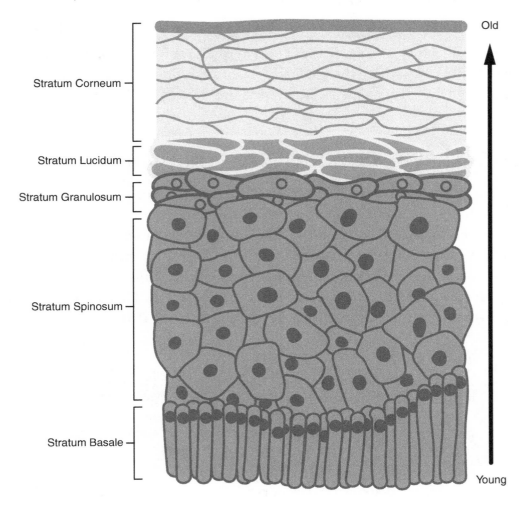

FOR EXAMPLE

The soles of the feet have five layers because they are exposed to a lot of friction as a person walks. The epidermis on the leg consists of only four layers.

Nerve endings and blood vessels are not found in the epidermis. Epidermal cells are found deep in the stratum basale and constantly undergo mitosis to make new cells. As new cells are made, they travel to the outer skin surface, producing the protein keratin. Epidermal cells fill with keratin and die upon reaching the skin's surface. When this happens, the leftover keratin from the dead cells help form the stratum corneum, which is the waterproof layer. These dead epidermal cells are gradually shed from the skin and replaced with new cells.

Example

How many epidermal layers make up the face?

A. 3   B. 4   C. 5   D. 6

The correct answer is **B**. The epidermis consists of either four or five layers. This depends on the part of the body where the epidermis is located. The soles of the feet and palms of the hand have five layers, and all other parts of the body, including the face, have four layers.

The Dermis Layer, Hypodermis, and Glands

The **dermis**, or dermal layer, is found directly under the epidermis. This deep, thick layer is made of tough connective tissue. It is connected to the epidermis by collagen fibers. Unlike the epidermis, nerve endings and blood vessels flow through the dermis. This means the dermal layer is responsible for a person feeling the sensations associated with touch, pain, heat, and cold. There are two major regions of the dermis: papillary region and reticular region. Both these regions provide elasticity to the skin, enabling it to stretch. This is helpful during physiological events like pregnancy, during which the abdominal area must stretch.

> **DID YOU KNOW?**
> The dermis layer of a young person is more elastic than that of an elderly person. This is because the dermis of elderly people has fewer elastic fibers. As the body ages, there is a reduction in physiological processes such as cell division, blood circulation, and muscle strength. These changes lead to a less elastic and thinner dermis.

Hair follicles and glands are also part of the dermis. Hair follicles are the sites where hair strands originate before protruding from the epidermal layer and onto the skin's surface. The two types of glands found in the dermis are detailed below:

- **Sweat glands:** These glands produce a fluid that contains water, salts, and other waste products. They are made of ducts that extend through the epidermis and look like pores on the skin's surface. There are two types of sweat glands:

  - **Apocrine:** These glands are found primarily in the armpits and groin area, where hair follicles are abundant. These glands are attached to hair follicles and create a watery fluid that contains proteins and fats. Apocrine glands are typically inactive until a person reaches puberty. They produce sweat when the body is anxious or experiencing stress.
  - **Eccrine:** These glands are found all over the body, primarily on the forehead, neck, palms, and soles of feet. They are not connected to hair follicles. They regulate body temperature with sweating if the body becomes too hot.

- **Sebaceous glands:** These oil-producing glands are typically attached to hair follicles. They release **sebum**, which is a fatty, oily substance. It waterproofs the hair and skin, preventing both structures from drying out. Sebum also has antimicrobial properties, which help the skin fight off infections.

DID YOU KNOW?
Sebaceous glands are found all over the body, but they are not found on the palms of the hands or soles of feet. The face and head contain the most sebum.

Right beneath the dermis is a third region of the integumentary system that contains subcutaneous tissue. This region is known as the **hypodermis**. It contains fat, or adipose tissue, that supplies energy for cells and provides insulation to regulate body temperature.

Example

Which structure produces sebum?

A. Hair follicles   B. Eccrine glands   C. Langerhans cells   D. D Sebaceous glands

The correct answer is **D**. The dermis is made of sebaceous glands and sweat glands. Eccrine and apocrine glands are two types of sweat glands, neither of which produce sebum. Sebaceous glands produce sebum, which is a fluid that flows through a hair follicle.

Hair and Nails

Nails and hair are accessory organs of the integumentary system. Fingernails and toenails are made of keratin, which is also found in the hair and skin. In addition to mechanical functions such as grasping things and picking up objects, nails prevent injuries to the ends of fingers. As shown in the image below, the nail is made of several parts.

The nail plate is the hard outer part of the nail. Adjoining the nail plate is the free edge, which overhangs the fingertip. This is the part of the nail that is commonly groomed and cut down. The nail bed is a layer of skin found under the nail plate. This layer of skin is comprised of epidermal cells. The white space between the nail bed and **cuticle** is called

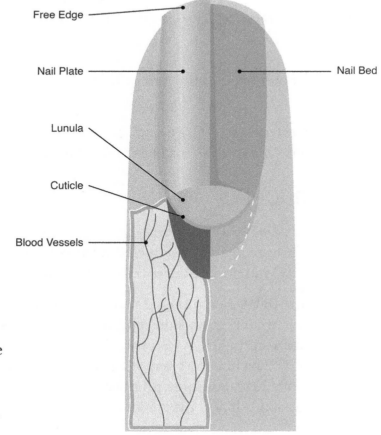

the **lunula**. The cuticle is a layer of dead skin cells that accumulate and form a thick overhang layer at the base of the nail and around the nail edge. During nail care, cuticles are removed. Beneath the cuticle is the **matrix**, which is a layer of tissue that contains blood vessels and nerves.

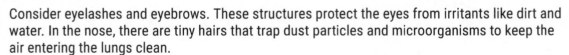

FOR EXAMPLE

Consider eyelashes and eyebrows. These structures protect the eyes from irritants like dirt and water. In the nose, there are tiny hairs that trap dust particles and microorganisms to keep the air entering the lungs clean.

Hair

Hair consists of dead keratinized cells and grows from the dermis out of the epidermis and onto the surface of the body. This accessory organ provides insulation for the body, especially for the head.

Recall that within the dermis is the hair follicle. This is where hair strands in the epidermis originate. The **hair shaft** is not attached to the follicle. It consists of the hair that is exposed on the surface of the body. The **hair root** is attached to

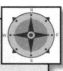

KEEP IN MIND

Aging affects the accessory organs. It causes hair and nails to thin over time.

the follicles and found beneath the skin's surface. Extending beyond the root, deep beneath the skin is the **hair bulb**, which contains actively dividing basal cells.

Example

What is the outer layer of the nail called?

A. Bed   B. Matrix   C. Plate   D. Shaft

The correct answer is **C**. The nail plate is the outer part of the nail that protects the edges of the finger. This structure is hard and connected to the free edge of the nail.

Skin Cancer

Skin cancer is the most common type of cancer that affects the integumentary system. There are many causes of skin cancer, including as genetics, but the strongest risk factor is exposure to ultraviolet (UV) radiation. Sources of UV radiation include sunlight and tanning beds.

Overexposure to UV radiation damages DNA in the body's cells. Exposure to UV radiation causes distinct mutations in skin cells. If the body does not repair the damage to these cells, the mutations accumulate. As a result, the cells can transform into cancerous cells and grow uncontrollably. The uncontrolled cell growth can lead to cancerous tumor formations. Most tumors are harmless, but some produce cells that can move away from the original site of DNA damage and establish new tumors in other organs. This process is called **metastasis**.

> **DID YOU KNOW?**
> There are different types of UV rays. UVA rays penetrate the dermis and can cause skin cancer. UVB rays penetrate the epidermis and cause damage to epidermal cells. UVB rays are responsible for sunburn and most skin cancers.

There are three types of skin cancer:

1. **Basal cell carcinoma:** This is the most common type of skin cancer that occurs in the basal cells of the epidermis. These cells are found in the stratum basale layer and divide to create keratinocytes. Basal cell carcinoma rarely spreads or undergoes metastasis.

2. **Squamous cell carcinoma:** This type of skin cancer occurs in the squamous cells of the epidermis. It affects the keratinocytes in the stratum spinosum. This is the second-most-common type of skin cancer. Because this type of skin cancer is more aggressive than basal cell carcinoma, if this carcinoma is not removed it can metastasize.

3. **Malignant melanoma:** This type of skin cancer occurs when there is an uncontrolled growth of melanocytes in the epidermis. Because melanocytes contribute to the pigmentation of the skin, melanoma is often associated with a dark patch on the body. It is the most dangerous and fatal type of skin cancer.

Example

What is a source of UV radiation?

A. Tanning bed

B. Indoor lighting

C. Topical products

D. Outdoor irritants

The correct answer is **A.** Tanning beds and overexposure to the sun are common sources of UV radiation. UVA and UVB rays are known to cause skin cancer in people.

Let's Review!

- The integumentary system is a body system composed of the skin, hair and nails.
- Skin is the largest organ of the body that primarily functions to protect the body and maintain homeostasis.
- The epidermis, dermis, and subcutaneous layer are the three layers of skin.
- The epidermis has four or five layers: the stratum basale, stratum granulosum, stratum lucidum, stratum spinosum, and stratum corneum.
- Two types of glands, sebaceous glands and sweat glands, are found in the dermis.
- Eccrine glands are found all over the body. Apocrine glands are found mainly in the armpits.
- Hair, nails, and skin all contain keratin, which hardens and toughens each structure.
- Exposure to UV radiation can cause three types of skin cancer.
- Aging affects the integrity and structure of the skin, hair, and nails.

CHAPTER 12 HUMAN ANATOMY AND PHYSIOLOGY: SUPPORT AND MOVEMENT PRACTICE QUIZ

1. Epidermal cells are found in the _____ before traveling to the skin's surface.

   A. stratum basale

   B. stratum lucidum

   C. stratum corneum

   D. stratum granulosum

2. Which layer contains nerve endings?

   A. Dermis

   B. Epidermis

   C. Stratum basale

   D. Subcutaneous tissue

3. Which is a characteristic of smooth muscle?

   A. Enables blood vessels to constrict

   B. Contributes to bone and joint flexibility

   C. Plays a role in how fast the heart contracts

   D. Consists of striated fibers that are branched

4. Which of the following organs contains cardiac muscle?

   A. Bladder

   B. Brain

   C. Heart

   D. Skin

5. Which organ does the vertebral column protect?

   A. Brain

   B. Heart

   C. Spinal cord

   D. Pelvic girdle

6. What does the skeletal system provide?

   A. Circulation

   B. Energy

   C. Immunity

   D. Support

Chapter 12 Human Anatomy and Physiology: Support and Movement Practice Quiz – Answer Key

1. **A.** Epidermal cells are found deep in the stratum basale. From there, they travel to the skin's surface, producing keratin along the way. This keratin creates the waterproof layer, or stratum corneum. **See Lesson: Integumentary System.**

2. **A.** The skin is comprised of three layers: epidermis, dermis, and subcutaneous tissue layer. The epidermis is the outermost layer and does not contain nerve endings. The dermis is the middle layer of skin that contains nerve endings. **See Lesson: Integumentary System.**

3. **A.** Smooth muscle is a non-striated muscle cell found in the internal walls of hollow organs like blood vessels. Under involuntary control, smooth muscle helps blood vessels contract and relax. **See Lesson: Muscular System.**

4. **C.** Cardiac muscle is a striated, branched type of muscle found only in the heart. Cardiac muscle is under involuntary control. **See Lesson: Muscular System.**

5. **C.** The vertebral column is part of the axial skeleton. It protects the spinal cord from external damage. **See Lesson: Skeletal System.**

6. **D.** The skeletal system serves many purposes, including providing support. Bones and cartilage help maintain body posture and comprise the framework of the skeletal system. **See Lesson: Skeletal System.**

Chapter 13 Human Anatomy and Physiology: Integration and Control

The Nervous System

This lesson introduces the anatomy of the nervous system, including its functions and divisions. It also explores the parts of neuron, neural conduction, and synaptic transmission.

What Is the Nervous System?

From perceptions to daily experiences, the **nervous system** controls many aspects of the human body. This system coordinates several activities in the body. It governs people's consciousness, their personalities, how they learn, and their ability to memorize. Working with the endocrine system, the nervous system regulates and maintains homeostasis.

The nervous system is anatomically divided into two parts:

1. **Central nervous system** (CNS): The central nervous system is comprised of the brain and spinal cord. It is where information processing and control occurs.
2. **Peripheral nervous system** (PNS): The peripheral nervous system is comprised of the nerves associated with the CNS. It connects all nerves of the body to the CNS. There are two types of fibers in the PNS: (a) **afferent fibers** that transmit impulses from organs and tissues of the body to the CNS; and (b) **efferent fibers** that transmit impulses from the CNS to the organs and tissues of the body.

The PNS is further divided into the somatic and autonomic nervous systems. The **somatic nervous system** primarily controls voluntary activities such as walking and riding a bicycle. Thus, this system sends information to the CNS and motor nerve fibers that are attached to skeletal muscle. The **autonomic nervous system** is responsible for activities that are non-voluntary and under unconscious control. Because this system controls glands and the smooth muscles of internal organs, it governs activities ranging from heart rate to breathing and digestion. The autonomic nervous system is further divided into the following:

- **Sympathetic nervous system:** The sympathetic nervous system focuses on emergency situations by preparing the body for fight or flight.
- **Parasympathetic nervous system:** The parasympathetic nervous system controls involuntarily processes unrelated to emergencies. This system deals with "rest or digest" activities.

Based on the activities of the nervous system, this system can be functionally divided into three parts:

1. **Sensory:** Information is gathered (both internally and externally) and carried to the CNS. The senses gather the information that the sensory nervous system transmits.
2. **Integrative:** The integrative nervous system is where the CNS process and interprets information received from the sensory nerves.
3. **Motor:** Motor nerves convey information that is processed by the CNS to muscles and glands.

The following flow chart summarizes the divisions of the nervous system:

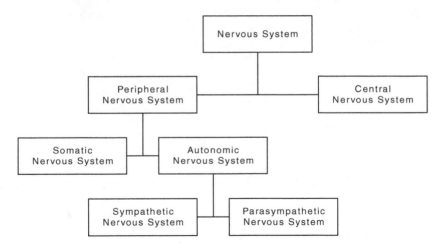

Examples

1. **Which organ is part of the central nervous system?**

   A. Brain   B. Heart   C. Lung   D. Stomach

   The correct answer is **A.** The nervous system is anatomically divided into two parts, the central and peripheral nervous systems. The central nervous system consists of the brain and spinal cord.

2. **What part of the nervous system controls blood vessel contraction?**

   A. Autonomic   B. Central   C. Somatic   D. Sympathetic

   The correct answer is **A.** The peripheral nervous system is divided into the somatic and autonomic nervous systems. The autonomic nervous system transmits neural signals to the smooth muscle found in the walls of internal organs and structures like blood vessels.

Anatomy of the Brain

The brain is a mass of tissue that is made of billions of nerve cells called neurons. This complex organ controls a wide range of processes and integrates information received from the five senses. Protected by the skull, the brain consists of four cavities called **ventricles**. These cavities are filled with **cerebrospinal fluid (CSF)**, which surrounds the CNS. This fluid serves many purposes such as protecting the brain from physical shocks and removing wastes from the neural tissue in the brain.

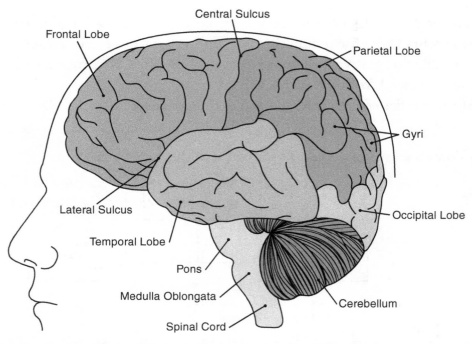

As shown in the above image, the brain is divided into the following three regions:

- **Cerebellum:** This is found beneath the cerebrum and behind the brainstem. It helps coordinate body movements, posture, and balance.
- **Brainstem:** This is found between the thalamus and the spinal cord. It is the lowest part of the brain that connects the brain with the spinal cord. Unconscious functions like breathing, heart rate, and blood pressure are controlled by the brainstem.
- **Cerebrum:** This part of the brain is the largest and part of the **forebrain**. The cerebrum controls higher-order functions such as interpreting touch, speech and language, reasoning, emotions, and fine motor control.

The **cerebral cortex** is **grey (or gray) matter** that surrounds the entire cerebrum. It is divided into a left and right hemisphere. The ridges of the cerebral cortex are called **gyri**, and the grooves are called **sulci**. The very large grooves are called **fissures**. The cerebral cortex is divided into four lobes: the frontal, parietal, temporal, and occipital

KEEP IN MIND

The lobes are named after the bones of the skull that protect each lobe. For example, the frontal bone protects the frontal lobe.

lobe. The cerebral cortex is the most complex part of the brain, and each lobe has specific functions that are outlined in the following table.

Lobe	Function
Frontal	Processes high-level cognitive skills, reasoning, concentration, motor skills, language, and functions as a control center for emotions.
Parietal	Integration site for visual perception and sensory information such as touch, pain, and pressure.
Temporal	Organizes sounds and processes language that is heard. Helps form memories, speech perception, and language skills.
Occipital	Interprets visual stimuli and information.

Example

What lobe helps a person interpret information received from the retinas of eyes?

A. Frontal   B. Occipital   C. Parietal   D. Temporal

The correct answer is **B**. The occipital lobe is part of the cerebrum. It interprets visual stimuli and information that comes from the eyes.

The Thalamus and Limbic System

Recall that the cerebral cortex is composed of grey matter. This mater is a type of neural tissue that contains three types of **neurons**, which are nerve cells that make up the nervous system:

- **Sensory neurons:** Afferent nerve cells that send information toward the CNS. This information is what is sensed, using the five senses, from the external environment.
- **Motor neurons:** Efferent nerve cells that carry impulses away from the CNS to the effectors, which are typically tissues and muscles of the body.
- **Interneurons:** Nerve cells that act as a bridge between motor and sensory neurons in the CNS. These neurons help form neural circuits, which helps neurons communicate with each other.

> **BE CAREFUL!**
> Grey matter is different from **white matter.** White matter is found in the spinal cord and surrounds the grey matter. It contains bundles of interneurons.

Another part of the forebrain incudes the **limbic system**, which controls emotions and memory. As shown in the image, this system is found right beneath the cerebral cortex and sits above the brainstem.

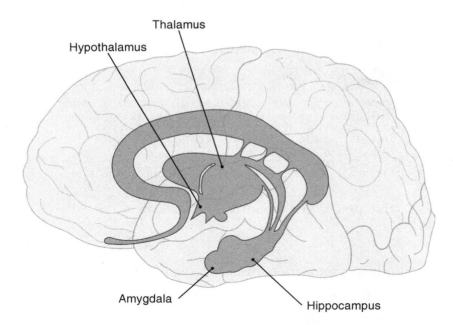

Four major structures of the brain comprise the limbic system:

- **Hypothalamus:** Found below the thalamus, this structure plays a role in regulating the autonomic nervous system. It is primarily concerned with homeostasis and regulates various activities such as hunger, anger, and the response to pain. The hypothalamus works with the pituitary gland from the endocrine system. This gland uses hormones, or chemical messengers, to generate responses in the body.
- **Amygdala:** Recognized as the aggression center, areas of this region produces feelings such as anger, violence, fear, and anxiety.
- **Thalamus:** Different sensory inputs come through the nerves and end at the thalamus, which directs this information to various parts of the cerebral cortex. The sense of smell is the only sense that bypasses the thalamus. Information related to movement is also processed by the thalamus.
- **Hippocampus:** Helps convert short-term memory to long-term memory. If the hippocampus is destroyed, new memories cannot be formed but old memories are retained.

DID YOU KNOW?
Kluver-Bucy syndrome is a condition that includes destruction of the amygdala. This means a person will present with erratic emotional behavior symptoms like hypersexuality, compulsive eating, and putting objects in the mouth.

Example

Which structure controls memory?

A. Amygdala   B. Hippocampus   C. Hypothalamus   D. Thalamus

The correct answer is **B.** All these structures are part of the limbic system and perform specific functions in the body. The hippocampus converts short-term memory into long-term memory.

Anatomy of a Neuron

Recall that the nervous system is comprised of specialized cells called neurons. A large network of neurons work together to quickly send and receive messages throughout the body. As shown in the following image, a neuron has several parts.

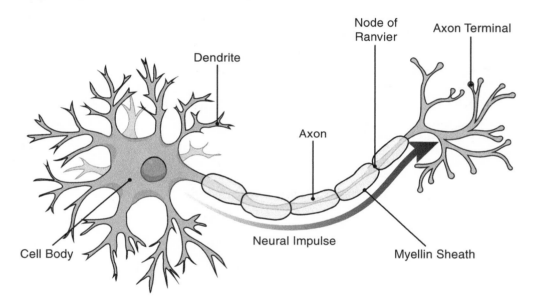

A neuron's structure is designed to transmit electric signals before they are transmitted as chemical signals to a target cell. The following three basic parts make up a single nerve cell:

- **Cell body:** This is the main part of the neuron that contains the nucleus of the nerve cell. Also called the soma, other organelles are also found in the cell body.
- **Dendrites:** These are appendages attached to the cell body that receive signals from other neurons.
- **Axon:** This is the long structure attached to the cell body. It conducts and transmits information to other cells. Branches at the end of the axon form **axon terminals**. These branches facilitate communication between neurons and target cells.

> **BE CAREFUL!**
>
> Do not confuse a neuron with a **neuroglial cell**. Neuroglial cells do not conduct nerve impulses like neurons. Rather, they provide support and protect neurons. Astrocytes, oligodendrocytes, microglial cell, and ependymal cells are the four major types of neuroglial cells in the CNS. Schwann and satellite cells are in the PNS.

Also shown in the image is a **myelin sheath** and **node of Ranvier**. The myelin sheath is a protein and lipid structure produced by a type of glial cell called a **Schwann cell**. This sheath functions like a blanket that provides a layer of insulation around the axon of a neuron, increasing the speed of electrical signal transmission. Regularly spaced gaps called nodes of Ranvier are found between the myleinated sheaths. Electric signals jump from one node to the next, thereby increasing the speed of signal transmission.

> **DID YOU KNOW?**
>
> Several diseases cause degeneration of the myelin sheath, or **demyelination**. One example is multiple sclerosis. When demyelination occurs, it can lead to severe neurological problems like motor and cognitive function. Demyelination reduces the speed at which neural impulses are transmitted along the axon.

Examples

1. **What structure receives information from another neuron?**

    A. Axon   B. Dendrite   C. Myelin   D. Soma

    The correct answer is **B**. Dendrites are appendages attached to the cell body, or soma, of a neuron. They receive information from other neurons and transmit this information to the cell body.

2. **How many types of neuroglia are found in the CNS?**

    A. 2   B. 4   C. 11   D. 17

    The correct answer is **B**. Neuroglia are cells that support neurons in the body. More neuroglia are present in the body than neurons. Four types are found in the CNS, and two types are found in the PNS.

Synaptic Transmission and Nerve Impulses

The electric signals neurons transmit are called **neural impulses**. Neurons must be excited to create a nerve impulse. A stimulus triggers excitation. At the resting state, the inside of the neuron is more negatively charged, while the outside of the neuron is more positively charged. This difference in electrical charge because of potassium and sodium ions establishes the **resting potential**.

DID YOU KNOW?

As a person ages, the rate of **neuroplasticity**, or ability for the brain to form neural connections through synapses, decreases. Neuroplasticity is important because it helps the brain adapt to new stimulation, damage, or changes in the environment.

During an **action potential**, a reverse in electrical charge occurs across the membrane of a neuron in its resting state. As shown in the following image, this happens when a neuron receives a neural impulse by way of a stimulus or a chemical signal from another neuron. The inside of the neuron becomes more positively charged, while the outside of the neuron becomes more negatively charged. This reverse in charge travels down the axon as an electric current.

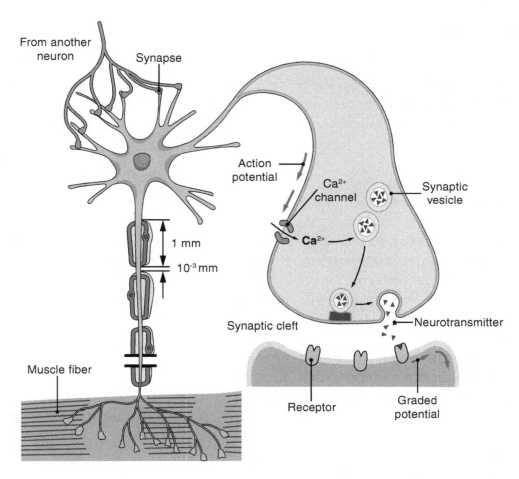

1. Once the action potential reaches the terminal bulbs of the axon terminal, the synaptic transmission process begins. The sequential numbers in the image outline the steps of synaptic transmission. The details of each numbered step are outlined below:An action potential travels down the axon and reaches the terminal branches of the axon. Voltage gated sodium gates open, causing sodium to enter the axon terminal bulb.
2. Voltage gated Ca2+ channels open at the same time.
3. Calcium ions move into the axon terminal bulb of the presynaptic neuron.

4. Calcium ions bind with proteins on synaptic vesicles that carry chemical messages called **neurotransmitters.**
5. This binding causes the vesicles to contract and move to the presynaptic membrane.
6. Neurotransmitters are released from the vesicles via exocytosis and diffuse across the **synaptic cleft**.
7. Neurotransmitters bind with receptors on the postsynaptic membrane of a neuron, gland, or muscle.
8. Depending on what the postsynaptic target cell is, the following responses will happen:

- Axon to dendrite: Action potential travels to next neuron.
- Axon and muscle cell: Muscle contraction.
- Axon and gland: Hormones released from gland.

Example

Which ion helps establish an action potential along an axon?

A. Barium   B. Calcium   C. Magnesium   D. Potassium

The correct answer is **D.** Electrical impulses travel along the axon of a neuron when the inside of a cell is positively charged and the outside of a cell is negatively charged. This difference in charge is due an exchange in the flow of sodium and potassium ions in and out the cell.

Let's Review!

- The nervous system is divided into the central nervous system (CNS) and peripheral nervous system (PNS).
- The somatic nervous system controls voluntary activities, while the autonomic nervous system is responsible for involuntary activities under unconscious control.
- The nervous system performs sensory, integrative, and motor functions.
- The three major regions of the brain are the cerebrum, brainstem, and cerebellum.
- Four lobes comprise the cerebral cortex, which is grey matter that surrounds the cerebrum.
- The limbic system consists of the hypothalamus, thalamus, hippocampus, and amygdala, each of which has different purposes.
- Neurons are made of dendrites, a cell body, an axon, and an axon terminal.
- Myelin sheaths insulate the axon of neuron, increasing the spread of electric signal transmission.
- A neuron must be excited from a stimulus to create a nerve impulse.
- Resting potentials are established when the outside of a nerve cell is more positively charged than the inside of a nerve cell.
- Action potentials are established when the reverse of a resting potential occurs.
- Synaptic transmission occurs in several steps and only occurs following an action potential.
- Neurotransmitters are chemical messengers released during an electrically stimulated synaptic transmission process.

THE ENDOCRINE SYSTEM

This lesson introduces the endocrine system and the role it plays in the maintenance of homeostasis.

Functions of the Endocrine System

The endocrine system works with the nervous system to regulate the activities critical to the maintenance of homeostasis. The following are the main functions of the endocrine system:

- Water balance
- Uterine contractions and milk release
- Growth, metabolism, and tissue maturation
- Ion regulation
- Heart rate and blood pressure regulation
- Blood glucose control
- Immune system regulation
- Reproductive functions control

Chemical Signals

Chemical signals, or **ligands**, are molecules released from one location that move to another location to produce a response. **Intracellular chemical signals** are produced in one part of a cell, such as the cell membrane, and travel to another part *of the same cell* and bind to receptors, either in the cytoplasm or in the nucleus. **Intercellular chemical signals** are released from one cell, are carried in the intercellular fluid, and bind to receptors that are found in *other* cells, but usually not in all cells of the body.

Intercellular chemical signals can be placed into functional categories on the basis of the tissues from which they are secreted and the tissues they regulate.

Autocrine chemical signals: These chemical signals are released by cells and have a local effect on the same cell type. Example: prostaglandin-like chemicals that are secreted in response to inflammation.

Paracrine chemical signals: These chemical signals are released by cells and have effects on other cell types. Example: somatostatin, secreted by the pancreas, inhibits the release of insulin by other cells in the pancreas.

Neuromodulators and neurotransmitters: These chemical signals are secreted by nerve cells and aid the nervous system. Example: acetylcholine produced during stressful encounters.

Pheromones: These chemical signals are secreted into the environment and modify the behavior and physiology of other individuals. Example: those produced by women can influence the length of the menstrual cycle of other women.

Example

Which chemical signal would respond to the redness caused by an infected wound?

A. Autocrines

B. Neuromodulators

C. Paracrines

D. Pheromones

The correct answer is **A**. Autocrine chemical signals include prostaglandin-like chemicals that are secreted in response to inflammation, which can indicate an infection.

Receptors

Chemical signals bind to proteins or glycoproteins called **receptor molecules** to produce a response. The shape and chemical characteristics of each receptor site allow only certain chemical signals to bind to it. This tendency is called **specificity**.

There are two major types of receptor molecules that respond to an intercellular chemical signal:

Intracellular receptors: These receptors are located in either the cytoplasm or the nucleus of the cell. Signals diffuse across the cell membrane and bind to the receptor sites on intracellular receptors.

Membrane-bound receptors: These receptors extend across the cell membrane, with their receptor sites on the outer surface of the cell membrane. They respond to intercellular chemical signals that are large, water-soluble molecules that do not diffuse across the cell membrane.

When an intercellular signal binds to a membrane-bound receptor, three general types of responses are possible:

Receptors that directly alter membrane permeability: For example, acetylcholine (adrenaline) from nerve fiber endings binds to receptors that are part of the membrane channels for sodium ions.

Receptors and G proteins: A G proteins (guanine nucleotide-binding proteins) are found on the inner surface of the plasma membrane and function as receptors of hormones. For example, chemical signals include cyclic adenosine monophosphate glycerol and inositol triphosphate that bind to receptor molecules in the cell and alter their activity to produce a response.

Receptors that alter the activity of enzymes: For example, increasing the activity of an enzyme responsible for the breakdown of glycogen into glucose makes glucose available as an energy source for muscle contractions.

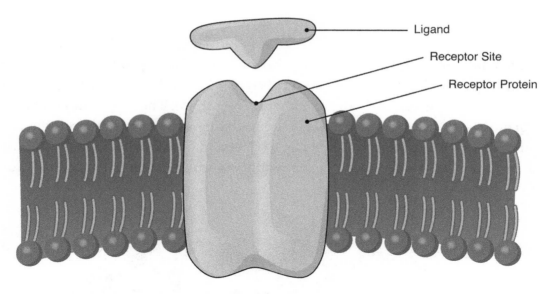

Receptor Protein

Some intercellular chemical signals diffuse across cell membranes and bind to intracellular receptors. Because these intracellular chemical signals are relatively small and soluble in lipids, they can diffuse through the cell membrane. The chemical signal and the receptor bind to DNA in the nucleus and increase specific messenger RNA synthesis in the nucleus of the cell. The messenger RNA then moves to the ribosomes, then to the cytoplasm, where new proteins are produced.

In contrast, intercellular chemical signals that bind to membrane-bound receptors produce rapid responses. For example, a few intercellular chemical signals can bind to their membrane-bound receptors, and each activated receptor can produce many intracellular chemical signal molecules that rapidly activate many specific enzymes inside the cell. This pattern of response is called the **cascade effect**.

Example

A friend is changing the tire on her car, and the jack breaks. Her hand is caught under the car. A passerby notices, runs over, and lifts the car off her hand. Which type of intercellular signal has responded?

> A. Receptors and G proteins
>
> B. Receptors that alter the activity of enzymes
>
> C. Receptors that directly alter membrane permeability
>
> D. Receptors that indirectly alter membrane permeability

The correct answer is **C**. Nerve fiber endings bind to receptors that are part of the membrane channels for sodium ions to enable adrenaline to respond.

Hormones

The term **endocrine** implies that intercellular chemical signals are produced within and secreted from endocrine glands, but the chemical signals have effects at locations that are away from, or separate from, the endocrine glands that secrete them. The intercellular chemical signals, or hormones, are transported in the blood to tissues some distance from the glands. **Hormones** are produced in minute amounts by a collection of cells to influence the activity of those tissues in a specific way. For example, **neurohormones** are hormones secreted from cells of the nervous system.

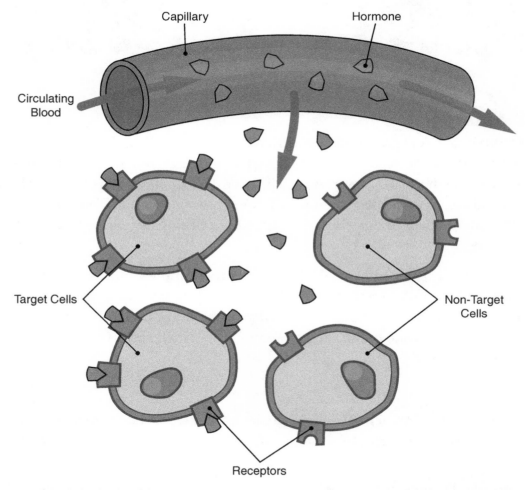

Hormones are distributed in the blood to all parts of the body, but only certain tissues, called **target tissues**, respond to each type of hormone. Target tissue is made up of cells that have receptor molecules for a specific hormone. Each hormone can only bind to its receptor molecules and cannot influence the function of cells that do not have receptor molecules for the hormone.

Regulation of Hormone Secretion

The secretion of hormones is controlled by negative-feedback mechanisms. Negative-feedback mechanisms keep the body functioning within a narrow range of values consistent with life. Hormone secretion is regulated in three ways:

1. **Blood levels of chemicals:** The secretion of some hormones is directly controlled by the blood levels of certain chemicals. For example, blood glucose levels control insulin secretion.
2. **Hormones:** The secretion of some hormones is controlled by other hormones. For example, hormones from the pituitary gland act on the ovaries and the testes, causing those organs to secrete sex hormones.
3. **Nervous system:** These hormones are controlled by the nervous system. For example, epinephrine is released from the adrenal medulla as a result of nervous system stimulation.

Example

The negative-feedback mechanism that regulates the level of glucose in a person's blood is an example of what type of hormone secretion regulation?

A. Hormone regulation

B. Nervous system regulation

C. Blood levels of chemicals regulation

D. Intercellular ion concentration regulation

The correct answer is **C.** The blood levels of certain chemicals, such as insulin, directly control the secretion of some hormones.

Endocrine Glands and Their Secretions

The endocrine system consists of ductless glands that secrete hormones directly into the blood. An extensive network of blood vessels supplies the endocrine glands. The following is a table of hormones secreted by the anterior pituitary gland.

Anterior Pituitary Gland		
Hormone	**Target**	**Response**
Growth hormone	Most tissues	Increases protein synthesis
Thyroid-stimulating hormone	Thyroid gland	Increases thyroid hormone secretion
Adrenocorticotropic	Adrenal cortex	Increases secretion of cortisol
Melanocyte-stimulating hormone	Melanocytes in skin	Increases melanin production to make skin darker
Luteinizing hormone	Females: ovaries Males: testes	Females: promotes ovulation Males: promotes sperm cell production

Follicle-stimulating hormone	Females: ovarian follicles Males: seminiferous tubules	Females: promotes follicle maturation Males: promotes sperm cell production
Prolactin	Ovary and mammary glands	Prolongs progesterone secretion

Additional common hormones are listed in the chart below.

Gland	Hormone	Target Tissue	Response	Under- or Overproduction of Hormone
Thyroid gland	Thyroid hormone	Most cells of the body	Increases metabolic rate	Hypothyroidism Hyperthyroidism
Adrenal medulla	Epinephrine	Heart, blood vessels, liver, adipose cells	Increases cardiac output and blood flow	Addison's disease
Pancreas	Insulin and glucagon	Liver, skeletal muscles, and adipose tissue	Insulin: increases uptake and use of glucose Glucagon: increases breakdown of glycogen	Diabetes

The Effects of Aging

The aging process affects hormone activity in one of three ways: their secretion can decrease, remain unchanged, or increase.

Hormones that decrease secretion include the following:

- Estrogen (in women)
- Testosterone (in men)
- Growth hormone
- Melatonin

In women, the decline in estrogen levels leads to menopause. In men, testosterone levels usually decrease gradually. Decreased levels of growth hormone may lead to decreased muscle mass and strength. Decreased melatonin levels may play an important role in the loss of normal sleep-wake cycles (circadian rhythms) with aging.

Hormones that usually remain unchanged or slightly decrease include the following:

- Cortisol
- Insulin
- Thyroid hormones

Hormones that may increase secretions levels include the following:

- Follicle-stimulating hormone
- Luteinizing hormone
- Norepinephrine
- Epinephrine, in the very old
- Parathyroid hormone

Example

Which of the following is an effect of aging on hormone secretion?

A. Weak teeth   B. Loss of appetite   C. Trouble sleeping   D. Loss of body hair

The correct answer is **C**. The reduction of melatonin can result in the inability to sleep.

Let's Review!

- The endocrine system functions with the nervous system to regulate the many activities critical to the maintenance of homeostasis.
- Chemical signals, or ligands, are molecules released from one location that move to another location to produce a response.
- Chemical signals bind to proteins or glycoproteins called receptor molecules to produce a response.
- A hormone is an intercellular chemical signal that is produced in minute amounts by collections of cells to influence the activity of those tissues in a specific way.
- Hormones are distributed in the blood to all parts of the body, but only certain tissues, called target tissues, respond to each type of hormone.
- Negative-feedback mechanisms control the secretion of hormones.
- The endocrine system consists of ductless glands that secrete hormones directly into the blood.
- The aging process affects hormone activity.

THE LYMPHATIC SYSTEM

This lesson introduces the structure and function of the lymphatic system, which is commonly referred to as the immune system. It also examines the common diseases and disorders of this system.

The Key Players in the Lymphatic System

Components of the lymphatic system are the spleen, tonsils, adenoids, appendix, thymus gland, and lymph nodes. The **spleen** helps fight certain types of bacteria. The **tonsils**, **adenoids**, and **appendix** were once believed to be vestigial organs, meaning they are remnants left over from human evolution. Now, scientists have found they have active functions. The **thymus gland** is located directly above the heart. It secretes hormones that stimulate the maturation of killer T cells. This gland is only active from birth through puberty. After puberty, it decreases in size and functionality.

The body initiates a battle as soon as a **pathogen**, or a foreign body, enters. Two types of **lymphocytes**, B cells and T cells, are white blood cells that target the pathogen. Macrophages, another type of white blood cell, join in the invasion.

Killer T cells attack and kill infected cells. **B cells** label invaders for later destruction by macrophages. **Helper T cells** activate killer T cells and B cells. **Macrophages** consume pathogens and infected cells. These four kinds of white blood cells exchange information and correlate their activities as an integrated system.

When someone comes down with the flu, influenza viruses enter the body in small water droplets inhaled into the respiratory system. If the mucous membranes do not ensnare them, they slip past patrolling macrophages and begin to infect and kill mucous membrane cells, which makes the person feel sick. Macrophages initiate an "alarm" signal that activates the helper T cells, which serve as the "generals" of the lymphatic system. Helper T cells activate killer T cells and B cells and produce defensive proteins.

The body now initiates a robust attack against the flu virus. Using a second chemical signal, the helper T cells call into action killer T cells, which recognize and destroy body cells that the virus has infected. The T cells have receptors that recognize tiny bits of the virus's proteins and release enzymes into the infected cells that encourage the cells to destroy themselves.

The protein the helper T cells releases also activates the B cells. Like killer T cells, B cells have receptor proteins called **antibodies** on their surfaces. The B cells can release copies of these antibodies into the bloodstream or attach them directly to pathogens, marking pathogens for destruction. These B cells also secrete antibodies that attach to any invading pathogen into the bloodstream.

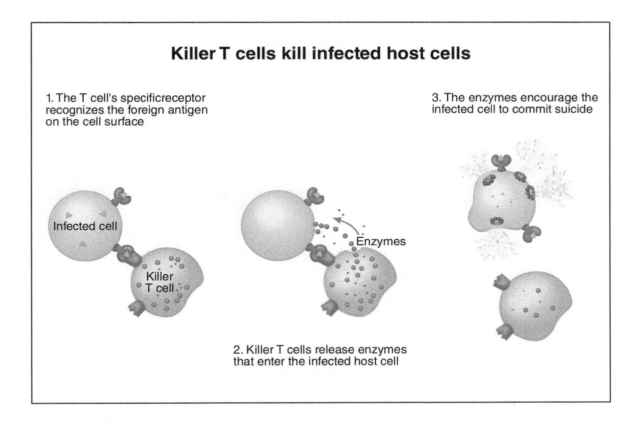

Killer T cells kill infected host cells

1. The T cell's specificreceptor recognizes the foreign antigen on the cell surface

3. The enzymes encourage the infected cell to commit suicide

Infected cell

Killer T cell

Enzymes

2. Killer T cells release enzymes that enter the infected host cell

Examples

1. **Which of the following is the correct series of the lymphatic system's defense mechanisms?**

    A. B cell and T cell → Macrophage → Helper T cell

    B. Helper T cell → T cell → B cell → Macrophage

    C. Macrophage → Helper T cell → B cell → T cell

    D. Macrophage → Helper T cell → B cell and T cell

    The correct answer is **D.** Once the macrophages sound the alarm, the helper T cells simultaneously activate the B cells and T cells.

2. **The B cells do not directly attack pathogens or infected cells. Instead, they**

    A. mark the pathogens for destruction by macrophages and B cells.

    B. mark the antibodies for destruction by B cells and natural killer cells.

    C. mark the antibodies for destruction by macrophages and killer T cells.

    D. mark the pathogens for destruction by macrophages and natural killer cells.

    The correct answer is **D.** The B cells do not directly attack pathogens or infected cells. Instead, they mark the pathogens for destruction by macrophages and natural killer cells.

When a B cell encounters a foreign microbe with a surface protein that matches the shape of its antibodies, it attaches an antibody to the microbe.

Types of Immunity

The four types of immunity are natural/passive, natural/active, artificial/passive, and artificial/active. The following are examples of these types of immunities:

- Natural/passive – Babies receive immunities from breastmilk.
- Natural/active – The body produces antibodies to combat an illness when a person becomes sick.
- Artificial/passive – This immunity is temporary and requires doses of serum to maintain the immunity.
- Artificial/active – A vaccination provides artificial/active immunity.

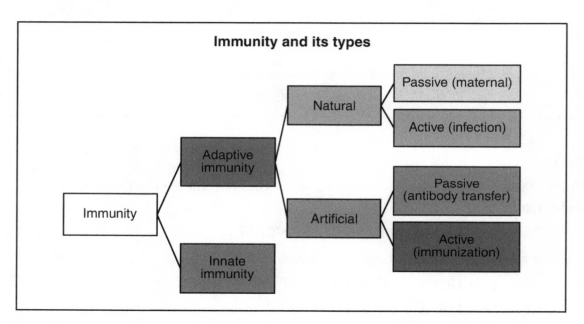

Example

When a child breastfeeds, that child is exposed to all the "germs" on the mother. As a result, what type of immunity is the child acquiring?

A. Artificial/active

B. Artificial/passive

C. Natural/active

D. Natural/passive

The correct answer is **D.** The child acquires this immunity without the baby's body experiencing an illness. The baby is not born with this immunity and does nothing to acquire it. Therefore, it is passive.

Vaccination Prepares the Lymphatic System

Vaccination is the introduction into the body of a dead or disabled pathogen or of a harmless microbe with the protein of a pathogen on its surface. Vaccination triggers the lymphatic system response against the pathogen without an infection occurring. Afterward, the bloodstream of the vaccinated person contains memory cells that are directed against the pathogen. The vaccinated person is immunized against the disease. Vaccinations have dramatically reduced the incidence of many bacterial and viral diseases, including polio, tetanus, and diphtheria. An intensive vaccination program led to the elimination of the deadly disease smallpox in the 1970s.

Example

Sometimes, people complain they have become sick because of a vaccination. Why is this impossible?

    A. The pathogen is dead.

    B. The pathogen was originally harmless.

    C. The pathogen is only viable for a short time.

    D. The pathogen has been disabled by sterilization.

The correct answer is **A**. Vaccination is the introduction into the body of a dead or disabled pathogen or of a harmless microbe with the protein of a pathogen on its surface.

Diseases and Disorders of the Lymphatic System

The ability of killer T cells and B cells to distinguish cells of the body from foreign cells is crucial to the fight against pathogens. In **autoimmune diseases**, this ability breaks down, causing the body to attack its own cells. The following chart gives examples of autoimmune conditions.

Diseases	Areas affected	Symptoms
Systemic Lupus Erythematosus	Connective tissue, joints, kidneys	Facial, skin rash; painful joints; fever; fatigue; kidney problems; weight loss
Type I Diabetes	Insulin-producing cells in the pancreas	Excessive urine production; blurred vision; weight loss; fatigue; irritability
Graves' Disease	Thyroid	Weakness; irritability; heat intolerance; increased sweating; weight loss; insomnia
Rheumatoid Arthritis	Joints	Crippling inflammation of the joints

Age

As people age, their bodies produce fewer B and T cells. As a result, their bodies' ability to defend themselves against viruses and bacteria lessens.

Allergies

Sometimes, the body's immune system works too well and attacks itself. This is known as an **allergy**. Hay fever is an example.

Mast cells, attached to white blood cells, line entrances to the body. When they encounter matching antibodies, they initiate an **inflammatory response**, which releases histamines. **Histamines** cause capillaries to swell and increase mucous membrane production.

HIV/AIDS: Lymphatic System Collapse

HIV/AIDS is a result of a mutation that occurred in a virus that affects chimpanzees. It destroys macrophages and helper T cells.

How Is HIV Transmitted?

Because there is no cure for AIDS, prevention is key. HIV/AIDS can only survive in blood or body fluids because macrophages are located there. The primary means of transmission is through sexual intercourse.

HIV is not transmitted through the air, on toilet seats, or by any other medium where a macrophage cannot survive. It cannot be transmitted through shaking hands, sharing food, or drinking from a water fountain because macrophages cannot be transmitted through casual contact.

Example

Why is AIDS a devastating disease?

A. It targets red blood cells.

B. It targets respiratory lining cells.

C. It targets many different types of cells.

D. It targets the cells in the lymphatic system that target pathogens.

The correct answer is **D**. A mutation arose in the chimpanzee virus that allowed it to recognize a human cell surface receptor on certain immune system cells, primarily the macrophages and helper T cells.

Let's Review!

- This lesson explored the lymphatic system's keys components and the major disease and disorders of the system.
- The lymphatic system provides immunity against pathogens.
- Several organs work together to make the lymphatic system efficient.
- Killer T cells recognize and destroy body cells that have been infected with a virus.

- B cells do not directly attack pathogens or infected cells.
- B cells have receptor proteins on their surface called antibodies.
- Vaccination is the introduction into the body of a dead or disabled pathogen or of a harmless microbe with the protein of a pathogen on its surface.
- In autoimmune diseases, the ability to distinguish cells of the body from foreign cells breaks down, causing the body to attack its own cells.
- Age has a negative effect on the lymphatic system.

CHAPTER 13 HUMAN ANATOMY AND PHYSIOLOGY: INTEGRATION AND CONTROL PRACTICE QUIZ

1. An area on a person's arm becomes inflamed. What type of response does this indicate?

   A. Autocrine

   B. Neuromodulator

   C. Paracrine

   D. Pheromone

2. Which of the following is one of the primary functions of the endocrine system?

   A. Blood glucose control

   B. Digestive system control

   C. Nervous system regulation

   D. Negative feedback initiation

3. Which of the following diseases exhibits symptoms such as weakness, irritability, heat intolerance, increased sweating, weight loss, and insomnia?

   A. Diabetes I

   B. Graves' disease

   C. Rheumatoid arthritis

   D. Systemic lupus erythematosus

4. _____ trigger the lymphatic system response against a pathogen without an infection occurring.

   A. B Cells   C. Vaccinations

   B. Antibodies   D. Helper T Cells

5. The nervous system works with the endocrine system to

   A. maintain internal homeostasis.

   B. filter wastes and toxins out the body.

   C. protect internal organs from getting damaged.

   D. supply oxygen to the cells and tissues in the body.

6. What is the purpose of motor function in the nervous system?

   A. Carry external information to the CNS

   B. Transmit information from the CNS to a muscle

   C. Process information received from sensory nerves

   D. Receive information after someone sees something

Chapter 13 Human Anatomy and Physiology: Integration and Control Practice Quiz – Answer Key

1. **A.** Autocrine chemical signals are released by cells and have a local effect on the same cell type. **See Lesson: The Endocrine System.**

2. **A.** Monitoring blood glucose levels is a vital function of the endocrine system. **See Lesson: The Endocrine System.**

3. **B.** The symptoms listed indicate Graves' disease. **See Lesson: The Lymphatic System.**

4. **C.** Vaccinations trigger the lymphatic system response against a pathogen without an infection occurring. **See Lesson: The Lymphatic System.**

5. **A.** The nervous system controls many parts of the body by coordinating activities. Its primary function with help from the endocrine system is to maintain homeostasis. **See Lesson: The Nervous System.**

6. **B.** Motor function involves the motor nerves, which send information from the CNS to glands or muscles. **See Lesson: The Nervous System.**

CHAPTER 14 LIFE AND PHYSICAL SCIENCES

An Introduction to Biology

This lesson introduces the basics of biology, including the process researchers use to study science. It also examines the classes of biomolecules and how substances are broken down for energy.

Biology and Taxonomy

The study or science of living things is called **biology**. Some characteristics, or traits, are common to all living things. These enable researchers to differentiate living things from nonliving things. Traits include reproduction, growth and development, **homeostasis**, and energy processing. Homeostasis is the body's ability to maintain a constant internal environment despite changes that occur in the external environment. With so many living things in the world, researchers developed a **taxonomy** system, which is used for classification, description, and naming. As shown below, there are seven classification levels in the classical Linnaean system.

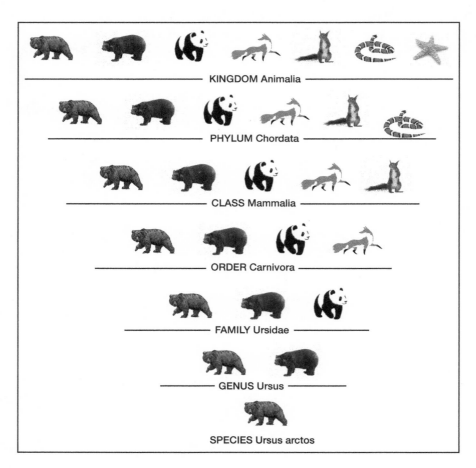

Specificity increases as the levels move from kingdom to species. For example, in the image the genus level contains two types of bears, but the species level shows one type. Additionally, organisms in each level are found in the level above it. For example, organisms in the order level are part of the class level. This classification system is based on physical similarities across living things. It does not account for molecular or genetic similarities.

> **DID YOU KNOW?**
> Carl Linnaeus only used physical similarities across organisms when he created the Linnaean system because technology was not advanced enough to observe similarities at the molecular level.

Example

A researcher classifies a newly discovered organism in the class taxonomy level. What other taxonomic level is this new organism classified in?

A. Order   B. Family   C. Species   D. Kingdom

The correct answer is **D.** Each level is found in the level above it. The levels above class are phylum and kingdom.

Scientific Method

To develop the taxonomic system, researchers had to ask questions. Researchers use seven steps to answer science questions or solve problems. These make up the **scientific method,** described below:

1. Problem: The question created because of an observation. *Example: Does the size of a plastic object affect how fast it naturally degrades in a lake?*
2. Research: Reliable information available about what is observed. *Example: Learn how plastics are made and understand the properties of a lake.*
3. Hypothesis: A predicted solution to the question or problem. *Example: If the plastic material is small, then it will degrade faster than a large particle.*
4. Experiment: A series of tests used to evaluate the hypothesis. Experiments consist of an **independent variable** that the researcher modifies and a **dependent variable** that changes due to the independent variable. They also include a **control group** used as a standard to make comparisons. *Example: Collect plastic particles both onshore and offshore of the lake over time. Determine the size of the particles and describe the lake conditions during this time period.*
5. Observe: Analyze data collected during an experiment to observe patterns. *Example: Analyze the differences between the numbers of particles collected in terms of size.*
6. Conclusion: State whether the hypothesis is rejected or accepted and summarize all results.
7. Communicate: Report findings so others can replicate and verify the results.

Sometimes, just a few steps of the scientific method are necessary to research a question. At other times, several steps may be repeated as needed. The goal of this method is to find a reliable answer to the scientific question.

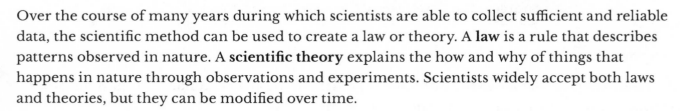

TEST TIP

Using the first letter in each of the steps, you can create a mnemonic device to remember the steps. For example: "**P**eople **R**eally **H**ave **E**lephants **O**n **C**ompact **C**ars." Try creating your own mnemonic device!

Over the course of many years during which scientists are able to collect sufficient and reliable data, the scientific method can be used to create a law or theory. A **law** is a rule that describes patterns observed in nature. A **scientific theory** explains the how and why of things that happens in nature through observations and experiments. Scientists widely accept both laws and theories, but they can be modified over time.

Example

In a study, a researcher describes what happens to a plant following exposure to a dry and hot environment. What step of the scientific method does this most likely describe?

A. Forming a hypothesis

B. Making an observation

C. Communicating findings

D. Characterizing the problem

The correct answer is **D**. The researcher is collecting qualitative data by describing what happens to the plant under specific conditions. This data collection corresponds to the observation step of the scientific method.

Water and Biomolecule Basics

From oceans and streams to a bottle, water is fundamental for life. Without water, life would not exist. Because of water's unique properties, it plays a specific role in living things. The molecular structure of water consists of an oxygen atom bonded to two hydrogen atoms. The structure of water explains some of its properties. For example, water is polar. The oxygen atom is slightly negatively charged, while both hydrogen atoms are slightly positively charged.

As shown below, a single water molecule forms **hydrogen bonds** with nearby water molecules. This type of bonding creates a weak attraction between the water molecules. Hydrogen bonding contributes to water's high boiling point. Water is necessary for biochemical processes like photosynthesis and cellular respiration. It is also a universal solvent, which means water dissolves many different substances.

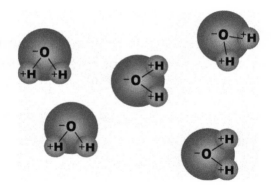

Only two water molecules are needed to show bonding. Remove the partial negative/positive signs and put a – sign next to the oxygen atom and a + sign next to each hydrogen (H) atom. Remove the solid lines between the H and O but keep the dashed line connecting one water molecule to the next.

> **KEEP IN MIND**
>
> It takes a lot of heat to create hot water. This is because of water's high specific heat capacity, which is the amount of heat required to raise the temperature of 1 kilogram of water by 1 degree Celsius. This property of water also makes it ideal for living things.

Biomolecules, or biological molecules, are found in living things. These organic molecules vary in structure and size and perform different functions. Researchers group the wide variety of molecules found in living things into four major classes for organizational purposes: proteins, carbohydrates, lipids, and nucleic acids. Each class of biomolecules has unique **monomers** and **polymers**. Monomers are molecules that covalently bond to form larger molecules or polymers. The table below lists characteristics of each class.

Biomolecule	Monomer(s)	Function	Example
Protein	Amino acid	A substance that provides the overall basic structure and function for a cell	Enzymes
Carbohydrate	Monosaccharides	A form of storage for energy	Glucose Cellulose Starch Disaccharides
Lipid	Glycerol and fatty acids	A type of fat that provides a long-term storage for energy	Fats Steroids Oils Hormones
Nucleic acid	Nucleotides	A substance that aids in protein synthesis and transmission of genetic information	DNA RNA

Example

During protein synthesis in a cell, the primary structure of the protein consists of a linear chain of monomers. What is another way to describe this structure?

 A. A linear chain of fatty acids that are hydrogen-bonded together

 B. A linear chain of nucleotides that are hydrogen-bonded together

 C. A linear chain of amino acids that are covalently bonded together

 D. A linear chain of monosaccharides that are covalently bonded together

The correct answer is **C**. The monomers of proteins include amino acids, which are covalently bonded together to form a protein.

The Metabolic Process

Just like water, energy is essential to life. Food and sunlight are major energy sources. Metabolism is the process of converting food into usable energy. This refers to all biochemical processes or reactions that take place in a living thing to keep it alive.

> **CONNECTIONS**
>
> Energy flows through living things. Energy from the sun is converted to chemical energy via photosynthesis. When living things feed on plants, they obtain this energy for survival.

A metabolic pathway is a series of several chemical reactions that take place cyclically to either build or break down molecules. An **anabolic pathway** involves the synthesis of new molecules. These pathways require an input of energy. **Catabolic pathways** involve the breakdown of molecules. Energy is released from a catabolic pathway.

Living things use several metabolic pathways. The most well-studied pathways include glycolysis, the citric acid cycle, and the electron transport chain. These metabolic pathways either release or add energy during a reaction. They also provide a continual flow of energy to living things.

1. **Glycolysis:** This is a catabolic pathway that uses several steps to break down glucose sugar for energy, carbon dioxide, and water. Energy that is released from this reaction is stored in the form of adenosine triphosphate (ATP). Two ATP molecules, two pyruvate molecules, and two NADH molecules are formed during this metabolic pathway.

> **BE CAREFUL!**
>
> Some of these metabolic pathways produce energy in different parts of the cell. Glycolysis takes place in the cytoplasm of the cell. But the citric acid cycle and oxidative phosphorylation occur in the mitochondria.

2. **Citric acid cycle:** The pyruvate molecules made from glycolysis are transported inside the cell's mitochondria. In this catabolic pathway, pyruvate is used to make two ATP molecules, six carbon dioxide molecules, and six NADH molecules.

3. **Electron transport chain and oxidative phosphorylation:** This also takes place in the cell's mitochondria. Many electrons are transferred from one molecule to another in this chain. At the end of the chain, oxygen picks up the electrons to produce roughly 34 molecules of ATP.

The following image provides an overview of **cellular respiration**. Glycolysis, the citric acid cycle, the electron transport chain, and oxidative phosphorylation collectively make up this process. Cellular respiration takes place in a cell and is used to convert energy from nutrients into ATP.

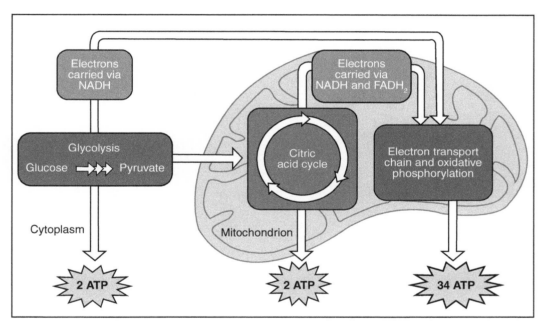

Example

Why are metabolic pathways cyclic?

    A. Metabolic reactions generally take place one at a time.

    B. All of the products created in metabolic reactions are used up.

    C. The reactions are continuous as long as reactants are available.

    D. Energy in the form of ATP is sent to different cells for various uses.

The correct answer is **C**. Metabolic reactions are cyclic, which means they keep occurring as long as enough starting materials are available to allow the reaction to proceed.

Let's Review!

- This lesson explored how living things are organized, what the scientific method is, and how biomolecules are classified. It also discussed how living things obtain energy via metabolism.
- Biology is the study of living things. Several characteristics distinguish living things from nonliving things.
- All living things are described, classified, and named using a taxonomic system.
- The scientific method uses seven steps to answer a question or solve a problem.
- Biomolecules are organic molecules that are organized into four classes: proteins, carbohydrates, lipids, and nucleic acids
- Living things rely on various metabolic pathways to produce energy and store it in the form of ATP.

CELL STRUCTURE, FUNCTION, AND TYPE

This lesson describes the cell structure and two different types of cells. The lesson also explores the functions of various cell parts.

Cell Theory and Types

All living things are made of cells. **Cells** are the smallest structural units and basic building blocks of living things. Cells contain everything necessary to keep living things alive. Varying in size and shape, cells carry out specialized functions. Robert Hooke discovered the first cells in the mid-eighteenth century. Many years later, after advancements in microscopy, the cell theory was formed. This theory, or in-depth explanation, about cells consists of three parts:

1. All living things are composed of one or more cells.
2. Cells are alive and represent the basic unit of life.
3. All cells are produced from preexisting cells.

DID YOU KNOW?

More than a trillion cells and at least 200 different types of cells exist in the human body!

Many different types of cells exist. Because of this, cells are classified into two general types: prokaryotic cells and eukaryotic cells. The following comparison table lists key differences between prokaryotes and eukaryotes:

Characteristic	Prokaryote	Eukaryote
Cell size	Around 0.2–2.0 mm in diameter	Around 10–100 mm in diameter
Nucleus	Absent	True nucleus
Organelles	Absent	Several present, ranging from ribosomes to the endoplasmic reticulum
Flagella	Simple in structure	Complex in structure

As shown in the image, prokaryotic cells lack nuclei. Their DNA floats in the **cytoplasm**, which is surrounded by a **plasma membrane**. Very simplistic in structure, these cells lack organelles but do have cell walls. **Organelles** are specialized structures with a specific cellular function. They also may have **ribosomes** that aid in protein synthesis. Also, these cells have a **flagellum** that looks like a tail attached to the cell. Flagella aid in locomotion. The **pili**, or hair-like structures surrounding the cells, aid in cellular adhesion. Bacteria and Archaea are the most common prokaryotes. Most prokaryotes are **unicellular**, or made of a single cell, but there are a few **multicellular organisms**.

Eukaryotic cells contain a membrane-bound nucleus where DNA is stored. Membrane-bound organelles also exist in eukaryotic cells. Similar to prokaryotic cells, eukaryotic cells have cytoplasm, ribosomes, and a plasma membrane. Eukaryotic organisms can be either unicellular or multicellular. Much larger than prokaryotes, examples of eukaryotic organisms include fungi and even people.

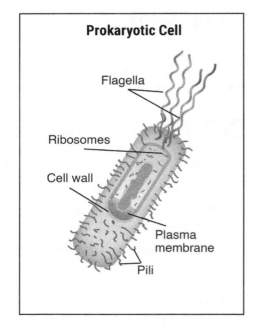

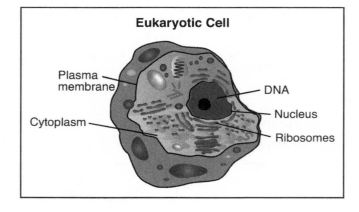

Example

What is an organelle?

A. The building block of all living things

B. A substance that is able diffuse inside a cell

C. The specific receptor found on a cell's surface

D. A membrane-bound structure with a special function

The correct answer is **D**. Organelles such as ribosomes and the nucleus are membrane-bound structures that have specific functions in a cell.

A Peek Inside the Animal Cell

Animal cells are eukaryotic cells. Cheek, nerve, and muscle cells are all examples of animal cells. Because there are many different types, each animal cell has a specialized function. But all animal cells have the same parts, or organelles. Use this image as a guide while going through following list, which describes the organelles found in a eukaryotic (or animal) cell.

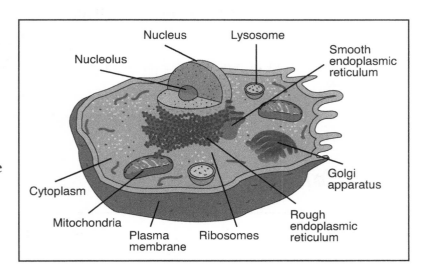

- **Cell membrane:** A double layer that separates the inside of the cell from the outside environment. It is semi-permeable, meaning it only allows certain molecules to enter the cell.
- **Nucleus:** A membrane-bound organelle that contains the genetic material, such as DNA, for a cell. Inside the nucleus is the **nucleolus** that plays a role in assembling subunits required to make ribosomes.

> **KEEP IN MIND!**
> Some of the organelles in animal cells are also present in plant cells. In addition, all organelles are found in the cytoplasm of the cell. The only exception is the nucleus, which it is separated from the cytoplasm because it has its own membrane.

- **Mitochondria:** The cell's powerhouses that provide energy to the cell for it to function. Much of the energy in the form of ATP is produced here.
- **Ribosomes:** The cell's protein factories that can be found floating in the cytoplasm or attached to the endoplasmic reticulum.
- **Vacuoles:** Small sacs in a cell that store water and food for survival. This organelle also stores waste material that is mostly in the form of water.
- **Endoplasmic reticulum:** A network of membranes that functions as a cell's transportation system, shuttling proteins and other materials around the cell. The **smooth endoplasmic reticulum** lacks ribosomes, and the **rough endoplasmic reticulum** has ribosomes.
- **Lysosomes:** Sac-like structures that contain digestive enzymes that are used to break down food and old organelles.
- **Golgi apparatus:** A stack of flattened pouches that plays a role in processing proteins received from the endoplasmic reticulum. It modifies proteins from the endoplasmic reticulum and then packages them into a vesicle that can be sent to other places in the cell.

Example

Which two organelles work together to facilitate protein synthesis?

A. Cytoplasm and lysosome

C. Nucleus and cell membrane

B. Vacuole and mitochondria

D. Ribosome and endoplasmic reticulum

The correct answer is **D**. After a protein is synthesized by ribosomes, it is shuttled to the endoplasmic reticulum, where it is further modified and prepared to be transported by vesicles to other places in the cell.

Plant Cells

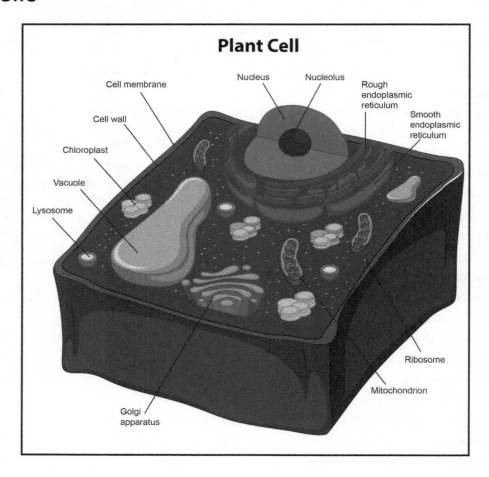

Plant Cell

Recall that plant cells are also eukaryotic cells. Structurally, these cells are similar to animal cells because some of the parts in a plant cell are also found in an animal cell. However, there are some notable differences. The following image shows the structure of a plant cell.

First, only plant cells have a **cell wall**. The purpose of this structure is to provide protection and support to plant cells. The cell wall also enforces the overall structural integrity of the plant cell, and it is found outside the cell membrane. The next organelle is a chloroplast. It is found in the cytoplasm of only plant cells. **Chloroplasts** are photosynthetic compounds used to make food for plant cells by harnessing energy from the sun. These organelles play a role in photosynthesis.

Chloroplasts and mitochondria are both designed to collect, process, and store energy for the cell. Thus, organisms are divided into autotrophs or heterotrophs based on how they obtain energy. **Autotrophs** are organisms that make energy-rich biomolecules from raw material in nature. They do this by using basic energy sources such the sun. This explains why most autotrophs rely on photosynthesis to transform sunlight into usable food that can produce energy necessary for life. Plants and certain species of bacteria are autotrophs.

Animals are **heterotrophs** because they are unable to make their own food. Heterotrophs have to consume and metabolize their food sources to absorb the stored energy. Examples of heterotrophs include all animals and fungi, as well as certain species of bacteria.

DID YOU KNOW?

More than 99% of all energy for life on Earth is provided through the process of photosynthesis.

Example

Kelp use chlorophyll to capture sunlight for food. What are these organisms classified as?

    A. Autotrophs   B. Chemotrophs   C. Heterotrophs   D. Lithotrophs

The correct answer is **A**. Kelp is an autotroph because it uses chlorophyll to trap energy from the sun to make food.

Let's Review!

- This lesson focused on the cell theory, different cell types, and the various cell parts found in plant and animal cells.
- The cell theory is an in-depth explanation, supported with scientific data, to prove a cell is a living thing and has unique characteristics.
- Cells are the basic building blocks of life. Coming in various sizes and shapes, cells have specialized functions.
- Two broad types of cells are prokaryotic and eukaryotic cells.
- Prokaryotes are single-celled organisms that lack a nucleus, while eukaryotes are multicellular organisms that contain a nucleus.
- Chloroplasts and cell walls are only found in plant cells.
- Both animal and plant cells have similar organelles such as ribosomes, mitochondria, and an endoplasmic reticulum.
- Living things can be classified as autotrophs or heterotrophs based on how they obtain energy.

CELLULAR REPRODUCTION, CELLULAR RESPIRATION, AND PHOTOSYNTHESIS

This lesson introduces basic processes including cellular reproduction and division, cellular respiration, and photosynthesis. These processes provide ways for cells to make new cells and to convert energy to and from food sources.

Cell Reproduction

Cells divide primarily for growth, repair, and reproduction. When an organism grows, it normally needs more cells. If damage occurs, more cells must appear to repair the damage and replace any dead cells. During reproduction, this process allows all living things to produce offspring. There are two ways that living things reproduce: asexually and sexually.

Asexual reproduction is a process in which only one organism is needed to reproduce itself. A single parent is involved in this type of reproduction, which means all offspring are genetically identical to one another and to the parent. All prokaryotes reproduce this way. Some eukaryotes also reproduce asexually. There are several methods of asexual reproduction.

Binary fission is one method. During this process, a prokaryotic cell, such as a bacterium, copies its DNA and splits in half. Binary fission is simple because only one parent cell divides into two daughter cells (or offspring) that are the same size.

Sexual reproduction is a process in which two organisms produce offspring that have genetic characteristics from both parents. It provides greater genetic diversity within a population than asexual reproduction. Sexual reproduction results in the production of **gametes**. These are reproductive cells. Gametes unite to create offspring.

Example

Binary fission is a method

A. where one daughter cell is produced.

B. required to produce reproductive cells.

C. that represents a form of asexual reproduction.

D. where two parent cells interact with each other.

The correct answer is **C**. Binary fission is a method organisms use to reproduce asexually. It involves a single parent cell that splits to create two identical daughter cells.

When the Cell Cycle Begins

For a cell to divide into more cells, it must grow, copy its DNA, and produce new daughter cells. The **cell cycle** regulates cellular division. This process can either prevent a cell from dividing or trigger it to start dividing.

> **KEEP IN MIND**
>
> The cell cycle is a circular process. This means after two daughter cells are made, they can participate in the cell cycle process, starting it over from the beginning.

The cell cycle is an organized process divided into two phases: **interphase** and the **M (mitotic) phase**. During interphase, the cell grows and copies its DNA. After the cell reaches the M phase, division and of the two new cells can occur. The G_1, S, and G_2 phases make up interphase.

- **G1:** The first gap phase, during which the cell prepares to copy its DNA
- **S:** The synthesis phase, during which DNA is copied
- **G2:** The second gap phase, during which the cell prepares for cell division

It may appear that little is happening in the cell during the gap phases. Most of the activity occurs at the level of enzymes and macromolecules. The cell produces things like nucleotides for synthesizing new DNA strands, enzymes for copying the DNA, and tubulin proteins for building the mitotic spindle. During the S phase, the DNA in the cell doubles, but few other signs are obvious under the microscope. All the dramatic events that can be seen under a microscope occur during the M phase: the chromosomes move, and the cell splits into two new cells with identical nuclei.

Example

For an organism, the cell cycle is needed for

A. competition.   B. dispersal.   C. growth.   D. parasitism.

The correct answer is **C**. The cell cycle is the process during which a cell grows, copies its own DNA, and physically separates into new cells. With help from the cell cycle, more cells can be provided to help an organism grow.

Mitosis

Mitosis is a form of cell division where two identical nuclei are produced from one nucleus. DNA contains the genetic information of the cell. It is stored in the nucleus. During mitosis, DNA in the nucleus must be copied, or replicated. Recall that this happens during the S phase of the cell cycle. During the M phase, this copied DNA is divided into two complete sets, one of which goes to a daughter cell.

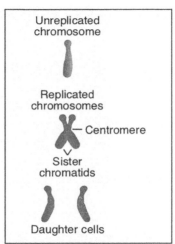

Unreplicated chromosome

Replicated chromosomes

Centromere

Sister chromatids

Daughter cells

When DNA replicates, it condenses to form **chromosomes** that resemble an X. The DNA forms chromosomes by wrapping around proteins called histones. As shown below, it takes two identical sister chromatids to form a chromosome. A **centromere** holds the sister chromatids together.

Four phases take place during mitosis to form two identical daughter cells:

1. **Prophase:** The nuclear membrane disappears, and other organelles move out of the way. The spindle, made of microtubules, begins to form. During **prometaphase**, the microtubules begin to attach to the centromeres at the center of the chromosome.
2. **Metaphase:** Spindle fibers line the chromosomes at the center of the cell. This is because they are pulled equally by the spindle fibers, which are attached to the opposite poles of the cell.
3. **Anaphase:** The chromosomes are pulled to the opposite poles of the cell.
4. **Telophase:** The chromosomes de-condense, the nuclear membrane reappears, and other parts of the cell return to their usual places in the cell.

The cell divides into two daughter cells by way of **cytokinesis**. The illustration below demonstrates the process of mitosis.

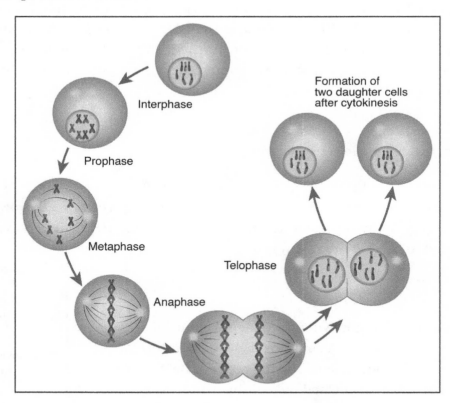

286

> **TEST TIP**
>
> There is a popular mnemonic to help remember the order of the phases for mitosis:
>
> *[Please] Pee on the MAT.*
>
> The "please" refers to prophase, while "pee" refers to prometaphase. MAT stands for metaphase, anaphase, and telophase, respectively.

Example

Before mitosis occurs

1. the spindle fibers must elongate.
2. DNA must wrap around histones.
3. chromosomes must split into chromatids.
4. the cell cycle process must be suspended.

The correct answer is **B**. After DNA replicates, it wraps around proteins called histones to form a chromosome. The chromosome must be formed for mitosis to occur.

Meiosis

Meiosis, sexual cell division in eukaryotes, involves two phases of mitosis that take place one after the other but without a second replication of DNA. This provides the reduction in chromosome number from $2n$ to n needed for fertilization to restore the normal $2n$ state. Diploid multicellular organisms use meiosis, which reduces the number of chromosomes by half. Then, when two haploid (n) sex cells (sperm, egg) unite, the normal number of chromosomes is restored. Diploid organisms, such as humans and oak trees, have two copies of every chromosome per cell ($2n$), as opposed to n, when one copy of every chromosome is present per cell.

> **DID YOU KNOW?**
>
> During prophase I of meiosis, **crossing over** occurs to increase genetic diversity. Corresponding chromosomes from the mother and the father of the organism undergoing meiosis are physically bound, and *X*-shaped structures called **chiasmata** form. These are where corresponding DNA from the different parental chromosomes are exchanged, resulting in increased diversity.

The process of meiosis is divided into two rounds of cell division: meiosis I and meiosis II. The phases that occur in mitosis (prophase, metaphase, anaphase, and telophase) also occur during each round of meiosis. Also, cytokinesis occurs after telophase during each round of cell division. However, DNA replication does not happen when meiosis I proceeds to meiosis II. The result of meiosis is one diploid cell that divides into four haploid cells, as shown in the following image.

Cytokinesis looks different in plant and animal cells. Plant cells build a new wall, or cell plate, between the two cells, while animal cells split by slowly pinching the membrane toward the center of the cell as the cell divides. Microtubules are more important for cytokinesis in plant cells, while the actin cytoskeleton performs the pinching-off operation during animal cytokinesis.

Example

How many rounds of cell division occur during meiosis?

A. 1   C. 3

B. 2   D. 4

The correct answer is **B**. A difference between mitosis and meiosis is that meiosis requires two rounds of cell division. At the end of both rounds, four haploid daughter cells have been produced.

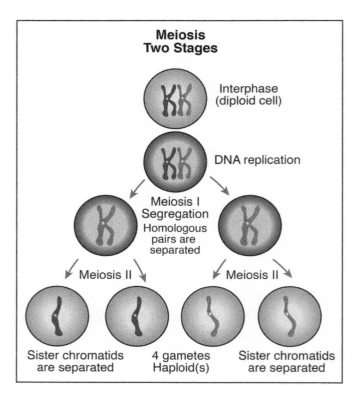

Meiosis Two Stages

Interphase (diploid cell)

DNA replication

Meiosis I Segregation Homologous pairs are separated

Meiosis II   Meiosis II

Sister chromatids are separated   4 gametes Haploid(s)   Sister chromatids are separated

---

KEY POINT

Meiosis and mitosis both require cytokinesis to physically separate a cell into daughter cells. Also, the sequence of events that occur in mitosis are the same in meiosis. However, there are two primary differences between the types of cell division: (1) meiosis has two rounds of cell division, and (2) daughter cells are genetically identical to the parent cell in mitosis but are not genetically identical in meiosis.

Cell Respiration

Once cells have been made, they need to be powered. Plants and some other cells can capture the energy of light and convert it into stored energy in ATP. However, most prokaryotic cells and all eukaryotic cells can perform a metabolic process called **cellular respiration**. Cellular respiration is the process by which the mitochondria of a cell break down glucose to produce energy in the form of ATP. The following is the general equation for cellular respiration:

$$O_2 + C_6H_{12}O_6 \rightarrow CO_2 + H_2O + ATP$$

Reactions during cellular respiration occur in the following sequence:

1. **Glycolysis:** One molecule of glucose breaks down into two smaller sugar molecules called **pyruvate**. This is an anaerobic process, which means it does not need oxygen to be present.

Glycolysis takes place in the cell's cytoplasm. End product yield from this reaction per one glucose molecule is

- two molecules of ATP
- two molecules of pyruvate
- two molecules of NADH

2. **Oxidation of pyruvate:** Pyruvate is converted into **acetyl coA** in the mitochondrial matrix. This transition reaction must happen for pyruvate to enter the next phase of cellular respiration. Pyruvate is **oxidized**, which means it loses two electrons and a hydrogen molecule. This results in the formation of NADH and loss of CO_2.

> **DID YOU KNOW?**
> The citric acid cycle is not identical for all organisms. Plants have some differences in terms of the enzymes used and energy carriers produced.

3. **Citric acid cycle:** Also called the **Krebs cycle**, during this cycle an acetyl group detaches from the coenzyme A in the acetyl coA molecule. This process is **aerobic**, which means it must occur in the presence of oxygen. The net yield per one glucose molecule is

- two molecules of ATP
- six molecules of NADH
- two molecules of $FADH_2$
- four molecules of CO_2

> **KEEP IN MIND**
> Cellular respiration requires oxygen, but there are forms of **fermentation** that extract energy from food without using oxygen. Fermentation can be either alcoholic (makes ethanol as an end product, like yeast in the brewing of beer) or lactic acid type. Lactic acid is produced in a person's muscles during strenuous activity when the body cannot move enough oxygen to the cells.

4. **Electron transport chain:** This process happens in the inner mitochondrial membrane. It consists of a series of enzymatic reactions. Both NADH and $FADH_2$ molecules are passed through a series of enzymes so that electrons and protons can be released from them. During this process, energy is released and used to fuel **chemiosmosis**. During chemiosmosis, protons are transported across the inner mitochondrial membrane to the outer mitochondrial compartment. This flow of protons drives the process of ATP synthesis. This step of cellular respiration creates an approximate net yield of 34 ATP per glucose molecule. Six molecules of water are also formed at the end of the electron transport chain.

Example

Before a molecule of glucose can be run through the citric acid cycle, it must experience

A. ATP production.

C. pyruvate oxidation.

B. NADH production.

D. oxygen deprivation.

The correct answer is **C.** A glucose molecule must first experience pyruvate oxidation because one CO_2 molecule must be removed from each pyruvate molecule after glycolysis and before the citric acid cycle.

Photosynthesis

Photosynthesis is the process plants use to make a food source from energy. This process can be thought of as the reverse of cellular respiration. Instead of glucose being broken down into carbon dioxide to create energy-containing molecules, energy is captured from the sun and used to turn carbon dioxide into glucose (and other organic chemicals the plant needs). The energy source is the sun. The reaction for photosynthesis is shown below:

$$CO_2 + H_2O \rightarrow C_6H_{12}O_6 + O_2$$

Energy is captured from the sun and used to turn carbon dioxide into glucose (and other organic chemicals). **Chloroplasts** are **organelles** in plants that contain green chlorophyll, which helps the plants absorb light from the sun.

The photosynthetic reaction involves two distinct phases: light reactions and dark reactions. Light-dependent reactions require light to produce ATP and NADPH. During dark reactions, also known as the **Calvin cycle**, light is not required. These reactions use ATP and NAPDH to produce sugar molecules like glucose.

> **DID YOU KNOW?**
> Some plants skip photosynthesis! These plants are parasites. They lack chlorophyll, so they attach to nearby plants, stealing water and sugar from their hosts.

Let's Review!

- Cells are needed for growth, repair, and reproduction.
- Mitosis is a form of cell division where one parent cell divides into identical two daughter cells.
- Meiosis involves two rounds of cell division to divide two parent cells into four haploid cells.
- Cells are powered by cellular respiration and photosynthesis, which make ATP and organic chemicals.
- Cellular respiration goes from glycolysis to the citric acid cycle to the electron transport chain.
- Photosynthesis proceeds from the light reactions to the dark reactions, which are known as the Calvin cycle.

GENETICS AND DNA

The lesson introduces genetics, which is the study of heredity. Heredity is the characteristics offspring inherit from their parents. This lesson also examines Gregor Mendel's theories of heredity and how they have affected the field of genetics.

Gregor Mendel and Garden Peas

From experiments with garden peas, Mendel developed a simple set of rules that accurately predicted patterns of heredity. He discovered that plants either **self-pollinate** or **cross-pollinate**, when the pollen from one plant fertilizes the pistil of another plant. He also discovered that traits are either **dominant** or **recessive**. Dominant traits are expressed, and recessive traits are hidden.

Mendel's Theory of Heredity

To explain his results, Mendel proposed a theory that has become the foundation of the science of genetics. The theory has five elements:

1. Parents do not transmit traits directly to their offspring. Rather, they pass on units of information called **genes**.
2. For each trait, an individual has two factors: one from each parent. If the two factors have the same information, the individual is **homozygous** for that trait. If the two factors are different, the individual is **heterozygous** for that trait. Each copy of a factor, or **gene**, is called an **allele**.
3. The alleles determine the physical appearance, or **phenotype**. The set of alleles an individual has is its **genotype**.
4. An individual receives one allele from each parent.
5. The presence of an allele does not guarantee that the trait will be expressed.

Punnett Squares

Biologists can predict the probable outcomes of a cross by using a diagram called a **Punnett square**. In the Punnett square illustrated at the right, the yellow pea pods are dominant, as designated by a capital Y, and the green pea pods are recessive, as designated with a lowercase y. In a cross between one homozygous recessive (yy) parent and a heterozygous dominant parent (Yy), the outcome is two heterozygous dominant offspring (Yy) and two homozygous recessive offspring (yy), which gives a ratio of 2:2.

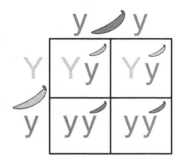

Example

In the Punnett square below, homozygous green pea pods are crossed with dominant yellow pea pods. What is the probability of a homozygous green pea pod?

A. 25%   C. 75%

B. 50%   D. 100%

The correct answer is **B**. There is a 2 out of 4, or 50%, chance of a homozygous green pea pod.

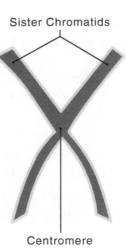

Chromosomes

A **gene** is a segment of DNA, deoxyribonucleic acid, which transmits information from parent to offspring. A single molecule of DNA has thousands of genes. A **chromosome** is a rod-shaped structure that forms when a single DNA molecule and its associated proteins coil tightly before cell division.

Chromosomes have two components:

- **Chromatids:** two copies of each chromosome
- **Centromeres:** protein discs that attach the chromatids together

Human cells have 23 sets of different chromosomes. The two copies of each chromosome are called **homologous** chromosomes, or homologues. An offspring receives one homologue from each parent. When a cell contains two homologues of each chromosome, it is termed **diploid (2n)**. A **haploid (n)** cell contains only one homologue of each chromosome. The only haploid cells humans are the sperm and eggs cells known as **gametes**.

Example

What is the difference between a diploid cell and a haploid cell?

A. A haploid cell is only found in skin cells.

B. A diploid cell is only found in heart cells.

C. A diploid cell has a full number of chromosomes, and a haploid cell does not.

D. A haploid cell has a full number of chromosomes, and a diploid cell does not.

The correct answer is **C**. Diploid cells have a full number of chromosomes, and haploid cells have half the number of chromosomes.

Deoxyribonucleic Acid

The **DNA molecule** is a long, thin molecule made of subunits called **nucleotides** that are linked together in a **nucleic acid** chain. Each nucleotide is constructed of three parts: a **phosphate group**, **five-carbon sugar**, and **nitrogen base**.

The four nitrogenous bases are

- adenine (A);
- guanine (G);
- thymine (T); and
- cytosine (C).

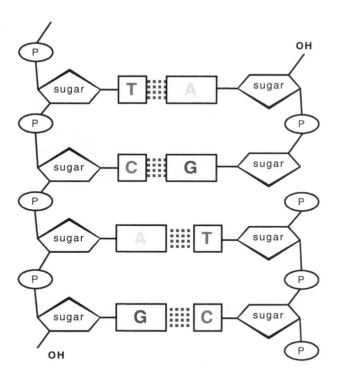

Adenine and guanine belong to a class of large, organic molecules called **purines**. Thymine and cytosine are **pyrimidines**, which have a single ring of carbon and nitrogen atoms. Base pairs are formed as adenine pairs with thymine and guanine pairs with cytosine. These are the only possible combinations.

DNA Replication

The process of synthesizing a new strand of DNA is called **replication**. A DNA molecule replicates by separating into two strands, building a complementary strand, and twisting to form a double helix.

Transcription

The first step in using DNA to direct the making of a protein is **transcription**, the process that "rewrites" the information in a gene in DNA into a molecule of messenger RNA. Transcription manufactures three types of RNA:

- Messenger RNA (mRNA)
- Transfer RNA (tRNA)
- Ribosomal RNA (rRNA)

Messenger RNA is an RNA copy of a gene used as a blueprint for a protein. In eukaryotes, transcription does not produce mRNA directly; it produces a pre-mRNA molecule. **Transfer RNA** translates mRNA sequences into amino acid sequences. **Ribosomal RNA** plays a structural role in ribosomes.

Transcription proceeds at a rate of about 60 nucleotides per second until the **RNA polymerase** (an enzyme) reaches a **stop codon** on the DNA called a **terminator** and releases the RNA molecule.

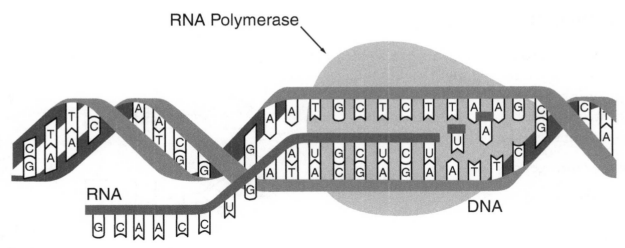

Translation

The components necessary for **translation** are located in the cytoplasm. Translation is the making of proteins by mRNA binding to a ribosome with the start codon that initiates the production of amino acids. A **peptide bond** forms and connects the amino acids together. The sequence of amino acids determines the protein's structure, which determines its function.

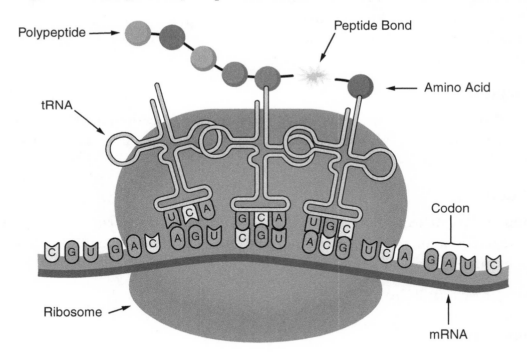

Example

Which type of RNA acts as an interpreter molecule?

A. mRNA   B. pre-mRNA   C. rRNA   D. tRNA

The correct answer is **D.** Transfer RNA (tRNA) acts as an interpreter molecule, translating mRNA sequences into amino acid sequences.

Let's Review!

- Gregor Mendel developed a simple set of rules that accurately predicts patterns of heredity.
- Mendel proposed a theory that has become the foundation of the science of genetics.
- Biologists can predict the probable outcomes of a cross by using a diagram called a Punnett square.
- A gene is a segment of DNA that transmits information from parent to offspring
- A chromosome is a rod-shaped structure that forms when a single DNA molecule and its associated proteins coil tightly before cell division.
- Deoxyribonucleic acid is a long, thin molecule made of subunits called nucleotides that are linked together in a nucleic acid chain.
- Replication is the process of synthesizing a new strand of DNA.
- Transcription is the first step in using DNA to direct the making of a protein.
- Translation is the process of making proteins.

CHAPTER 14 LIFE AND PHYSICAL SCIENCES PRACTICE QUIZ

1. **Which discovery is Robert Hooke credited with?**

   A. Finding the first cell

   B. Developing the cell theory

   C. Describing organelles in a cell

   D. Identifying prokaryotes in nature

2. **Which organelle is DNA found in?**

   A. Nucleus

   B. Ribosome

   C. Mitochondrion

   D. Endoplasmic reticulum

3. **Someone experiences a cut on the finger. Cell division is used during this situation for the purposes of**

   A. energy.   C. repair.

   B. growth.   D. reproduction.

4. **During which phase of the cell cycle is DNA copied?**

   A. Mitotic   C. Synthesis

   B. First Gap   D. Second Gap

5. **What is replication?**

   A. Twisting DNA into a double helix

   B. Synthesizing a new strand of DNA

   C. Altering the lagging and leading strands of DNA

   D. Repeating codons needed to manufacture specific proteins

6. **Which of the following is a segment of DNA that transmits information from parent to offspring?**

   A. Centromere   C. Chromosome

   B. Chromatid   D. Gene

7. **What is a theory?**

   A. A rule that describes patterns observed in nature

   B. A widely accepted explanation that is not modifiable

   C. A single experiment that is capable of being repeated

   D. A well-supported explanation about why things happen

8. **What is the scientific method?**

   A. A process used to answer a question or address a problem

   B. An approach that is used to create theories or laws in science

   C. A collection of metabolic reactions that occur in cyclic fashion

   D. An outdated technique that researchers use to study phenomena

CHAPTER 14 LIFE AND PHYSICAL SCIENCES PRACTICE QUIZ — ANSWER KEY

1. A. English scientist Robert Hooke is credited with discovering the first cell in a piece of cork. He described the cell as a resembling a tiny box or honeycomb shape. **See Lesson: Cell Structure, Function, and Type.**

2. A. The nucleus is a membrane-bound organelle found only in eukaryotic cells. It contains the genetic information for a cell, or DNA. **See Lesson: Cell Structure, Function, and Type.**

3. C. Cells were killed when they were cut. Thus, cells are needed to replace the damaged or dead cells and facilitate wound healing. **See Lesson: Cellular Reproduction, Cellular Respiration, and Photosynthesis.**

4. C. After the first and second gap phases, DNA of the cell is replicated during the synthesis (or S) phase. **See Lesson: Cellular Reproduction, Cellular Respiration, and Photosynthesis.**

5. B. Replication is the process of synthesizing a new strand of DNA. **See Lesson: Genetics and DNA.**

6. D. A gene is a segment of DNA that transmits information from the parent to the offspring. **See Lesson: Genetics and DNA.**

7. D. The culmination of research and findings can be used to support an explanation about something that occurs in nature. This explanation is a theory, which can be refined over time as more data become available. **See Lesson: An Introduction to Biology.**

8. A. The scientific method is a process researchers use to answer a question or solve a problem. This process helps researchers form theories and laws. **See Lesson: An Introduction to Biology.**

SECTION V. FULL-LENGTH PRACTICE EXAMS

KNAT Practice Exam 1

Section I. Writing

1. They _____ lunch together yesterday.

   A. eit
   B. ate
   C. aet
   D. eight

2. Which of the following is correct?

   A. senate
   B. congress
   C. White House
   D. Supreme court

3. Which of the following sentences is correct?

   A. The woman was intelligent kind and strong.
   B. The woman had intelligence-kindness-and-strength.
   C. The woman was; intelligent, kind, and strong
   D. The woman had three qualities: intelligence, kindness, and strength.

4. Choose the correct plural noun to complete the following sentence.

   It was surprising to suddenly see some _____ as we drove along the deserted road.

   A. mooses
   B. churchs
   C. cactuses
   D. passersby

5. Select the pronoun that could be used in the following sentence.

   I recognized two people, one of _____ I had worked with before.

   A. him
   B. who
   C. them
   D. whom

6. Which word in the following sentence is an adverb?

   That racecar is incredibly fast!

   A. That
   B. is
   C. incredibly
   D. fast

7. Which is <u>not</u> a prepositional phrase?

   Let's meet at 3:00 in the guest lounge of the airport.

   A. Let's meet
   B. at 3:00
   C. in the guest lounge
   D. of the airport

8. Which exclamation contains a verb?

   A. Oh no!
   B. Not me!
   C. So true!
   D. That's great!

9. Which of the following options would complete the sentence below to make it a compound sentence?

   Good doctors are _____.

   A. attentive and busy
   B. attentive yet busy
   C. attentive, and they are busy
   D. attentive even though they are busy

10. Fill in the blank with the correct coordinating conjunction.

    Desert climates are hot and dry, _____ many plants grow there.

    A. so
    B. yet
    C. for
    D. and

11. **What is the verb in the following sentence?**

It's time for lunch.

A. It   C. time

B. is   D. lunch

12. **Which word or phrase in the following sentence is not a modifier?**

The woman found her lost earring yesterday.

A. found   C. lost

B. her   D. yesterday

13. **Identify the likely misplaced modifier in the following sentence.**

Earlier this week, the young fishermen caught twenty fish, who were out all day.

A. Earlier this week   C. twenty

B. young   D. who were out all day

14. **Select the verb that acts on the underlined direct object in the following sentence.**

James Madison and Thomas Jefferson were among the men who helped to write the Constitution.

A. were   C. helped

B. among   D. write

15. **What part of speech correctly describes the underlined phrase in the following sentence?**

Leo watched his older brother walk to the bus stop on the first day of school.

A. Direct object

B. Indirect object

C. Subject

D. Object of the preposition

16. **What is the best definition of the word postscript?**

A. A summary   C. An introduction

B. A foreword

D. An afterword

17. **Which of the following prefixes means "too much"?**

A. sub-   C. mis-

B. non-   D. over-

18. **Select the word from the following sentence that has more than one meaning.**

Phillip watched excitedly as the racecars sped around the track.

A. Excitedly   C. Racecars

B. Watched   D. Track

19. **Select the context clue from the following sentence that helps you define the multiple meaning word pupils.**

The doctor had to dilate the patient's pupils, so she could examine his eyes.

A. "doctor"   C. "examine"

B. "patient's"   D. "eyes"

20. **Facile : Simplistic :: Effusive :**

_____

A. Adoring   C. Supportive

B. Astounded   D. Demonstrative

21. **Which of the following words in the list of synonyms shows the strongest degree in meaning?**

A. Upset   C. Distraught

B. Gloomy   D. Melancholy

Section II. Mathematics

1. **Evaluate the expression 1,004 + 110.**

   A. 2,104

   B. 1,411

   C. 1,204

   D. 1,114

2. **What is the difference between natural numbers and whole numbers?**

   A. They are the same.

   B. The whole numbers include zero, but the natural numbers exclude zero.

   C. The natural numbers only go to 10, but the whole numbers have no limit.

   D. The whole numbers include negative numbers, but the natural numbers do not.

3. **Evaluate the expression $15 \times (-15)$.**

   A. -225

   B. -30

   C. -1

   D. 0

4. **What is the quotient of a number divided by itself?**

   A. -1

   B. 0

   C. 1

   D. Not enough information

5. **How many prime numbers are less than 20 but greater than 0?**

   A. 8

   B. 9

   C. 10

   D. 11

6. **Which number is prime?**

   A. 4

   B. 27

   C. 49

   D. 61

7. **Convert 15,000 grams to metric tons.**

   A. 0.00015 metric ton

   B. 0.0015 metric ton

   C. 0.015 metric ton

   D. 0.15 metric ton

8. **Convert 0.75 kilograms to grams.**

   A. 0.0075 grams

   B. 0.075 grams

   C. 75 grams

   D. 750 grams

9. **Which decimal is the greatest?**

   A. 4.04

   B. 4.404

   C. 4.44

   D. 4.044

10. **Which decimal is the least?**

    A. 0.786

    B. 0.876

    C. 0.687

    D. 0.768

11. **Multiply $\frac{6}{7} \times \frac{7}{10}$.**

    A. $\frac{1}{17}$

    B. $\frac{1}{3}$

    C. $\frac{3}{5}$

    D. $\frac{13}{17}$

12. **Multiply $3\frac{1}{5} \times \frac{5}{8}$.**

    A. 1

    B. 2

    C. 3

    D. 4

13. **Solve the inequality for the unknown, $3(4x-1) > 5(2x + 3)$.**

    A. $x > 2$

    B. $x > 9$

    C. $x > 10$

    D. $x > 18$

14. **Solve the equation for the unknown, $\frac{x}{2} + 5 = 8$.**

    A. $\frac{3}{2}$

    B. $\frac{5}{2}$

    C. 6

    D. 26

15. Solve the system of equations,
    $2y + x = -20$
    $y = -x - 12$.

    A. (4, 8)   C. (-4, 8)

    B. (4, -8)   D. (-4, -8)

16. Solve the system of equations,
    $x + 3y = 34$
    $-3x + y = -12$.

    A. (-7, -9)   C. (7, 9)

    B. (-9, -7)   D. (9, 7)

17. Eric buys $2\frac{2}{5}$ pounds of apples each week for four weeks. How many total pounds does he buy?

    A. $7\frac{3}{5}$ C. $9\frac{3}{5}$

    B. $8\frac{2}{5}$ D. $10\frac{2}{5}$

18. An even roll of a number cube results in +2 points, and an odd roll of a number cube is –3 points. If there are 14 even numbers and 11 odd numbers, then how many points are scored?

    A. –61   C. 5

    B. –5   D. 61

19. A person has $250 in a checking account and writes checks for $70, $85, $60, and $100. There is also a fee of $20. What is the balance of the account?

    A. –$335   C. $335

    B. –$85   D. $685

20. Solve the equation by any method,
    $2x^2 - 70 = 2$.

    A. ±2   C. ±6

    B. ±4   D. ±8

21. Solve the equation by completing the square, $x^2 - 2x - 37 = 0$.

    A. $-1 \pm \sqrt{37}$ C. $-1 \pm \sqrt{38}$

    B. $1 \pm \sqrt{37}$ D. $1 \pm \sqrt{38}$

22. Solve the equation by factoring,
    $x^2 + 3x - 88 = 0$.

    A. –8, –11   C. 8, –11

    B. –8, 11   D. 8, 11

23. Multiply, $(5x - 3)(5x + 3)$.

    A. $25x^2 - 9$

    B. $25x^2 + 9$

    C. $25x^2 + 30x - 9$

    D. $25x^2 + 30x + 9$

24. Apply the polynomial identity to rewrite $x^3 + 125$.

    A. $(x + 5)(x^2 - 5x + 25)$

    B. $(x - 5)(x^2 - 10x + 25)$

    C. $(x + 5)(x^2 + 5x + 25)$

    D. $(x - 5)(x^2 + 10x + 25)$

25. Which is different from the others?

    A. 6.4%

    B. $\frac{8}{125}$

    C. 128:2000

    D. All of the above are equal.

26. Which is different from the others?

    A. 0.5   C. $\frac{1}{2}$

    B. 1:2   D. 1:2 odds

27. Solve $x^3 = -216$.

    A. –6   C. 4

    B. –4   D. 6

28. Simplify $\left(\frac{x^0}{y^2}\right)^2$.

    A. $\frac{1}{y^4}$ C. y^4

    B. $\frac{x}{y^4}$ D. $x^4 y^4$

SECTION III. READING

Please read the text below and answer questions 1-3.

It is perhaps unsurprising that school dress codes are becoming more common in American public schools. In our high-status-driven society, students feel the pressure to keep up with the most current fashion trends. The additional anxiety of wanting to "fit in" with peers can distract students from performing their best academically. In addition, some fashion trends are downright inappropriate and can be distracting to other students! Enforcing a dress code can allow schools to offer guidelines for clothing options that are suitable for school. Some school administrators are in favor of requiring students to wear a specific school uniform. Others suggest this may not be the most advantageous option as cost could still be a factor for some students, resulting in the same level of anxiety. Instead, they argue, offering simple guidelines that afford students the ability to meet their school's dress code requirements with maximum flexibility.

1. The topic of this paragraph is:
   A. fashion trends.
   B. dress codes.
   C. school uniforms.
   D. academic excellence.

2. The topic sentence of this paragraph is:
   A. In our high-status-driven society, students feel the pressure to keep up with the most current fashion trends.
   B. Enforcing a dress code can allow schools to offer guidelines for clothing options that are suitable for school.
   C. Some school administrators are in favor of requiring students to wear specific a school uniform.
   D. Others suggest this may not be the most advantageous option as cost could still be a factor for some students, resulting in the same level of anxiety.

3. If the author added a description of a student who wore inappropriate outfits to school and ended up distracting other students, what type of information would this be?
   A. A main idea
   B. A topic sentence
   C. A supporting detail
   D. An off-topic sentence

Read the following text and then answer questions 4-6.

Preheat your oven to 350 degrees. Get out all your equipment and ingredients. In a large bowl, combine flour, baking powder, sugar, and salt. Then soften 1 cup of butter. Next add the butter and the eggs to the dry mixture and stir until all the ingredients are mixed. Mix in the chocolate chips. Using a tablespoon, spoon out the batter onto a pre-greased cookie sheet. Bake in the oven for 12 minutes. Allow cookies to cool before serving.

4. **Which of the following words from the text indicate sequence?**

    A. Preheat, Mix

    B. Then, Next

    C. Using, Bake

    D. Get, In

5. **What does the term "pre-greased cookie sheet" tell you?**

    A. That you are supposed to grease the cookie sheet right after you spoon out the batter

    B. That you are supposed to grease the cookie sheet at some time before putting the batter onto it

    C. That you are supposed to grease the cookie sheet after preheating the oven

    D. That you are supposed to grease the cookie sheet after the baking the cookies

6. **What sequence word would best fit at the beginning of this sentence from the text?**

    Allow cookies to cool before serving.

    A. Then

    B. Last

    C. After

    D. Next

Read the following passage and answer questions 7-9.

Are you tired of your children not listening to you? Do they seem distracted every time you ask them to do something? Are you met with a glossy-eyed stare every time you say something to them? Part of the problem is too much screen time.

Technology has its benefits, but it does a lot to ruin our children's focus. There are too many flashes of light, too many colors, too many hyperlinks to navigate – it's a wonder our children can even focus at all!

Limiting your children's screen time would do wonders for them. Make more time to have face-to-face conversations. This will allow your children to actually practice good listening *and* communication skills. Hand them a book! This will help them sit still and focus on *one* thing for a period of time.

Technology won't be going away anytime soon, but you can set limits for your children to help them focus, listen, and better engage with you.

7. **This article is written for:**

    A. parents.

    B. children.

    C. teachers.

    D. policymakers.

8. **The author of this article assumes that:**

    A. parents are frustrated by their children not listening to them.

    B. parents are on screens more than their children are.

    C. children do not like to be told what to do by their parents.

    D. children would rather talk and read books than be on screens.

9. **Which conclusion is *not* supported by the article?**

   A. The author thinks kids are on their screens too much.

   B. The author thinks technology is negatively impacting children.

   C. The author thinks parents do not know how to discipline their children.

   D. The author thinks parents need to do more to help draw kids away from technology.

10. **Which of the following sentences uses the MOST informal language?**

    A. My puppy isn't potty trained yet.

    B. The heat in the summer is unbearable.

    C. I want to take a vacation to the beach.

    D. The dramatic TV show was extremely suspenseful.

11. **Which of the following sentences uses the MOST formal language?**

    A. What's up?   C. How's it going?

    B. How are you?   D. How's your day?

Read the following passage and answer questions 12-14.

When Dr. Kingston Hussein saw an announcement for a conference titled Ethics of Human

Embryonic Research, he booked his tickets six months in advance.

"We need to stop and reflect on the ramifications of every new development in our research," said Dr. Hussein, the lead researcher in embryology at the Dampson Crockett Institute in Lewiston, Maine. "Every researcher in our field

feels the weight of responsibility here. It's what we talk about when we go out for drinks after work."

Attitudes like Dr. Hussein's stand in stark contrast to common public perceptions of embryonic research. "These guys think they're gods," said Liz Goode, chairwoman of The Center for Ethical and Dignified Humanity, an organization that opposes all research on human embryos. "They want to get rich selling designer babies to billionaires. It's a nightmare."

An outside observer might expect a researcher like Dr. Hussein to avoid all contact with an activist like Goode. On the contrary, Dr. Hussein wrote to the organizers of the conference and requested that they invite Goode to host a panel. "We need dialogue," he said. "We need to hear what makes the public uncomfortable." He chuckled. "We also need to inform them about what we're actually doing."

And what *are* embryonic researchers doing? "Not building designer babies," he said. Dr. Hussein uses words like "run-of-the-mill medical" to describe his research goals. For instance, he is seeking causes and treatments for a variety of neurological disorders.

12. **Which adjective most accurately describes the author's tone?**

    A. Scathing   C. Negative

    B. Objective   D. Ironic

13. **Reread the following quotation from the passage:**

"Every researcher in our field feels the weight of responsibility here. It's what we talk about when we go out for drinks after work."

Which adjective most accurately describes Dr. Hussein's tone?

A. Scathing   C. Earnest

B. Apathetic   D. Ironic

14. **Reread the following quotation from the passage:**

"These guys think they're gods...They want to get rich selling designer babies to billionaires. It's a nightmare."

Which adjective most accurately describes Liz Goode's tone?

A. Harsh   C. Earnest

B. Tolerant   D. Ironic

Read the passages below and answer questions 15-16.

Electroconvulsive therapy was pioneered in the 1930s as a method for combatting severe psychiatric symptoms such as intractable depression and paranoid schizophrenia. This procedure, which involves delivering a deliberate electrical shock to the brain, was controversial from the beginning because it caused pain and short-term memory loss. It fell strongly out of public favor after the 1962 publication of Ken Kesey's novel *One Flew Over the Cuckoo's Nest*, which featured an unprincipled nurse using electroconvulsive therapy as a means of control over her patients. Paradoxically, medical advances at the time of the novel's publication made electroconvulsive therapy significantly safer and more humane.

Although the public is still generally opposed to electroconvulsive therapy, it remains a genuine option for psychiatric patients whose symptoms do not improve with medication. Medical professionals who offer this option should be especially careful to make clear distinctions between myth and reality. On this topic, unfortunately, many patients tend to rely on fiction rather than fact.

*

We were led into a stark exam room, where three doctors positioned themselves so Mama and I had no direct path to the door. The one in charge cleared his throat and told me my mother needed electroshock. My brain buzzed—almost as if it was hooked up to some crackpot brainwashing machine—as Big Doctor droned on about his sadistic intentions. I didn't hear any of it. All I could think was that these people wanted to tie my mother down and stick wires in her ears.

When Big Doctor was finished, he flipped through the papers on his clipboard and asked if I had questions. I mumbled something noncommittal. Then, when he and his silent escort left, I grabbed Mama and beat it out of that wacko ward as fast as I could make her go.

15. **What is the purpose of the first paragraph of Passage 1?**

A. To inform   C. To persuade

B. To distract   D. To entertain

16. **What is the purpose of the second paragraph of Passage 1?**

    A. To inform   C. To persuade

    B. To distract   D. To entertain

Read the following paragraph and answer questions 17-18.

The idea of raising children in prison is controversial, but well-run prison nursery programs can actually be beneficial. A study of preschool age children showed that anxiety and depression are common among young children who are separated from their mothers at birth and reunited later. In contrast, babies who spent brief sentences of two years or less behind bars with their mothers showed greater resilience and stronger attachments.

According to a nationwide analysis of women who participated in prison nursery programs, the benefits for mothers are even clearer than the benefits to children. Women who were allowed to remain with their infants during prison sentences were less likely to be convicted of another crime and less likely to use drugs in the five years after release. They were more likely to continue their education in prison and more likely to find employment on the outside. Mothers involved in prison nursery programs also reported better mental health and greater confidence in their own parenting skills.

17. **Which statement expresses an opinion?**

    A. A study of preschool age children showed that anxiety and depression are common among young children who are separated from their mothers at birth and reunited later.

    B. The idea of raising children in prison is controversial, but well-run prison nursery programs can actually be beneficial.

    C. Mothers involved in prison nursery programs also reported better mental health and greater confidence in their own parenting skills.

    D. Women who were allowed to remain with their infants during prison sentences were less likely to be convicted of another crime and less likely to use drugs after release.

18. **Consider the following sentence from the passage:**

    Mothers involved in prison nursery programs also reported better mental health and greater confidence in their own parenting skills.

    Is this statement a fact or an opinion? Why?

    A. An opinion because it shares information about confidence, which is an emotion

    B. A fact because it states verifiable information about how women reported they felt

    C. A fact because it focuses on information from medical records rather than faulty memories

    D. An opinion because it relies on human input rather than objective sources like computer records

Read the map below and answer questions 19-20.

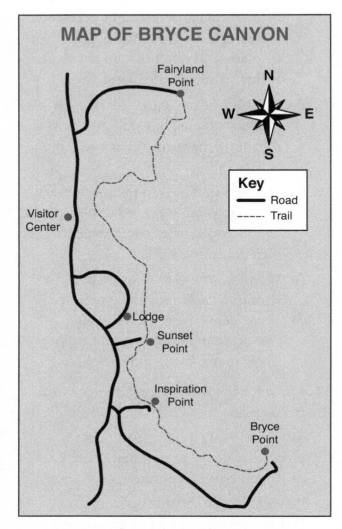

MAP OF BRYCE CANYON

19. A person could get from the Lodge to Fairyland Point by:

A. driving east on the road.

B. driving west on the road.

C. walking north on the Rim Trail.

D. walking south on the Rim Trail.

20. Which feature on the map is between Sunset Point and Bryce Point?

A. Sunrise Point

B. Fairyland Point

C. Visitor's Center

D. Inspiration Point

Read the following text and answer questions 21-22.

When my mother was a teenager, most kids didn't have cell phones. If she wanted to talk to her friends after school, she had to call their landline. Sometimes a friend's mom or dad answered, and she had to ask to talk to their kid. She says that was awkward. Also, if she and a friend talked on the phone for a long time, the whole family's phone line was busy, so nobody else could get calls. Parents got mad at kids for tying up the phone too long.

Today, every kid I know has a smartphone. We talk and text whenever we want, and none of us ever have awkward conversations with our friends' parents. But in some ways, parents today have more control. A lot of parents check kids' phone records and read their texts, so they can tell if their kids are up to no good. Families don't all rely on one phone line, so when kids talk for a long time, we don't prevent anyone else in the family from communicating with their friends. But parents today still get mad—mainly because kids' phone habits cost too much money.

21. What category of writing is this?

A. Narrative   C. Expository

B. Technical   D. Persuasive

22. The structure of the passage is:

A. description.

B. cause/effect.

C. problem-solution.

D. compare/contrast.

SECTION IV. SCIENCE

1. The term *anatomical position* refers to a person standing erect with the feet forward, arms hanging to the sides, and _____.

   A. eyes looking down

   B. eyes looking forward

   C. palms facing forward

   D. palms facing the body

2. Exchanges of substances like gases and nutrients occurs at the

   A. arteries.

   B. capillaries.

   C. veins.

   D. venules.

3. After the trachea, the first branch that leads toward the lungs is the

   A. alveolus.

   B. bronchi.

   C. larynx.

   D. pharynx.

4. Which of the following diseases causes localized inflammatory degeneration that causes the wall of the small intestine to thicken?

   A. Peptic ulcers

   B. Crohn's disease

   C. Ulcerative colitis

   D. Malabsorption syndrome

5. Menopause occurs _____.

   A. earlier in males than in females

   B. in females at an average age of 51

   C. just after the end of embryogenesis

   D. during the second week of each menstrual cycle

6. After urine flows through one sphincter at the start of the bladder, this fluid flows through the

   A. urethra naturally because of gravity.

   B. urethra after two sphincters contract.

   C. second sphincter under voluntary control.

   D. collecting ducts at the base of the renal tubule.

7. What is a characteristic of compact bone?

   A. Site of hematopoiesis

   B. Made of dense connective tissue

   C. Contains the osteocyte bone cells

   D. Consists of several openings or pores

8. A characteristic of all muscles is that they recoil after stretching, or are known to be _____.

   A. elastic

   B. relaxing

   C. excitable

   D. contractile

9. What is a characteristic of malignant melanoma?

   A. Most common form of skin cancer

   B. Affects keratinocytes during mitosis

   C. Presents as dark patches on the skin

   D. Occurs in basal cells of the epidermis

10. An axon binds to a _____ to release hormones in the body.

   A. gland

   B. dendrite

   C. cell body

   D. muscle cell

11. Which two hormones promote sperm cell production in males?

    A. Growth and thyroid-stimulating

    B. Follicle-stimulating and prolactin

    C. Luteinizing and follicle-stimulating

    D. Thyroid-stimulating and luteinizing

12. Why does blood provide a vehicle for transmitting AIDS?

    A. Blood contains oxygen.

    B. Blood contains glucose.

    C. Blood contains proteins.

    D. Blood contains many macrophages.

13. Which is part of the monomer structure of a nucleic acid?

    A. DNA   C. Thymine

    B. Glucose   D. Cellulose

14. Which of the following helps differentiate a non-living thing from a living thing?

    A. Energy processing

    B. Behavior in nature

    C. Occurrence in nature

    D. Description of habitat

15. Which organism would most likely be labeled as a consumer?

    A. Archaea   C. Heterotroph

    B. Autotroph   D. Prokaryote

16. Chromosomes contain all of the information necessary to run a cell and pass on a cell's hereditary traits to new cells. Where are these structures found in a cell?

    A. Nucleus   C. Cytoplasm

    B. Ribosome   D. Golgi
                            apparatus

17. Which organism most likely produces offspring asexually?

    A. Bacteria   C. Humans

    B. Birds   D. Lions

18. Sister chromatids and centromeres are found in a _____ chromosome.

    A. replicated

    B. duplicated

    C. histone absent

    D. loosely condensed

19. Adenine is a nucleotide base that pairs with _____.

    A. guanine   C. uracil

    B. cytosine   D. thymine

20. Which of the following directly plays a role in protein synthesis?

    A. Messenger RNA

    B. DNA Replication

    C. DNA polymerase

    D. Nitrogenous base

KNAT PRACTICE EXAM 1
ANSWER KEY WITH EXPLANATORY ANSWERS

Section I. Writing

1. B. *Ate* is the correctly spelled form of the past tense of eat. **See Lesson: Spelling.**

2. C. White House. The White House is capitalized because it is an important governmental building. **See Lesson: Capitalization.**

3. D. *The woman had three qualities: intelligence, kindness, and strength.* Colons are used to introduce a list. **See Lesson: Punctuation.**

4. D. *Passersby* is the only correct plural form offered. It is the plural of the noun *passerby*. **See Lesson: Nouns.**

5. D. The pronoun *whom* should be used as the object of the preposition *of*. **See Lesson: Pronouns.**

6. C. *Incredibly* is an adverb that describe the adjective *fast*. **See Lesson: Adjectives and Adverbs.**

7. A. *Let's meet* does not contain a preposition. *At, in*, and *of* are prepositions. **See Lesson: Conjunctions and Prepositions.**

8. D. *That's great* contains the contraction *That is*. *Is* is a verb. **See Lesson: Verbs and Verb Tenses.**

9. C. This option would make the sentence a compound sentence. **See Lesson: Types of Sentences.**

10. B. Yet. It is the only conjunction that fits within the context of the sentence. **See Lesson: Types of Clauses.**

11. B. *It's* is a contraction of *it is*. The verb is *is*. **See Lesson: Subject and Verb Agreement.**

12. A. *Found* is the main verb in this sentence; it is not a modifier. **See Lesson: Modifiers.**

13. D. *Who were out all day* most likely refers to *fishermen*, so it should be placed after that word, not after *fish*. **See Lesson: Modifiers.**

14. D. *The Constitution* is a direct object of the verb *write*. **See Lesson: Direct Objects and Indirect Objects.**

15. A. *His older brother* is a direct object of the verb *watched* in this sentence. **See Lesson: Direct Objects and Indirect Objects.**

16. D. The root *post* means "after," so *postscript* means something that was written after something else. **See Lesson: Root Words, Prefixes, and Suffixes.**

17. D. The prefix that means "too much" is *over*. **See Lesson: Root Words, Prefixes, and Suffixes.**

18. D. The word "track" has more than one meaning. **See Lesson: Context Clues and Multiple Meaning Words.**

19. D. The meaning of <u>pupils</u> in this context is "the dark circular opening at the center of the eyes." The word "eyes" helps you figure out which meaning of <u>pupils</u> is being used. **See Lesson: Context Clues and Multiple Meaning Words.**

20. D. *Facile* and *simplistic* are synonyms in the same way that *effusive* and *demonstrative* are synonyms. **See Lesson: Synonyms, Antonyms, and Analogies.**

21. C. *Distraught* is the word that shows the strongest degree in the list of synonyms. **See Lesson: Synonyms, Antonyms, and Analogies.**

Section II. Mathematics

1. D. The correct solution is 1,114. Use the addition algorithm or note the two numbers never have nonzero digits in the same place. This fact allows addition by inspection. **See Lesson: Basic Addition and Subtraction.**

2. B. The correct solution is the whole numbers include zero, but the natural numbers exclude zero. The natural or "counting" numbers are 1, 2, 3, 4,.... To get the whole numbers, just include 0 with the natural numbers. **See Lesson: Basic Addition and Subtraction.**

3. A. When multiplying signed numbers, remember that the product of a negative and a positive is negative. Other than the sign, the process is the same as multiplying whole numbers. **See Lesson: Basic Multiplication and Division.**

4. C. Since division yields a positive quotient when the signs of the dividend and divisor are the same, the answer must be positive. Pick any nonzero number: $231 \div 231$, for example. The quotient is always 1. **See Lesson: Basic Multiplication and Division.**

5. A. Start by eliminating 1, which is not a prime number. The number 2 is the only even prime; the other even numbers are composite. Therefore, consider only odd numbers greater than 2. The prime numbers less than 20 but greater than 0 are 2, 3, 5, 7, 11, 13, 17, and 19. The total is eight. **See Lesson: Factors and Multiples.**

6. D. A prime number has only 1 and itself as factors. One approach is to start at 2 and test each successive whole number to determine whether it is a factor by dividing. If the quotient is a whole number, it is a factor. Alternatively, recall the multiplication table: 4, 27, and 49 are all products of various whole numbers (2×2, 3×9, and 7×7, respectively). Therefore they are all composite, leaving 61 by elimination. **See Lesson: Factors and Multiples.**

7. C. The correct solution is 0.015 metric ton. $15{,}000 \text{ g} \times \frac{1 \text{ kg}}{1{,}000 \text{ g}} \times \frac{1 \text{ t}}{1{,}000 \text{ kg}} = \frac{15{,}000}{1{,}000{,}000} = 0.015 \text{ t}$. **See Lesson: Standards of Measure.**

8. D. The correct solution is 750 grams. $0.75 \text{ kg} \times \frac{1{,}000 \text{ g}}{1 \text{ kg}} = 750 \text{ g}$. **See Lesson: Standards of Measure.**

9. C. The correct solution is 4.44 because 4.44 contains the largest values in the tenths and hundredths places. **See Lesson: Decimals and Fractions.**

10. C. The correct solution is 0.687 because 0.687 contains the smallest value in the tenths place. **See Lesson: Decimals and Fractions.**

11. C. The correct solution is $\frac{3}{5}$ because $\frac{6}{7} \times \frac{7}{10} = \frac{42}{70} = \frac{3}{5}$. **See Lesson: Multiplication and Division of Fractions.**

12. B. The correct solution is 2 because $\frac{16}{5} \times \frac{5}{8} = \frac{80}{40} = 2$. **See Lesson: Multiplication and Division of Fractions.**

13. B. The correct solution is $x > 9$.

$12x - 3 > 10x + 15$	Apply the distributive property.
$2x - 3 > 15$	Subtract $10x$ from both sides of the inequality.
$2x > 18$	Add 3 to both sides of the inequality.
$x > 9$	Divide both sides of the inequality by 2.

See Lesson: Equations with One Variable.

14. C. The correct solution is 6.

$\frac{x}{2} = 3$	Subtract 5 from both sides of the equation.
$x = 6$	Multiply both sides of the equation by 2.

See Lesson: Equations with One Variable.

15. D. The correct solution is (-4, -8).

	The second equation is already solved for y.
$2(-x - 12) + x = -20$	Substitute $-x - 12$ in for y in the first equation.
$-2x - 24 + x = -20$	Apply the distributive property.
$-x - 24 = -20$	Combine like terms on the left side of the equation.
$-x = 4$	Add 24 to both sides of the equation.
$x = -4$	Divide both sides of the equation by -1.
$y = -(-4) - 12$	Substitute -4 in the second equation for x.
$y = 4 - 12 = -8$	Simplify using order of operations.

See Lesson: Equations with Two Variables.

16. C. The correct solution is (7, 9).

$x = -3y + 34$	Solve the first equation for x by subtracting $3y$ from both sides of the equation.
$-3(-3y + 34) + y = -12$	Substitute $-3y + 34$ in for x in the second equation.
$9y-102 + y = -12$	Apply the distributive property.
$10y-102 = -12$	Combine like terms on the left side of the equation.
$10y = 90$	Add 102 both sides of the equation.
$y = 9$	Divide both sides of the equation by 10.
$x + 3(9) = 34$	Substitute 9 in the first equation for y.
$x + 27 = 34$	Simplify using order of operations.
$x = 7$	Subtract 27 from both sides of the equation.

See Lesson: Equations with Two Variables.

17. C. The correct solution is $9\frac{3}{5}$ because $2\frac{2}{5} \times 4 = \frac{12}{5} \times \frac{4}{1} = \frac{48}{5} = 9\frac{3}{5}$ pounds of apples. **See Lesson: Solving Real-World Mathematical Problems.**

18. B. The correct solution is -5 because $14(2) + 11(-3) = 28 + (-33) = -5$ points. **See Lesson: Solving Real-World Mathematical Problems.**

19. B. The correct solution is $-\$85$ because $250-(70 + 85 + 60 + 100+ 20) = 250 - 335 = -\$85$. **See Lesson: Solving Real-World Mathematical Problems.**

20. C. The correct solutions are ± 6. Solve this equation by the square root method.

$2x^2 = 72$	Add 70 to both sides of the equation.
$x^2 = 36$	Divide both sides of the equation by 2.
$x = \pm 6$	Apply the square root to both sides of the equation.

See Lesson: Solving Quadratic Equations.

21. D. The correct solutions are $1 \pm \sqrt{38}$.

$x^2-2x = 37$	Add 37 to both sides of the equation.
$x^2-2x + 1 = 37 + 1$	Complete the square, $(\frac{2}{2})^2 = 1^2 = 1$.
	Add 1 to both sides of the equation.
$x^2-2x + 1 = 38$	Simplify the right side of the equation.
$(x-1)^2 = 38$	Factor the left side of the equation.
$x-1 = \pm\sqrt{38}$	Apply the square root to both sides of the equation.
$x = 1 \pm \sqrt{38}$	Add 1 to both sides of the equation.

See Lesson: Solving Quadratic Equations.

22. C. The correct solutions are 8 and −11.

$(x + 11)(x–8) = 0$ Factor the equation.

$(x + 11) = 0 \text{ and } (x–8) = 0$ Set each factor equal to 0.

$x + 11 = 0$ Subtract 11 from both sides of the equation to solve for the first factor.

$x = –11$

$x–8 = 0$ Add 8 to both sides of the equation to solve for the second factor.

$x = 8$

See Lesson: Solving Quadratic Equations.

23. A. The correct solution is $25x^2–9$.

$(5x–3)(5x + 3) = 5x(5x + 3)–3(5x + 3) = 25x^2 + 15x–15x–9 = 25x^2–9$

See Lesson: Polynomials.

24. A. The correct solution is $(x + 5)(x^2–5x + 25)$. The expression $x^3 + 125$ is rewritten as $(x + 5)(x^2–5x + 25)$ because the value of a is x and the value of b is 5. **See Lesson: Polynomials.**

25. D. All of the answer choices are equal. Although answer C is not in lowest terms, it is equal to $\frac{8}{125}$, which is equal to 0.064 or 6.4%. **See Lesson: Ratios, Proportions, and Percentages.**

26. D. The decimal 0.5 is equal to $\frac{1}{2}$, which is also equal to the ratio 1:2. But 1:2 odds are different because odds use colon notation in a different manner. **See Lesson: Ratios, Proportions, and Percentages.**

27. A. The correct solution is –6 because the cube root of –216 is –6. **See Lesson: Powers, Exponents, Roots, and Radicals.**

28. C. The correct solution is y^4 because $\left(\frac{x^0}{y^{-2}}\right)^2 = \frac{x^{0\times2}}{y^{-2\times2}} = \frac{x^0}{y^{-4}} = \frac{1}{y^{-4}} = y^4$. **See Lesson: Powers, Exponents, Roots, and Radicals.**

Section III. Reading

1. B. The topic of this paragraph is dress codes. Enforcing a specific school uniform is related to this topic, but is not covered in detail in this passage. **See Lesson: Main Ideas, Topic Sentences, and Supporting Details.**

2. A. The first sentence of this paragraph leads the reader toward the main idea, which is expressed next in a topic sentence about the benefits of school dress codes. **See Lesson: Main Ideas, Topic Sentences, and Supporting Details.**

3. C. A description of a student wearing clothing that does not meet dress code requirements would function as a supporting detail in this paragraph about the school dress codes. **See Lesson: Main Ideas, Topic Sentences, and Supporting Details.**

4. B. The words "Then" and "Next" indicate sequence because they tell you when to do a step. **See Lesson: Summarizing Text and Using Text Features.**

5. B. The prefix "pre" in the word "pre-greased" means "before," so the cookie sheet needs to be greased sometime before putting the batter onto it. **See Lesson: Summarizing Text and Using Text Features.**

6. B. Since this is the final step, you would use the word "last" to indicate it is the final step in the directions. **See Lesson: Summarizing Text and Using Text Features.**

7. A. From phrases like "your children," you can infer that the intended audience of this passage is parents. **See Lesson: Understanding Primary Sources, Making Inferences, and Drawing Conclusions.**

8. A. The author assumes that many parents have the problem of their children not listening to them or being able to focus well. **See Lesson: Understanding Primary Sources, Making Inferences, and Drawing Conclusions.**

9. C. The author does not suggest parents do not know how to discipline their children. This article is about setting limits on technology. It is not about disciplining children. **See Lesson: Understanding Primary Sources, Making Inferences, and Drawing Conclusions.**

10. A. My puppy isn't potty trained yet. The sentence has contractions and words that are informal and less polite. **See Lesson: Formal and Informal Language.**

11. B. How are you? It is the only sentence that does not have a contraction and does not use slang. **See Lesson: Formal and Informal Language.**

12. B. The author of this passage is reporting on a controversial issue with an objective or impartial tone. **See Lesson: Tone, Mood, and Transition Words.**

13. C. Dr. Hussein's words show that he cares deeply about the responsibility of his position. His tone could be described as earnest or concerned. **See Lesson: Tone, Mood, and Transition Words.**

14. A. Liz Goode is highly critical of embryonic research. Her tone could be described as harsh, scathing, or critical. **See Lesson: Tone, Mood, and Transition Words.**

15. A. Passage 1 is intended to inform readers about electroconvulsive therapy. **See Lesson: Understanding the Author's Purpose, Point of View, and Rhetorical Strategies.**

16. C. The second paragraph of passage 1 makes opinion statements about what doctors should do. This is a sign of persuasive writing. **See Lesson: Understanding the Author's Purpose, Point of View, and Rhetorical Strategies.**

17. B. The argument that prison nursery programs can be beneficial is an opinion statement because it makes a judgment. **See Lesson: Facts, Opinions, and Evaluating an Argument.**

18. B. The statement makes a factual statement about how people said they felt. This makes it a fact even though it contains opinion information. **See Lesson: Facts, Opinions, and Evaluating an Argument.**

19. C. The Rim Trail is the dotted line running generally north-south past the Lodge in the middle. Fairyland Point is in the far north, so a walk north on the trail would get you there. **See Lesson: Evaluating and Integrating Data.**

20. D. Inspiration Point is between Sunset Point and Bryce Point along the Rim Trail. **See Lesson: Evaluating and Integrating Data.**

21. C. This passage is an explanation of phone habits in two eras. Although it uses a few time words, it does not describe narrative scenes. It is an expository piece. **See Lesson: Types of Passages, Text Structures, Genre and Theme.**

22. D. The passage describes phone use in two eras, highlighting similarities and differences. This makes it a compare/contrast piece. **See Lesson: Types of Passages, Text Structures, Genre and Theme.**

Section IV. Science

1. C. The term *anatomical position* refers to a person standing erect with the feet forward, arms hanging to the sides, and palms facing forward. **See Lesson: Organization of the Human Body.**

2. B. Classified as the thinnest blood vessels with the largest surface areas, the structure of capillaries facilitates exchanges of substances between blood and body tissues. **See Lesson: Cardiovascular System.**

3. B. The trachea branches into bronchi, which branch into bronchioles before terminating at the alveolar region of the lung. **See Lesson: The Respiratory System.**

4. B. Crohn's disease causes localized inflammatory degeneration that causes the walls of the small intestine to thicken. **See Lesson: Gastrointestinal System.**

5. B. Menopause is caused by age-related, fundamental hormonal changes in the female body. It marks the end of the regular menstrual cycle. The age of menopause varies widely, but it usually occurs from the mid-40s to the mid-50s, with the average age in the United States being about 51. **See Lesson: Reproductive System.**

6. C. There are two sphincters in the urinary system, one at the beginning of bladder and the other at the end of the bladder. The sphincter at the end of the bladder pushes urine to the urethra, where it can be excreted. This sphincter is under voluntary control. **See Lesson: The Urinary System.**

7. B. Compact bone is a dense type of bone tissue that is comprised of units called osteons. It provides the hard, outer surface of bone and creates a tough protective layer around the soft, spongy bone. **See Lesson: Skeletal System.**

8. A. All muscles are elastic because they are flexible. That is, they can recoil and shorten after being stretched. **See Lesson: Muscular System.**

9. C. Malignant melanoma is the most dangerous type of skin cancer. It occurs when melanocytes experience uncontrolled cell growth and causes dark patches or lesions to form on the skin's surface. **See Lesson: Integumentary System.**

10. A. If a presynaptic neuron forms a synapse with the postsynaptic membrane of a gland, and a neurotransmitter binds to receptors on a gland, this will stimulate a release of hormones from that gland. **See Lesson: The Nervous System.**

11. C. Both luteinizing hormones and follicle-stimulating hormones promote sperm cell production in males. **See Lesson: Endocrine System.**

12. D. AIDS is transmitted through macrophages, and blood contains many macrophages. **See Lesson: The Lymphatic System.**

13. C. Adenine and thymine bond with each other to form a nucleotide. This nucleotide is the monomer of the nucleic acid DNA. **See Lesson: An Introduction to Biology.**

14. A. There are several features that scientists use to identify living things. These features include: how living things process energy, growth and development, reproduction, and homeostasis. **See Lesson: An Introduction to Biology.**

15. C. A consumer is any living thing that must consume or feed on another living thing to obtain energy. A consumer is also known as a heterotroph. **See Lesson: Cell Structure, Function, and Type.**

16. A. The nucleus is where genetic information is found in a cell. This genetic information, or DNA, is packaged into chromosomes. **See Lesson: Cell Structure, Function, and Type.**

17. A. Prokaryotes like bacteria participate in asexual reproduction. This means they can create offspring using a single parent. **See Lesson: Cellular Reproduction, Cellular Respiration, and Photosynthesis.**

18. D. When two sister chromatids come together, they are bound by a centromere; this enables them to form a loosely condensed chromosome. **See Lesson: Cellular Reproduction, Cellular Respiration, and Photosynthesis.**

19. D. There are four nucleotide base pairs in DNA. These bases form unique covalent bonds with each other. Specifically, adenine pairs with thymine and guanine pairs with cytosine. **See Lesson: Genetics and DNA.**

20. A. After DNA is replicated, with the help of DNA polymerase, this strand is transcribed into messenger RNA. The messenger RNA molecule is used as a template to make a protein. Nitrogenous bases are used to create a strand of DNA. **See Lesson: Genetics and DNA.**

KNAT Practice Exam 2

Section I. Writing

1. **What is the correct plural of *chair*?**

   A. Chair   C. Chaires

   B. Chairs   D. Chairies

2. **Which of the following is correct?**

   A. Rome, Italy   C. rome, italy

   B. rome, Italy   D. Rome, italy

3. **What is the mistake in the following sentence?**

   In history, people and dates are important, but three things are important in English, punctuation, spelling, and grammar.

   A. There should be no comma after *history*.

   B. The comma after *English* should be a colon.

   C. There should be no comma after *important*.

   D. There should be a semicolon after *important*.

4. **What type of error can be found in the following sentence?**

   Mr. and Mrs. Hughes are alumnuses of Georgetown University.

   A. Verb tense   C. Capitalization

   B. Punctuation   D. Plural formation

5. **What part of speech are the underlined words?**

   <u>My</u> boss asked <u>me</u> to work late tonight, so <u>I</u> won't be able to go to <u>your</u> party.

   A. Nouns   C. Pronouns

   B. Articles   D. Prepositions

6. **How many adverbs are in the following sentence?**

   Your apple pie is perfect!

   A. 0   C. 2

   B. 1   D. 3

7. **Select another conjunction with the same meaning as the underlined conjunction.**

   <u>Because</u> we arrived early, we were able to end our shift early.

   A. Since   C. Nor

   B. Nevertheless   D. Although

8. **Which movie title contains a verb?**

   A. *Annie Hall*

   B. *Midnight in Paris*

   C. *Play it Again, Sam*

   D. *The Purple Rose of Cairo*

9. Which sentence combines all of the information below using a parallel structure?

    Dental care requires brushing. You should also floss. Rinse with a fluoride wash.

    A. Dental care requires to brush, floss, and rinsing.

    B. Dental care requires brushing, to floss, and rinse.

    C. Dental care requires brushing, flossing, and rinse.

    D. Dental care requires brushing, flossing, and rinsing.

10. Identify the independent clause in the following sentence.

    The mother could not take her kids to school because it snowed all night.

    A. The mother could not take her kids

    B. It snowed all night

    C. Because it snowed all night

    D. The mother could not take her kids to school

11. Which part of the following sentence is the predicate?

    My granddaughter was born on January 18.

    A. My granddaughter

    B. was

    C. was born on January 18

    D. January 18

12. Which modifier could not be added before the underlined word?

    The workers ate lunch.

    A. hungrily   C. laughing

    B. hungry   D. uniformed

13. Which word does the underlined modifier describe?

    The puppy, who hadn't eaten all day, whined until we fed him.

    A. puppy   C. eaten

    B. who   D. whined

14. Identify the indirect object in the following sentence.

    The dressmaker made Selena a lovely gown.

    A. dressmaker   C. lovely

    B. Selena   D. gown

15. Which of the following verbs can take a direct object?

    A. Go   C. Buy

    B. Sneeze   D. Die

16. Which of the following suffixes means "having characteristics of"?

    A. -ic   C. -er

    B. -ed   D. -ist

17. Which of the following suffixes means "act, process"?

    A. -able   C. -less

    B. -tion   D. -ible

18. Select the correct definition of the underlined word that has multiple meanings in the sentence.

    The loud crack of thunder frightened the children.

    A. Space   C. Joke

    B. Bang   D. Attempt

19. **Select the meaning of the underlined word in the sentence based on the context clues.**

    The landscape of the tundra was <u>stark</u> and contained nothing but flat, open land.

    A. Vast   C. Bright

    B. Plain   D. Beautiful

20. **Quaff : Beverage :: Garnish :**
    _____

    A. Plate   C. Canvas

    B. Closet   D. Garden

21. **Which of the following words in the list of synonyms shows the weakest degree of meaning?**

    A. Blissful   C. Content

    B. Ecstatic   D. Delighted

SECTION II. MATHEMATICS

1. **What is the sum of two negative numbers?**

   A. Negative number

   B. Positive number

   C. Zero

   D. Not enough information

2. **Which statement is true?**

   A. A numeral is a symbol that represents a number.

   B. A number is a symbol that represents a numeral.

   C. Numerals and numbers are the same.

   D. None of the above.

3. **What is $762 \div 127$?**

   A. 4   C. 8

   B. 6   D. 9

4. **Which expression yields a quotient with no remainder?**

   A. $5 \div 5$ C. $81 \div 40$

   B. $26 \div 5$ D. $365 \div 87$

5. **Which number is prime?**

   A. 34   C. 191

   B. 106   D. 208

6. **Which number is a prime factor of 108?**

   A. 3   C. 11

   B. 7   D. 13

7. **Convert 9 meters to yards.**

   A. 4.09 yards   C. 9.84 yards

   B. 8.23 yards   D. 12.28 yards

8. **Convert 1,000 fluid ounces to gallons.**

   A. 7.8125 gallons   C. 31.25 gallons

   B. 15.625 gallons   D. 62.5 gallons

9. **Write $\frac{7}{9}$ as a percent.**

   A. $0.\overline{7}\%$ C. $77.\overline{7}\%$

   B. $7.\overline{7}\%$ D. $777.\overline{7}\%$

10. **Write $83.\overline{3}\%$ as a decimal.**

    A. $8.\overline{3}$ C. $0.08\overline{3}$

    B. $0.8\overline{3}$ D. 0.0083

11. **Multiply $\frac{2}{3} \times \frac{4}{15}$.**

    A. $\frac{3}{20}$ C. $\frac{8}{45}$

    B. $\frac{1}{6}$ D. $\frac{1}{3}$

12. **Multiply $2 \times \frac{3}{4}$.**

    A. $\frac{1}{4}$ C. $1\frac{1}{2}$

    B. $\frac{3}{8}$ D. $2\frac{3}{4}$

13. **Solve the equation for the unknown, $\frac{x}{4} + 8 = 6$.**

    A. -8 C. 2

    B. -2 D. 8

14. **Solve the equation for the unknown, $\frac{3}{4}(x + 3) - 2 = 3 - \frac{2}{3}(x + 1)$.**

    A. $\frac{6}{5}$ C. $\frac{8}{5}$

    B. $\frac{25}{17}$ D. $\frac{28}{17}$

15. **Solve the system of equations,**
    $-4x + 3y = 30$
    $3x + 4y = 15$.

    A. $(3, -6)$ C. $(-3, -6)$

    B. $(-3, 6)$ D. $(3, 6)$

16. Solve the system of equations,
$y = -x$
$x^2 + y^2 = 8$.

    A. (1, 1) and (-1, -1)

    B. (1, -1) and (-1, 1)

    C. (2, 2) and (-2, -2)

    D. (2, -2) and (-2, 2)

17. In a game, positive and negative points can be scored. For 10 turns, the point total is −5, +4, −7, −2, 0, +3, +5, −6, −4, +2. What is the average point total?

    A. −2   C. 1

    B. −1   D. 2

18. In a state, the highest elevation is 1,450 feet and the lowest elevation is −80 feet. What is the difference in the elevations in feet?

    A. 1,370   C. 1,530

    B. 1,430   D. 1,570

19. A teacher buys 4 bottles of water for class. Each bottle of water contains 3 liters. Each cup holds $\frac{2}{3}$ of a liter. How many cups can be filled?

    A. 12   C. 42

    B. 30   D. 60

20. Solve the equation by any method, $x^2 - 23x + 125 = 0$.

    A. −8.81 and −14.2   C. 8.81 and −14.2

    B. 8.81 and 14.2   D. −8.81 and 14.2

21. Solve the equation by completing the square, $x^2 + 12x + 10 = 0$.

    A. $6 \pm \sqrt{26}$ C. $6 \pm \sqrt{10}$

    B. $-6 \pm \sqrt{26}$ D. $-6 \pm \sqrt{10}$

22. Solve the equation by the quadratic formula, $12x^2 + x - 3 = 0$.

    A. −0.46 and −0.54

    B. 0.46 and −0.54

    C. −0.46 and 0.54

    D. 0.46 and 0.54

23. Apply the polynomial identity to rewrite $27x^3 - 8$.

    A. $(3x-2)(9x^2-6x+4)$

    B. $(3x-2)(9x^2+6x+4)$

    C. $(3x-2)(9x^2+6x-4)$

    D. $(3x-2)(9x^2-6x-4)$

24. Perform the operation,
$(-2x^2 + 8x) + (3x^3 - 4x^2 + 1)$.

    A. $3x^3 - 6x^2 + 8x + 1$

    B. $3x^3 - 2x^2 + 8x + 1$

    C. $3x^3 + 6x^2 + 8x + 1$

    D. $3x^3 + 2x^2 + 8x + 1$

25. Which expression is different from the others?

    A. 2:5   C. 40%

    B. $\frac{2}{5}$ D. 0.04

26. Which expression is different from the others?

    A. 4:9   C. 44%

    B. 0.44   D. $\frac{9}{4}$

27. Simplify $5^6 \times 5^{-3}$.

    A. 5   C. 125

    B. 15   D. 625

28. Solve $x^2 = 225$.

    A. −5, 5   C. −15, 15

    B. −10, 10   D. −20, 20

325

Section III. Reading

Please read the text below and answer questions 1-3.

In the past 10-15 years, koalas have been repeatedly harmed or killed in traffic accidents. When the animals cross busy roads, highways, and intersections to get to their food source, the eucalyptus tree, many of them meet a terrible fate. Australian developers have been taking over koala habitats to keep up with the country's booming population. This has resulted in the endangerment of the country's most beloved animal. Concerned individuals have taken action by creating koala "pathways," routes traveling over roads, highways, and intersections to ensure koalas keep safe. In addition, koala hospitals have been established in these areas to rehabilitate the injured animals.

1. **Which phrase best describes the topic of the group of sentences above?**

    A. An analysis of animal behavior in the wild

    B. An account of human impact on an animal species

    C. A description of a building development plan

    D. An examination of the ways humans help animals

2. **Which of the following sentences would best function as a topic sentence to unite the information above?**

    A. Over 4,000 koalas are hurt or injured each year by automobiles.

    B. Koalas spend most of their time in trees but need to occasionally travel across roads to move around.

    C. Human encroachment on natural habitats has negatively impacted the koala population.

    D. Australia's building development projects have tripled over the past decade.

3. **Which sentence provides another supporting detail to address the topic of the sentences above?**

    A. Kangaroos, emus, and wombats are other popular animals in Australia.

    B. Australia has a diverse population of citizens from various countries throughout the world.

    C. Koalas are not bears but marsupials, mammals that carry their young in a pouch.

    D. Australia has erected over 500 koala pathways over the past two years.

Read the following text and then answer questions 4-6.

In the late morning, Cynthia met Max at the state park where he had been waiting. They went on a hike. They followed a path that first led them through the deep, lush woods. The path then took them past a beautiful, serene lake. They were beginning to get thirsty, so they stopped to sit on a large rock to drink some water. Next, they continued hiking and came upon a clearing, Cynthia was astonished to see a picnic blanket all set up with plates and a picnic basket.

"Max!" she exclaimed.

Max had set up the picnic to surprise Cynthia.

4. **According to the paragraph, which event happened first?**

    A. Cynthia met Max at a state park in the late morning.

    B. Max set up the picnic for him and Cynthia.

    C. Cynthia and Max walked past a lake.

    D. Cynthia and Max stopped to drink water on a rock.

5. **Which word clues help you understand that this event happened first?**

    A. "had set up"

    B. "first went"

    C. "beginning to get"

    D. "in the late morning"

6. **Which of the following words from the passage is *not* a sequence word?**

    A. First   C. Next

    B. Then   D. Beginning

Read the following passage and answer questions 7-9.

Manny looked out the window.

"Not yet," he mumbled to himself.

He walked into the kitchen to try to distract himself. He was about to open the cookie jar when he heard a car motor.

"Now?" he ran to the window.

"Ugh," he sighed, "it is just Mr. Mendez."

Suddenly he saw it. The small, white truck he was searching for.

He burst through the door and breathlessly greeted Stanley.

Stanley smiled as he handed a stack of envelopes to Manny.

"Is this what you're looking for, son?" Stanley said with a smile.

Manny looked at the return address. *Michigan State University.*

"Yes! Thank you!" Manny cried as he bolted into his house.

"Good luck, Manny!" Stanley yelled after him.

7. **From the text above, you can infer that Manny is:**

    A. best friends with Stanley.

    B. anxiously awaiting the mail.

    C. very hard on himself.

    D. not a fan of Mr. Mendez.

8. **Which detail does *not* provide evidence to back up the conclusion that Manny is eager for the mail to come?**

   A. He mumbles "not yet" to himself.

   B. He is about to open the cookie jar.

   C. He sighs when he sees Mr. Mendez.

   D. He bursts through the door and greets Stanley.

9. **Which detail from the text supports the inference that Stanley knows Manny pretty well?**

   A. He drives up in his truck.

   B. He hands him a stack of envelopes.

   C. He asks if an envelope is what he is looking for.

   D. He smiles at Manny.

10. **In which of the following situations would you use formal language?**

    A. Writing a letter

    B. A family road trip

    C. Going to the beach

    D. Talking to the doctor

11. **Which of the following sentences uses the MOST formal language?**

    A. This essay claims that sugar is bad for people.

    B. I think that sugar is bad for people.

    C. I believe that sugar is bad for people.

    D. I say that sugar is bad for people.

Read the passage and answer questions 12-14.

Dear Mr. O'Hara,

I am writing to let you know how much of a positive impact you have made on our daughter. Before being in your algebra class, Violet was math phobic. She would shut down when new concepts would not come to her easily. As a result, she did not pass many tests. Despite this past struggle, she has blossomed in your class! Your patience and dedication have made all the difference in the world. Above all, your one-on-one sessions with her have truly helped her in ways you cannot imagine. She is a more confident and capable math student, thanks to you. We cannot thank you enough.

Fondly,

Bridgette Foster

12. **Which adjective best describes the tone of this passage?**

    A. Arrogant   C. Friendly

    B. Hopeless   D. Appreciative

13. **Which phrase from the passage has an openly appreciative and warm tone?**

    A. I am writing to let you know

    B. you have made on our daughter

    C. made all the difference

    D. We cannot thank you enough

14. **What mood would this passage most likely evoke in the math teacher, Mr. O'Hara?**

    A. Calm

    B. Grateful

    C. Sympathetic

    D. Embarrassment

Read the following text and answer questions 15-16.

Wizard WiFi is a digital application that allows you to manage your home WiFi network and connected devices. Wizard WiFi is easy to install and set up! Once installed Wizard WiFi enables you to find your WiFi password, know who is online, troubleshoot issues and manage family members' online experiences. You will be a tech-savvy genius in no time!

Concerned about creating healthy tech-usage habits? Wizard WiFi allows you to create individualized WiFi usage limits and alert family members when they are nearing their daily quota, set a "Bedtime Mode" to create an optimal "tech-free" nighttime environment, and ensure age-appropriate, safe Web surging with features like Pause and Parental Controls. It is the best technology management system on the market!

If you are a Wizard Internet subscriber with a SuperWiz Gateway, you can access the Wizard WiFi experience at no additional cost through a mobile app, website or an app on the SuperWiz TV Box.

New Wizard Internet subscribers can access Wizard WiFi once their SuperWiz Gateway is activated. Existing subscribers with eligible SuperWiz Gateways can log into the Wizard WiFi portal immediately.

Top-level high-tech executives, like Pear Technology CEO Rusty Bartlett, rely on Wizard WiFi to manage the safety and security of their home WiFi network systems. Shouldn't you do the same?

15. **The purpose of this passage is to:**

A. decide. C. persuade.

B. inform. D. entertain.

16. **With which statement would the author of this passage most likely agree?**

A. People who have home WiFi networks use excessive technology and do not value spending quality time with family members.

B. Parents who do not buy WiFi monitoring devices are unable to have confidence in the security of their household network.

C. The best way to achieve a healthy tech environment is to create family rules for technology usage and avoid monitoring apps.

D. Consumers want help managing their home technology systems to create healthy habits and ensure a secure and safe online environment for family members.

Read the following passage and answer questions 17-18.

Most people under age 35 spend too much time on social media. Statistics show that over nine out of ten teens go online using a mobile device daily, and seven out of ten use more than one major social media site. This is too much. Teens and young adults must limit their use of social media or face deteriorating relationships in real life. You know how frustrating it feels to try to talk to someone who constantly disengages to check a phone. Interacting online can be fun, but it never provides as much satisfaction as talking with actual human beings. Social media shouldn't be the primary social outlet for young people because people who rely mainly on the Internet for social interaction are unhappy and unfulfilled.

17. **What is the primary argument in the passage?**

    A. All young people face emotional and social problems.

    B. Teens and young adults should limit their social media use.

    C. People under age 35 have never known life without the Internet.

    D. Disengaging to check a phone can damage real-life social interactions.

18. **Which excerpt from the text, if true, is a fact?**

    A. Most people under age 35 spend too much time on social media.

    B. Statistics show that over nine out of ten teens go online using a mobile device daily.

    C. Teens and young adults must limit their use of social media or face deteriorating relationships in real life.

    D. Interacting online can be fun, but it never provides as much satisfaction as talking with actual human beings.

Study the following label and answer questions 19-20.

Nutrition Facts

Serving Size 20 crackers (38g)
Servings Per Container 5

Amount Per Serving

Calories 150   Calories from Fat 45

	% Daily Value*
Total Fat 9g	**12%**
Saturated Fat 4g	**20%**
Trans Fat 0g	
Cholesterol 0mg	**0%**
Sodium 160mg	**7%**
Total Carbohydrate 16g	**6%**
Dietary Fiber Less than 1g	**2%**
Sugars Less than 1g	**0%**
Protein 1g	
Vitamin D	0%
Calcium	5%
Iron	20%
Potassium	8%

* Percent Daily Values are based on a 2,000 calorie diet. Your Daily Values may be higher or lower depending on your calorie needs:

	Calories:	2,000	2,500
Total Fat	Less than	65g	80g
Saturated Fat	Less than	20g	25g
Cholesterol	Less than	300mg	300mg
Sodium	Less than	2,400mg	2,400mg
Total Carbohydrate		300g	375g
Dietary Fiber		25g	30g

19. **How many calories are in one serving of this product?**

    A. 5   C. 150

    B. 20   D. 3750

20. Germain ate 60 crackers out of this box. How many servings did he consume?

A. 1

B. 3

C. 5

D. 10

Read both of the following texts and answer questions 21-22.

1. Once when a Lion was asleep a little Mouse began running up and down upon him; this soon wakened the Lion, who placed his huge paw upon him, and opened his big jaws to swallow him. "Pardon, O King," cried the little Mouse: "forgive me this time, I shall never forget it: who knows but what I may be able to do you a turn some of these days?" The Lion was so tickled at the idea of the Mouse being able to help him, that he lifted up his paw and let him go. Sometime after the Lion was caught in a trap, and the hunters who desired to carry him alive to the King, tied him to a tree while they went in search of a wagon to carry him on. Just then the little Mouse happened to pass by, and seeing the sad plight in which the Lion was, went up to him and soon gnawed away the ropes that bound the King of the Beasts. "Was I not right?" said the little Mouse.

Little friends may prove great friends.

2. Beast left his mark on the fence.

It was lime green and slate gray and beautiful, so of course my father was outraged. If Beast hadn't had talent, Dad would have left it a while, but as it was, he got two of his parishioners to paint the thing over. Within the hour, the fence was back to being as white as the everlasting soul. My father's anger lasted longer than the tag.

The funny thing was, Beast loved my father. I don't know why. Life had knocked that kid down so hard so often he should have hated everything with the name of God stamped on it. But he loved my preacher father more than anyone else in the world. Maybe it was the dark suits and the white collars. Beast liked a pretty picture.

So there was my dad, ministering to the people in the worst parts of town, charging straight into drug dens and whorehouses to save people when they called him. He acted like he had no fear whatsoever. Plenty of the neighbors, the hardest-put ones, hated him for that. Lots of times he came close to getting his throat cut. More than once it was Beast who saved him.

And every time Beast saved my dad, he left his mark on the fence.

Dad couldn't stand it.

21. What type of writing is used in the passages?

A. Both are narrative.

B. Passage 1 is narrative and passage 2 is expository.

C. Passage 1 is expository and passage 2 is narrative.

D. Both are expository.

22. Which term describes the structure of both passages?

A. Sequence

B. Description

C. Cause/effect

D. Problem-solution

SECTION IV. SCIENCE

1. The hip is _____ to the thigh.

   A. anterosuperior   C. proximal

   B. deep   D. superficial

2. Which blood group does NOT display A and B antibodies in the plasma?

   A. A   C. B

   B. AB   D. O

3. Which substance determines a person's blood pH level?

   A. Carbonic acid

   B. Carbon dioxide

   C. Carbon monoxide

   D. Carbonic anhydrase

4. What is the first enzyme that functions in the digestive system?

   A. Amylase   C. Maltase

   B. Lactase   D. Sucrase

5. Which of the following is generally true regarding human newborns?

   A. Newborns require a large amount of parental care.

   B. Newborns enter the first stages of puberty within a few weeks of birth.

   C. Newborns are capable of sexually reproducing within a few months of birth.

   D. Newborns are able to visually track objects with their eyes moments after delivery.

6. What is one side effect of aging as it relates to the urinary system?

   A. Increased bladder elasticity

   B. Weakened bladder muscles

   C. Replaced nephrons in the kidneys

   D. Improved signaling between ADH and the kidneys

7. The tibia is connected to the _____.

   A. tarsals   C. clavicle

   B. Ischium   D. ulna

8. What body system must the muscular system work with to help the body move?

   A. Cardiovascular

   B. Digestive

   C. Respiratory

   D. Skeletal

9. The lunula is the _____ found near the nail bed.

   A. area of white space

   B. thick overhang layer

   C. region of epidermal cells

   D. collection of keratinized cells

10. Neuroglia are different from neurons because they

    A. participate in synaptic transmission.

    B. maintain sustained action potentials.

    C. transmit electric signals as messages.

    D. provide a form of protection and support.

11. Hormones from the pituitary gland act on the ovaries and the testes, causing those organs to secrete sex hormones. Which of the following is a function of sex hormones?

    A. Decrease acne

    B. Initiate puberty

    C. Increase adipose

    D. Produce sweating

12. Why is it crucial for killer T cells and B cells to distinguish cells of a person's own body from foreign cells?

    A. They can divide and conquer.

    B. They develop more antibodies.

    C. They will only attack cancer cells.

    D. They will not attack the body's cells.

13. A researcher characterizes a polymer that consists of glycerol molecules. What does she write in her notes about this polymer?

    A. These molecules will form lipid biomolecules.

    B. This polymer is capable of storing very little energy.

    C. The glycerol molecules are covalently bonded together.

    D. This polymer will help transmit genetic information in a cell.

14. What standard is used to make comparisons in experiments?

    A. Sample size

    B. Control group

    C. Dependent variable

    D. Independent variable

15. Which organelles work together to ensure plant cells have enough energy to use?

    A. Ribosome and nucleus

    B. Chloroplast and mitochondria

    C. Cell membrane and cytoplasm

    D. Golgi apparatus and endoplasmic reticulum

16. Which cell part stores material in the cell?

    A. Chloroplast   C. Ribosome

    B. Nucleus   D. Vacuole

17. If someone needs ATP desperately and has run out of oxygen, what could help?

    A. Meiosis

    B. Calvin cycle

    C. Fermentation

    D. Electron transport chain

18. A child falls down and punctures his skin. What biological process must occur to repair the damaged skin?

    A. Glycolysis

    B. Cell respiration

    C. Gluconeogenesis

    D. Cell reproduction

19. Samantha uses a Punnett Square to estimate what a litter of puppies will look like. She crosses homozygous dominant trait of brown fur with a homozygous recessive trait for curly fur. Which of the following most likely designates the dominant trait in this Punnett Square?

    A. F   C. ff

    B. FF   D. f

20. Which of the following is a component
    of a chromosome?

    A. Centromere   C. Homologue

    B. Gamete   D. Ribose

KNAT Practice Exam 2
Answer Key with Explanatory Answers

Section I. Writing

1. B. For words ending in most consonants, add -s. **See Lesson: Spelling.**

2. A. Rome, Italy. Cities and countries are capitalized. **See Lesson: Capitalization.**

3. B. *The comma after English should be a colon.* Colons are used to introduce lists. **See Lesson: Punctuation.**

4. D. *Alumni* is the plural of *alumnus.* **See Lesson: Nouns.**

5. C. These words are pronouns. **See Lesson: Pronouns.**

6. A. None of these words are adverbs. **See Lesson: Adjectives and Adverbs.**

7. A. *Since* has the same meaning as *because* in this sentence. **See Lesson: Conjunctions and Prepositions.**

8. C. *Play* is a verb. **See Lesson: Verbs and Verb Tenses.**

9. D. This sentence combines the information using parallel structure. **See Lesson: Types of Sentences.**

10. D. The mother could not take her kids to school. It is independent because it has a subject, verb, and expresses a complete thought. **See Lesson: Types of Clauses.**

11. C. The subject is *my granddaughter,* and the predicate is *was born on January 18.* **See Lesson: Subject and Verb Agreement.**

12. A. *Hungrily* is an adverb that could modify *ate.* It could not be placed before *workers.* **See Lesson: Modifiers.**

13. D. *Until we fed him* is an adverb phrase that describes *whined.* **See Lesson: Modifiers.**

14. B. *Gown* is the direct object of the verb made, and *Selena* is the indirect object. **See Lesson: Direct Objects and Indirect Objects.**

15. C. *Buy* is the only verb here that can take a direct object. The other verbs are intransitive. **See Lesson: Direct Objects and Indirect Objects.**

16. A. The suffix that means "having characteristics of" is *-ic.* **See Lesson: Root Words, Prefixes, and Suffixes.**

17. B. The suffix that means "capable of" is *-tion*. **See Lesson: Root Words, Prefixes, and Suffixes.**

18. B. The meaning of <u>crack</u> in the context of this sentence is "a sudden sharp and loud noise." **See Lesson: Context Clues and Multiple Meaning Words.**

19. B. The meaning of <u>stark</u> in the context of this sentence is "plain." **See Lesson: Context Clues and Multiple Meaning Words.**

20. A. Quaff is an action that you do with a beverage in the same way that garnish is an action you do with a plate of food. **See Lesson: Synonyms, Antonyms, and Analogies.**

21. C. *Content* is the word that shows the weakest degree in the list of synonyms. **See Lesson: Synonyms, Antonyms, and Analogies.**

Section II. Mathematics

1. A. The correct solution is a negative number. Try a few examples: $(-1) + (-1)$, $(-8) + (-2)$. By the rule $(-x) + (-y) = -(x + y)$, the sum is always negative. **See Lesson: Basic Addition and Subtraction.**

2. A. The correct solution is a numeral is a symbol that represents a number. Recall that numbers are abstract quantities, but a numeral is a symbol that represents a number. **See Lesson: Basic Addition and Subtraction.**

3. B. Use the division algorithm. Because 127 is greater than 7 and 76, the process begins with all three digits in the dividend. **See Lesson: Basic Multiplication and Division.**

4. A. By inspection, $5 \div 5 = 1$, so it has no remainder. Using the division algorithm on the other expressions produces a remainder. **See Lesson: Basic Multiplication and Division.**

5. C. A prime number has only 1 and itself as factors. All even numbers (except 2) are composite because they have 2 as a factor. By elimination, only answer C is a prime number. **See Lesson: Factors and Multiples.**

6. A. To determine whether a number is a factor of another number, divide the second number by the first number. If the quotient is whole, the first number is a factor. In this case, all the numbers are prime, but 108 is only divisible by 3. **See Lesson: Factors and Multiples.**

7. C. The correct solution is 9.84 yards. $9 \text{ m} \times \frac{3.28 \text{ ft}}{1 \text{ m}} \times \frac{1 \text{ yd}}{3 \text{ ft}} = \frac{29.52}{3} = 9.84$ yd. **See Lesson: Standards of Measure.**

8. A. The correct solution is 7.8125 gallons. $1{,}000 \text{ fl oz} \times \frac{1 \text{ pt}}{16 \text{ fl oz}} \times \frac{1 \text{ qt}}{2 \text{ pt}} \times \frac{1 \text{ gal}}{4 \text{ qt}} = \frac{1{,}000}{128} = 7.8125$ gal. **See Lesson: Standards of Measure.**

9. C. The correct answer is $77.\overline{7}\%$ because $\frac{7}{9}$ as a percent is $\frac{7}{9} = 0.\overline{7} \times 100 = 77.\overline{7}\%$. **See Lesson: Decimals and Fractions.**

10. B. The correct answer is $0.8\overline{3}$ because $83.\overline{3}\%$ as a decimal is $0.8\overline{3}$. **See Lesson: Decimals and Fractions.**

11. C. The correct solution is $\frac{8}{45}$ because $\frac{2}{3} \times \frac{4}{15} = \frac{8}{45}$. **See Lesson: Multiplication and Division of Fractions.**

12. C. The correct solution is $1\frac{1}{2}$ because $\frac{2}{1} \times \frac{3}{4} = \frac{6}{4} = 1\frac{2}{4} = 1\frac{1}{2}$. **See Lesson: Multiplication and Division of Fractions.**

13. A. The correct solution is -8.

$\frac{x}{4} = -2$	Subtract 8 from both sides of the equation.
$x = -8$	Multiply both sides of the equation by 4.

See Lesson: Equations with One Variable.

14. B. The correct solution is $\frac{25}{17}$.

$9(x+3)-24 = 36-8(x+1)$	Multiply all terms by the least common denominator of 12 to eliminate the fractions.
$9x + 27-24 = 36-8x-8$	Apply the distributive property.
$9x + 3 = 28-8x$	Combine like terms on both sides of the equation.
$17x + 3 = 28$	Add $8x$ to both sides of the equation.
$17x = 25$	Subtract 3 from both sides of the equation.
$x = \frac{25}{17}$	Divide both sides of the equation by 17.

See Lesson: Equations with One Variable.

15. B. The correct solution is $(-3, 6)$.

$-12x + 9y = 90$	Multiply all terms in the first equation by 3.
$12x + 16y = 60$	Multiply all terms in the second equation by 4.
$25y = 150$	Add the equations.
$y = 6$	Divide both sides of the equation by 25.
$3x + 4(6) = 15$	Substitute 6 in the second equation for y.
$3x + 24 = 15$	Simplify using order of operations.
$3x = -9$	Subtract 24 from both sides of the equation.
$x = -3$	Divide both sides of the equation by 3.

See Lesson: Equations with Two Variables.

16. D. The correct solutions are $(2, -2)$ and $(-2, 2)$.

$x^2 + (-x)^2 = 8$	Substitute $-x$ in for y in the second equation.
$x^2 + x^2 = 8$	Apply the exponent.
$2x^2 = 8$	Combine like terms on the left side of the equation.

$x^2 = 4$	Divide both sides of the equation by 2.
$x = \pm 2$	Apply the square root to both sides of the equation.
$y = -2$	Substitute 2 in the first equation.
$y = -(-2) = 2$	Substitute -2 in the first equation and multiply.

See Lesson: Equations with Two Variables.

17. B. The correct solution is –1 because the sum of the scores is –10. The average is –10 divided by 10, or –1 point. **See Lesson: Solving Real-World Mathematical Problems.**

18. C. The correct solution is 1,530 because $1,450-(-80) = 1,450 + 80 = 1,530$ feet. **See Lesson: Solving Real-World Mathematical Problems.**

19. B. The correct solution is 30 because $4(3) \div \frac{2}{5} = 12 \div \frac{2}{5} = \frac{12}{1} \times \frac{5}{2} = \frac{60}{2} = 30$ cups of water. **See Lesson: Solving Real-World Mathematical Problems.**

20. B. The correct solutions are 8.81 and 14.2. The equation can be solved by the quadratic formula.

$x = \dfrac{-(-23) \pm \sqrt{(-23)^2 - 4(1)(125)}}{2(1)}$	Substitute 1 for a, –23 for b, and 125 for c.
$x = \dfrac{23 \pm \sqrt{529 - 500}}{2}$	Apply the exponent and perform the multiplication.
$x = \dfrac{23 \pm \sqrt{29}}{2}$	Perform the subtraction.
$x = \dfrac{23 \pm 5.39}{2}$	Apply the square root.
$x = \dfrac{23 + 5.39}{2}, x = \dfrac{23 - 5.39}{2}$	Separate the problem into two expressions.
$x = \dfrac{28.39}{2} = 14.2, x = \dfrac{17.61}{2} = 8.81$	Simplify the numerator and divide.

See Lesson: Solving Quadratic Equations.

21. B. The correct solutions are $-6 \pm \sqrt{26}$.

$x^2 + 12x = -10$	Subtract 10 from both sides of the equation.
$x^2 + 12x + 36 = -10 + 36$	Complete the square, $(\frac{12}{2})^2 = 6^2 = 36$.
	Add 36 to both sides of the equation.
$x^2 + 12x + 36 = 26$	Simplify the right side of the equation.
$(x + 6)^2 = 26$	Factor the left side of the equation.
$x + 6 = \pm\sqrt{26}$	Apply the square root to both sides of the equation.
$x = -6 \pm \sqrt{26}$	Subtract 6 from both sides of the equation.

See Lesson: Solving Quadratic Equations.

22. B. The correct solutions are 0.46 and -0.54.

$$x = \frac{-1 \pm \sqrt{1^2 - 4(12)(-3)}}{2(12)}$$ Substitute 12 ifor a, 1 for b, and -3 for c.

$$x = \frac{-1 \pm \sqrt{1 - (-144)}}{24}$$ Apply the exponent and perform the multiplication.

$$x = \frac{-1 \pm \sqrt{145}}{24}$$ Perform the subtraction.

$$x = \frac{-1 \pm 12.04}{24}$$ Apply the square root.

$$x = \frac{-1 + 12.04}{24}, x = \frac{-1 - 12.04}{24}$$ Separate the problem into two expressions.

$$x = \frac{11.04}{24} = 0.46, x = \frac{-13.04}{24} = -0.54$$ Simplify the numerator and divide.

See Lesson: Solving Quadratic Equations.

23. B. The correct solution is $(3x-2)(9x^2 + 6x + 4)$. The expression $27x^3 - 8$ is rewritten as $(3x-2)(9x^2 + 6x + 4)$ because the value of a is $3x$ and the value of b is 2. **See Lesson: Polynomials.**

24. A. The correct solution is $3x^3 - 6x^2 + 8x + 1$.

$$(-2x^2 + 8x) + (3x^3 - 4x^2 + 1) = 3x^3 + (-2x^2 - 4x^2) + 8x + 1 = 3x^3 - 6x^2 + 8x + 1$$

See Lesson: Polynomials.

25. D. The expression 0.04 is different from the others. The expression in answer A is a fraction, and it is equal to the ratio in answer B. Dividing 2 by 5 yields 0.4, which is equal to 40%. The option left is 0.04, which is different from the others. **See Lesson: Ratios, Proportions, and Percentages.**

26. D. Converting answers A and D to decimals yields (approximately) 0.44 and 2.25, respectively. Answers B and C are both equal to 0.44, so answer D differs from the others. **See Lesson: Ratios, Proportions, and Percentages.**

27. C. The correct solution is 125 because $5^6 \times 5^{-3} = 5^{6+(-3)} = 5^3 = 125$. **See Lesson: Powers, Exponents, Roots, and Radicals.**

28. C. The correct solution is -15, 15 because the square root of 225 is 15. The values of -15 and 15 make the equation true. **See Lesson: Powers, Exponents, Roots, and Radicals.**

Section III. Reading

1. B. All of the sentences are related in some way to the text, but the topic is specifically about an account of human impact on an animal species. **See Lesson: Main Ideas, Topic Sentences, and Supporting Details.**

2. C. The best topic sentence to unite the above information would be the one about human encroachment negatively impacting the koala population. The others would be additional supporting details. **See Lesson: Main Ideas, Topic Sentences, and Supporting Details.**

3. D. Each of the above sentences is related in some way to the passage, but the detail about the number of koala pathways that have been built is the best fit for the topic of the text. **See Lesson: Main Ideas, Topic Sentences, and Supporting Details.**

4. B. Even though the detail about Max setting up the picnic came at the end, it was the event that happened first since he had to have set up before Cynthia came to the park because it was there before they arrived. **See Lesson: Summarizing Text and Using Text Features.**

5. A. The word clues "had set up" indicates that Max set up the picnic earlier so that it would be a surprise for Cynthia when they got to the clearing. **See Lesson: Summarizing Text and Using Text Features.**

6. D. Even though the word "beginning" seems like a sequence word indicating something that comes first, in the context of the passage it means they "started to" get thirsty. The other words are sequence words, which indicate the order of events. **See Lesson: Summarizing Text and Using Text Features.**

7. B. Manny is anxiously awaiting the mail. You know this because he "looked out the window," says, "not yet," and bursts "through the door" after he sees the "small, white truck." **See Lesson: Understanding Primary Sources, Making Inferences, and Drawing Conclusions.**

8. B. Manny opening the cookie jar does not explicitly show that he is eager for the mail to come. **See Lesson: Understanding Primary Sources, Making Inferences, and Drawing Conclusions.**

9. C. When Stanley shows Manny the envelope from Michigan State and says with a smile, "Is this what you're looking for, son?" it shows that he knows Manny is eagerly waiting to hear from colleges. This proves that he knows Manny pretty well since he knows what's going on in his life. **See Lesson: Understanding Primary Sources, Making Inferences, and Drawing Conclusions.**

10. D. Talking to the doctor. Using formal language with a doctor is best, because it shows respect and he or she is probably not a close friend. **See Lesson: Formal and Informal Language.**

11. A. This essay claims that sugar is bad for people. In academic writing, pronouns such as I should not be used. **See Lesson: Formal and Informal Language.**

12. D. The tone of this letter is appreciative as the author openly thanks the teacher for all he has done for her daughter. **See Lesson: Tone, Mood, and Transition Words.**

13. D. The author of the letter uses a lot of respectful and admiring language, but the line "We cannot thank you enough" has an especially appreciative and warm tone. **See Lesson: Tone, Mood, and Transition Words.**

14. B. A teacher receiving a note like this would likely feel grateful. **See Lesson: Tone, Mood, and Transition Words.**

15. C. This is an advertisement. Although it includes some information its primary purpose is to convince you to buy something. This makes it a persuasive text. **See Lesson: Understanding the Author's Purpose, Point of View, and Rhetorical Strategy.**

16. D. Writers of advertisements are tasked with selling a product, therefore, It is difficult to know much about the true feelings. However, it is a fair bet that advertising writers believe people will pay money for products presented the way they describe. **See Lesson: Understanding the Author's Purpose, Point of View, and Rhetorical Strategy.**

17. B. This passage argues that teens and young adults spend too much time on social media. **See Lesson: Facts, Opinions, and Evaluating an Argument.**

18. B. Factual information is verifiable and not based on personal beliefs or feelings. The statistic about the number of teens who go online daily is a fact. **See Lesson: Facts, Opinions, and Evaluating an Argument.**

19. C. The label shows the number of calories per serving: 150. **See Lesson: Evaluating and Integrating Data.**

20. B. The label shows that there are 20 calories per serving. 60 crackers would be three servings. **See Lesson: Evaluating and Integrating Data.**

21. A. Both passages tell stories. That makes this narrative writing. **See Lesson: Types of Passages, Text Structures, Genre and Theme.**

22. A. Both passages say what happened first, second, third, and so on, in chronological order. This is a sequential structure. **See Lesson: Types of Passages, Text Structures, Genre and Theme.**

Section IV. Science

1. A. The term *anterosuperior* means "in front of" or "above." The hip is above the thigh. **See Lesson: Organization of the Human Body.**

2. D. Blood group O is the universal donor that does not display A or B antigens on the surface of red blood cells. **See Lesson: Cardiovascular System.**

3. B. Blood pH levels are determined by analyzing the concentration of carbon dioxide in blood. **See Lesson: The Respiratory System.**

4. A. Amylase is secreted in the mouth, and it is the first enzyme that goes into action. **See Lesson: Gastrointestinal System.**

5. A. Newborn humans require a great deal of parental care. Visual tracking of objects usually begins around three months of age; puberty does not start for several years; and reproductive capability does not start until the end of puberty. **See Lesson: Reproductive System.**

6. B. As the body ages, so do the bladder and kidneys. Nephron loss occurs, and the bladder loses its elasticity. When this decreased elasticity is coupled with weakened bladder muscles, a person may have trouble urinating voluntarily. **See Lesson: The Urinary System.**

7. A. The tibia belongs to the appendicular system, which consists of the upper and lower extremities. The tibia is found in the leg. It is connected to the femur, or thighbone, and the tarsals, which make up the ankle and foot. **See Lesson: Skeletal System.**

8. D. The skeletal system consists of all the bones of the body. Bones alone are unable to move; but when attached to muscles, bones can move. **See Lesson: Muscular System.**

9. A. Between the nail bed and cuticle is the lunula. This is an area of white space that is lighter than the nail plate. **See Lesson: Integumentary System.**

10. D. Neuroglia provide protection and support for neurons. They do not participate in the generation of a neural impulse, which means they are unable to transmit electric signals or generate action potentials. **See Lesson: The Nervous System.**

11. B. The production of sex hormones causes the onset of puberty. **See Lesson: Endocrine System.**

12. D. The ability of killer T cells and B cells to distinguish cells of the body from foreign cells is crucial to the fight against pathogens. In autoimmune diseases, this ability breaks down, causing the body to attack its own cells. **See Lesson: The Lymphatic System.**

13. C. This polymer is a carbohydrate, so it must consist of several glycerol molecules that are covalently bonded together. **See Lesson: An Introduction to Biology.**

14. B. A control group is a factor that does not change during an experiment. Due to this, it is used as a standard for comparison with variables that do change such as a dependent variable. **See Lesson: An Introduction to Biology.**

15. B. The chloroplast traps sunlight energy for a plant cell to make food via photosynthesis. Mitochondria convert stored energy from food into a usable form that the cell can use. **See Lesson: Cell Structure, Function, and Type.**

16. D. Found in both plant and animal cells, a vacuole functions as a storage site for many substances in the cell. **See Lesson: Cell Structure, Function, and Type.**

17. C. Fermentation is a metabolic process that produces ATP in the absence of oxygen. Thus, it is an anaerobic form of respiration. **See Lesson: Cellular Reproduction, Cellular Respiration, and Photosynthesis.**

18. D. Cell reproduction is the process where cells grow and differentiate to create offspring or new cells. When the skin is damaged, new skin cells are needed which are created through cell reproduction. **See Lesson: Cellular Reproduction, Cellular Respiration, and Photosynthesis.**

19. B. Dominant traits are designated by a capital letter in a Punnett square and a homozygous trait is indicated by two of the same facto, or letter. FF would represent a homozygous dominant genotype and homozygous recessive would be indicated by ff. **See Lesson: Genetics and DNA.**

20. A. The protein disc that holds two sister chromatids together is what collectively makes a chromosome. **See Lesson: Genetics and DNA.**